College of American Pathologists
Practical Guide to
Gynecologic Cytopathology

Morphology, Management, and Molecular Methods

David C. Wilbur, MD
Michael R. Henry, MD
Editors

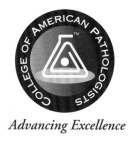

Advancing Excellence

Library of Congress Control Number: 2008940536

ISBN: 978-0-930304-94-2

Printed in the United States of America

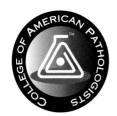

Advancing Excellence

College of American Pathologists
325 Waukegan Road
Northfield, Illinois 60093
800-323-4040

Contributors

David C. Wilbur, MD
Massachusetts General Hospital
Department of Pathology
Boston, Massachusetts

Michael R. Henry, MD
Mayo Clinic
Department of Laboratory Medicine and Pathology
Rochester, Minnesota

Joel S. Bentz, MD
University of Utah
Department of Pathology
Salt Lake City, Utah

George G. Birdsong, MD
Department of Pathology and Laboratory Medicine
Emory University School of Medicine
Department of Anatomic Pathology
Grady Health System
Atlanta, Georgia

Christine Noga Booth, MD
Cleveland Clinic
Department of Anatomic Pathology
Cleveland, Ohio

Karen M. Clary, MD
Rochester General Hospital
Department of Pathology
Rochester, New York

Amy C. Clayton, MD
Mayo Clinic
Department of Laboratory Medicine and Pathology
Rochester, Minnesota

Camilla J. Cobb, MD
Loma Linda University Medical Center
Department of Pathology
Loma Linda, California

Terence J. Colgan, MD
Mount Sinai Hospital
Department of Pathology and Laboratory Medicine
Toronto, Ontario, Canada

Teresa M. Darragh, MD
University of California, San Francisco
Departments of Pathology and Ob/Gyn
San Francisco, California

Diane D. Davey, MD
Department of Medical Education
University of Central Florida College of Medicine
Orlando, Florida

Barbara S. Ducatman, MD
West Virginia University Health Sciences Center
Department of Pathology
Morgantown, West Virginia

Paul A. Elgert, CT(ASCP)
Cytopathology Laboratory
Department of Pathology
Bellevue Hospital Center
New York University School of Medicine
New York, New York

Lisa A. Fatheree, SCT(ASCP)
College of American Pathologists
Northfield, Illinois

Jonathan H. Hughes, MD, PhD
Laboratory Medicine Consultants Ltd
Las Vegas, Nevada

Rodolfo Laucirica, MD
Baylor College of Medicine
Department of Pathology
Houston, Texas

Dina R. Mody, MD
The Methodist Hospital
Department of Pathology
Houston, Texas

Ann T. Moriarty, MD
AmeriPath Indiana
Indianapolis, Indiana

Margaret Havens Neal, MD
KWB Pathology Associates
Tallahassee, Florida

Marianne Unger Prey, MD
Chesterfield, Missouri

Andrew A. Renshaw, MD
Homestead Hospital
Homestead, Florida

Mary R. Schwartz, MD
The Methodist Hospital
Department of Pathology
Houston, Texas

Susan E. Spires, MD
University of Kentucky Healthcare Systems
Good Samaritan Hospital
Lexington, Kentucky

William D. Tench, MD
Palomar Medical Center Laboratory
Escondido, California

Theresa M. Voytek, MD
Hartford Hospital
Department of Pathology
Hartford, Connecticut

Nancy A. Young, MD
Albert Einstein Medical Center
Department of Pathology and Laboratory Medicine
Philadelphia, Pennsylvania

Sue Zaleski, MA, HT(ASCP), SCT
University of Iowa Health Care
Department of Pathology
Iowa City, Iowa

Contents

6. Glandular Epithelial Abnormalities 97

7. Look-Alikes and Morphologic Spectrums of Change   145

Preface

CLIA = 1988
→ Prof. test (started 2005)

There are many monographs, textbooks, and atlases available having to do with morphology and methods in gynecologic cytology. However, with the advent of individual proficiency testing (PT) in 2005, as mandated in the Clinical Laboratory Improvement Amendments of 1988, the need for an updated practical manual covering both the basics and advanced gynecologic cytology practice has grown. Practitioners, especially those who have been away from the field for long periods or who practice gynecologic cytology as only a small piece of their overall practice, need an image-intense guide with cogent explanations that is applicable to both their daily work and to "brush-up" prior to the proficiency test itself.

The Cytopathology Resource Committee of the College of American Pathologists was an ideal body to take on the task of building such a practical manual. The Committee has been responsible for the development and maintenance of the CAP's longstanding educational and laboratory accreditation programs in gynecologic cytology. It has published extensively regarding performance of practitioners in these exercises, and more recently in the PT setting. Finally, it maintains a very large stock of glass slides used in the programs and has been intimately involved in the regulatory and quality management issues faced by the field in recent years.

The Committee took it upon itself to conceptualize what topics would be most needed for a practical guide to gynecologic cytology, and what presentation format would be most efficient in helping practitioners review the basic concepts and cement their knowledge base. This process has evolved into the present manual. It is designed to extensively cover the basic principals of gynecologic cytology, including an approach to the evaluation of a patient and their accompanying specimen, criteria to determine specimen adequacy, normal elements, and an extensive review of the morphology of the vast majority of entities, both benign and malignant, that will routinely be identified in Pap tests. The morphology-based chapters are heavy on "look-alikes" and "spectrums" of cellular changes because the Committee felt that this type of approach would provide a more realistic presentation of the relationships between biologic entities that commonly cause problems in diagnosis. This approach better expresses the real-life variability seen in these specimens than would presentation of only "classic" illustrations of unequivocal and therefore seemingly static entities, and acknowledges the fact that the morphology of gynecologic cytology always represents a spectrum of change without sharp cutoffs between entities. This feature of the manual is unique among monographs on this subject available today. In addition, the Committee felt strongly that it was essential to present background material relevant to the understanding of basic cervical carcinogenesis, including the role of human papillomavirus and its vaccines, to both new students of the field and mature practitioners who may not have been exposed to such material in their initial training.

To provide a complete resource, the basic principals relevant to the management of the laboratory were also added to the manual. These include the sometimes-cryptic rules for coding of specimens, the basic tenets and practical issues behind quality assurance in the laboratory, and some tips for effective personnel management.

This effort has been a collaborative one. We wish to thank the members of the Cytopathology Resource Committee, past and present, for their work as contributors of chapters and images, and for their support, ideas, and comments in the long task of bringing this project to completion. A special thank you goes out to CAP staff for the Committee, including Lisa Fatheree, Beth Anne Chmara, Jennifer Haja, Barbara Blond; and also to Caryn Tursky, in the Publications Department—we could not have achieved this result without the assistance of this splendid group.

David C. Wilbur, MD, FCAP, Boston, Massachusetts
Michael R. Henry, MD, FCAP, Rochester, Minnesota

Gynecologic Cytology: Approach to the Slide and Normal Morphology

David C. Wilbur, MD

Introduction

Gynecologic cytology (the Pap test) is the most successful cancer screening program ever devised—that despite a test sensitivity as low as 50% sensitivity for the detection of cervical abnormalities. The test has been successful in screened populations because annual screening intervals give patients multiple "shots" at the detection of a neoplastic process. Furthermore, the generally slow progression of the preneoplastic process leading to invasive carcinoma allows multiple attempts to intervene at each step in this progression. In effect, the principle is that with annual screening, preinvasive lesions will be caught prior to the development of cancer, with no untoward effects. The high false-negative rate of the Pap test is multifactorial, including inadequate sampling, particularly of small lesions; incomplete transfer (and hence loss) of abnormal cells from those collected on the sampling device to a glass slide (typically in conventional smears); poor preparation; screening errors; and misinterpretation of abnormal cells identified on screening. The introduction of modern sampling devices, liquid-based specimen preparation, and computerized screening devices has helped to improve false-negative rates for a variety of reasons. However, 100% sensitivity is unlikely to ever be achieved without a concomitant loss of necessary specificity.

This monograph is intended to provide a comprehensive and user-friendly source of biologic and morphologic information related to Pap testing, to provide important information on quality assurance and cytology laboratory management, and to predict future developments, including the introduction of vaccines against the human papil-

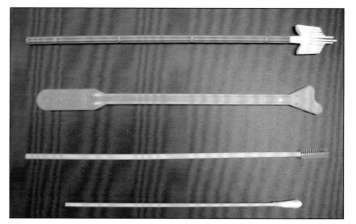

Figure 1-2. The sampling devices utilized for the taking of Pap test specimens. The broom device (top) is used as a single sampling device. The combination of endocervical brush and spatula (the next two sampling devices, moving down) are used for sampling the endocervix and exocervix, respectively. The cotton swab (bottom) is not recommended for use at present because it poorly samples cells from the transformation zone and does not transfer cells adequately to either conventional smears or liquid-based transport media.

lomavirus (HPV) and the introduction of new methods of screening.

In order to reliably and accurately identify abnormal cells and patterns in Pap tests, a practitioner must possess a thorough knowledge of the ranges of normal and benign reactive patterns. Criteria need to be utilized to distinguish the often very subtle differences separating reactive entities from neoplastic lesions. This opening chapter will present an approach to interpretation of a Pap test and the basic facts regarding the normal cells and cell patterns that are routinely seen in the Pap test, and will include a discussion of specimen adequacy and common reporting terminology.

Preanalytical Examination of the Specimen

Specimen Type (Figure 1-1)

Is the slide a conventionally prepared Pap smear or a liquid-based cytology specimen (The ThinPrep® Pap Test, SurePath™ Pap, or MonoPrep®)? Judging specimen adequacy will be different, and subtle morphology differences will be present between these types of specimens (see chapter 11).

Sampling Device Utilized (Figure 1-2)

Is a modern sampling device (eg, broom or combination spatula/endocervical brush) utilized? Specimens obtained with spatula only or in combination with the cotton swab will often be less than optimal due to poor sampling of the

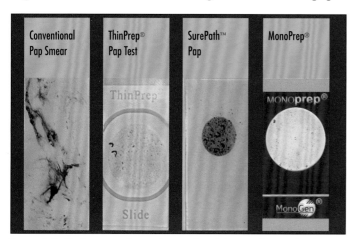

Figure 1-1. The four types of gynecologic cytology slides. From left to right, the specimens are the conventional smear, ThinPrep, SurePath, and MonoPrep preparations.

transformation zone and poor cell transfer. Was the device utilized properly? Adequate training of clinicians is important because results obtained will be directly proportional to proper use (eg, broom devices require multiple rotations in a given direction, brush devices require only quarter turns in the os).

Integration of Requisition Information into the Analysis

Prior to analysis of the slide, the cytologist should integrate critical clinical information. Cytologic patterns may differ depending on clinical circumstances, and hence the latter should be known in advance. In addition, the time from the last menstrual period, use of drugs (particularly estrogen/progesterone types), and prior history of Paps (both normal and abnormal) should be sought. With regard to information provided on the requisition, it is always good practice to assume that information is incomplete (often it is) and, if possible, search your own laboratory information system (LIS) or clinical information database looking for more complete information. In Pap tests performed for the follow-up of a known premalignant or malignant entity, such information is vital to proper/complete evaluation. An example of a requisition format is illustrated in Figure 1-3.

Specimen Reporting Format

Laboratories operating under the regulations of the Clinical Laboratory Improvement Amendments of 1988 (CLIA '88) must use a descriptive terminology for reporting Pap test results. The Papanicolaou classification scheme (Class I-V) is unacceptable, as the nonspecificity of this scheme can lead to misunderstandings of what entity is actually being reported. The most common method of reporting (although not the only method) is the use of the 2001 Bethesda System,[1] which breaks the report into a series of categories that include:

❖ Specimen type: conventional versus liquid-based versus other

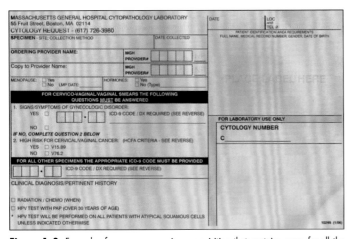

Figure 1-3. Example of a one-page specimen requisition that contains space for all the patient identifiers and clinical information needed for the evaluation of a Pap test specimen.

❖ Specimen adequacy: satisfactory or unsatisfactory for evaluation
❖ General categorization: essentially normal or abnormal, and of what general type
❖ Interpretation/result (specific result)
❖ Results of ancillary testing (if applicable): for example HPV/Gonococcus/Chlamydia testing
❖ Automated review (if applicable): for use of a computerized scanning device
❖ Educational notes and suggestions (optional)

All of these specific categories convey information that is useful to clinicians/patients and to cytologists reviewing subsequent material, and document exactly how a specimen was processed and hence how the final interpretation was determined. Reports should contain each element if it applies, but, at a minimum, all reports should contain information about specimen type, specimen adequacy, general categorization, and interpretation/result.[1]

Specimen Adequacy

In the Bethesda System, there are two categories for reporting specimen adequacy; either a specimen is satisfactory or it is unsatisfactory for interpretation. For an unsatisfactory designation, there are two routes: (1) a specimen could not be processed, meaning it was not properly labeled, was received broken, or could not be processed for other reason; or (2) it was fully processed and evaluated but could not be interpreted due to some limitation in the nature of the specimen itself. The most common reasons for unsatisfactory specimens of the latter type are lack of squamous cellularity, obscuration by inflammation and blood, or a technical artifact, such as air-drying. The former is most commonly a cause for unsatisfactory specimens in liquid-based cytology, whereas the latter two categories are typically noted only in conventionally prepared specimens. Currently, it is recommended that patients with unsatisfactory specimens obtain repeat examinations within a short time period.

The criteria for a satisfactory specimen are nicely illustrated in the Bethesda System manual. Essentially, all that is required for this category is an adequate number of well-presented squamous cells (5000 for liquid-based and 8000 to 12,000 for conventional cytology specimens). Actual cell counting is not implied by these numbers, and methods for rapid visual assessments are given in the manual.[1]

The presence of transformation zone (TZ) sampling for specimen adequacy is somewhat controversial. In the Bethesda System, evidence of TZ sampling is not explicitly required for a satisfactory sample. Studies are conflicting as to the sensitivity of the Pap test for the detection of abnormality in the presence and absence of TZ components. However, most recent data suggest that if modern sampling devices designed to cover the endocervical canal are utilized, disease detection is similar whether there is, or is not, evidence of TZ sampling on the slide.[2] Therefore, the Bethesda System does not require that TZ components be present on the slide for a fully satisfactory specimen. However laboratories may elect to comment on the absence of TZ components under a "quality indicators (QI)" section of the report. As such, the Bethesda System no longer recognizes an intermediate category of adequacy (ie, "satisfactory but limited by....") as it did in the first version of the terminology.

Transformation zone sampling can be of either endocervical or metaplastic cells, and there should be at least 10 such cells, either in groups or isolated. In cases where a QI of lack of TZ component is given in the report, clinicians should be counseled that this does not require an immediate repeat of the specimen unless there is some risk of missed disease specific to that patient. In "normal" risk individuals, an annual repeat is appropriate in this circumstance.

Normal Cells Identified From the Vagina, Cervix, Transformation Zone, Endocervix, and Endometrium

Vaginal and Exocervical Mucosa

The vaginal and exocervical mucosa are similar and contain native squamous epithelial cells. There are three presentations of native squamous cells from these areas, as follows:

Superficial Squamous Cells. These are the most mature cell normally found in the vagina or exocervix. Superficial cells have an abundant, polygonally shaped cytoplasm, which is generally dense or "glassy," and can be colored either orange or blue/green in the Pap stain, depending on the degree of maturation of the keratin cytoskeleton (ie, the most mature keratins stain orange). The nuclei are pyknotic and small, generally measuring about 15 to 20 μm² in area (Figure 1-4).

Intermediate Squamous Cells. These are cells of "intermediate" differentiation that are found just below the superficial cell in the normal, fully mature, native squamous epithelium. The cytoplasmic configuration is polygonal, similar to superficial cells, but it may have more "rounded" edges. Intermediate cells contains less mature keratins, hence they are almost always blue/green and dense to slightly granular in texture. The nucleus is larger than the superficial cell (typically about 35 μm² [see Figure 1-5 for presentation of nuclear size illustration]) and has a less dense, "open" chromatin that is evenly distributed and finely granular (Figure 1-6).

Parabasal Squamous Cells. These cells represent the least mature cells in the native squamous epithelium. They are not normally identified in a fully mature epithelium, as the Pap test typically samples only the top three to four layers of cells. Therefore, parabasal cells are only identified in Pap tests from women who have immature epithelia due to lack of estrogenic stimulation (eg, postmenopausal women). Parabasal cells are overall smaller and have a higher nuclear to cytoplasmic ratio and round to oval cytoplasm. The cytoplasm is of greater density than intermediate cells and may be more granular in texture. Parabasal

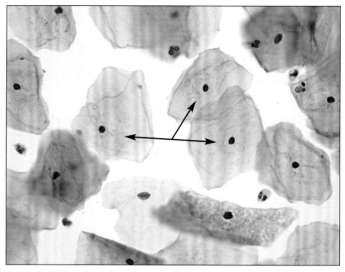

Figure 1-4. Normal superficial squamous cells (arrows).

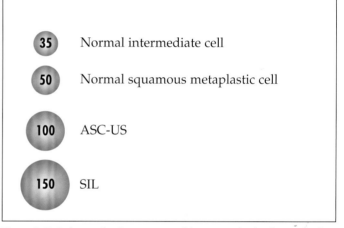

Figure 1-5. Evaluation of nuclear size is a useful exercise in the classification of cells in Pap test specimens. This chart illustrates the average nuclear sizes for the common reference cells present in gynecologic cytology samples. Abbreviations: ASC-US, atypical squamous cells of undetermined significance; SIL, squamous intraepithelial lesion.

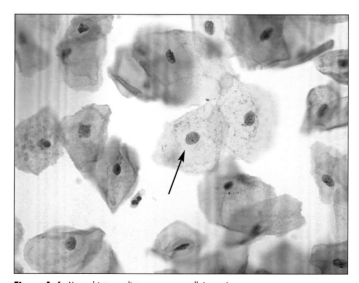

Figure 1-6. Normal intermediate squamous cell (arrow).

3

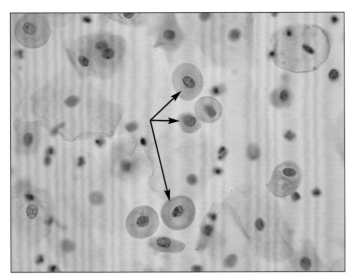

Figure 1-7. Normal parabasal squamous cells (arrows).

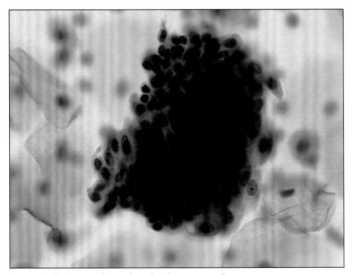

Figure 1-8. A group of normal parabasal squamous cells.

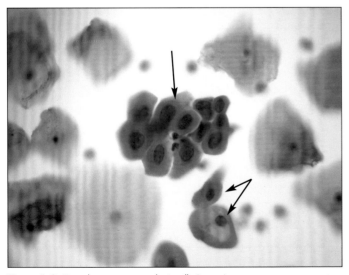

Figure 1-9. Normal squamous metaplastic cells (arrows).

cell cytoplasm appears blue/green with the Pap stain. The nuclei are larger than their intermediate cell counterparts, typically about 50 μm². The nuclei have evenly distributed, finely granular chromatin. Parabasal cells may also present in groups, particularly in atrophic specimens (Figures 1-7 and 1-8).

Transformation Zone Mucosa

The transformation zone consists of the area just above the exocervical native squamous epithelium, which originally consists of endocervical epithelium but, over the course of time, changes to a squamous epithelium via the process referred to as squamous metaplasia. This area can be identified on cervical biopsies either by the presence of endocervical epithelium abutting squamous epithelium or by mature or metaplastic squamous epithelium overlying endocervical glands deep in the cervical stroma.

Squamous Metaplastic Cells

These are cells that are in the process of maturing from reserve cells (the least differentiated squamous precursor found at the very base of the normal squamous epithelium) to ultimately become intermediate and superficial squamous cells. Their appearance is very reminiscent of, and often indistinguishable on an individual cell basis from, parabasal cells. They represent a spectrum of change from the undifferentiated to the intermediate cell, but on average show round to oval cytoplasm that is dense, may be granular, and, with the Pap stain, is colored blue/green. Small cytoplasmic vacuoles may be noted. Metaplastic cells have a higher nucleus to cytoplasm ratio than do intermediate cells, and the nuclear size is larger, approximately 50 μm². The chromatin pattern is evenly dispersed and finely granular (Figure 1-9).

Because of the similarity of the appearances of metaplastic and parabasal cells, differentiation is often based on the pattern they present in the total smear—meaning small numbers of these types of cell scattered in the background of a well-estrogenized (ie, dominant intermediate/superficial cell mature pattern) indicate that these are most likely of metaplastic origin and are derived from the transformation zone. Cells of similar morphology which dominate the overall pattern are most likely to represent parabasal cells—an indication of an atrophic or nonestrogenized pattern. On the other hand, if the overall pattern shows many of these cells with only intermediate cells in addition (nonestrogenized, immature), then it is most likely that the cells are parabasal in origin.

Endocervical Cells

These are the simple, columnar, mucus-producing cells that normally line the endocervical canal. They are found proximal to the TZ (higher in the canal). Native endocervical epithelial cells maintain a columnar configuration when traumatically sampled. They are tall and contain a frothy mucus cap. Nuclei are basally located, round to oval, about 35 μm² in area, have smooth envelopes, and have evenly

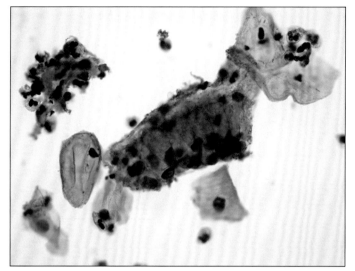

Figure 1-10. Normal endocervical cells showing the "picket-fence" columnar cell arrangement.

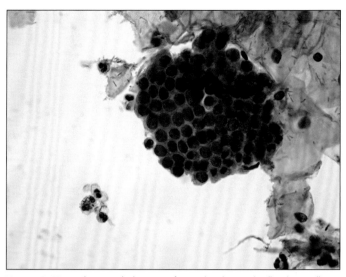

Figure 1-11. A "honeycombed" group of normal endocervical cells. These cells are viewed "on end," down the long axis of the columnar cells.

distributed, finely granular chromatin and a characteristic small, dot-like, round nucleolus. If endocervical cells are spontaneously exfoliated, their appearance may change to a more rounded cell, still containing the frothy cytoplasm and similar nucleus. In some cases, it may be difficult to distinguish rounded up endocervical cells from squamous metaplastic cells; some cytologists have utilized the term "metacervical" to describe such cells having ambiguous morphologic features. When in groups, endocervical cells exhibit architectural patterns of the "picket-fence" when viewed from the side (Figure 1-10) and the "honeycomb" when viewed on end (Figure 1-11). In the former, the cells are arranged in a side-by-side columnar fashion, with basilar placed nuclei and mucus caps. In the latter, the cells take on a rigid structure of evenly spaced nuclei with minimal overlapping, well-defined cytoplasmic boundaries, and a three-dimensional depth of focus that allows the nucleus to be in the plane at one point and the mucus cap to be present at a different focusing point.

Higher in the endocervical canal, variants of the native endocervical epithelium can be seen, most commonly recapitulating the epithelium of the fallopian tube, a pattern referred to as "tubal metaplasia." This consists of columnar cells with terminal bars and cilia, goblet cells, and slender "intercalated" cells (Figure 1-12). These cells are often arranged in a pseudostratified manner and can morphologically mimic neoplastic processes such as endocervical adenocarcinoma in situ. This entity will be discussed in much greater detail in the section on glandular lesions of the cervix (see chapter 6).

Endometrial Cells

Similar to endocervical cells, endometrial cells, in their native state, are a columnar epithelium with a pseudostratified architecture. However, in Pap specimens, endometrial cells only take on this appearance if directly sampled (eg, lower uterine segment sampling). In most cases, endometrial cells present in Pap tests will be from actively shed

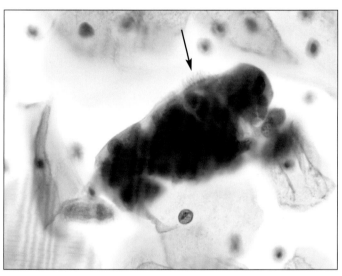

Figure 1-12. A strip of tubal metaplastic cervical epithelium. Note the ciliated luminal border (arrow). In distinction to the native endocervical epithelium (Figure 1-10), the nuclei are pseudostratified, as opposed to predominantly basal.

endometrium during menses or at other times in dysfunctional uterine bleeding. In this form, they will not present as two-dimensional sheets but will reflect conformational changes that take place when the groups are "suspended" in the endocervical blood and mucous—hence, rounded up, three-dimensional groupings (Figure 1-13). Shed endometrial cells are typically small (total cell size is 35 μm^2 on average) with round, oval, or reniform nuclei, often showing degenerative changes, including gritty heterogenous chromatin and apoptotic bodies. They may have associated inflammation within the groups. Typical appearance at the end of the menstrual flow period (days 5 to 10) may show a characteristic two-layered "ball" consisting of a central core of densely packed endometrial stroma and an external layer of endometrial glandular cells. This pattern has been referred to as an "exodus" pattern, referring to the end of menstrual flow (Figure 1-14). Especially in liquid-

5

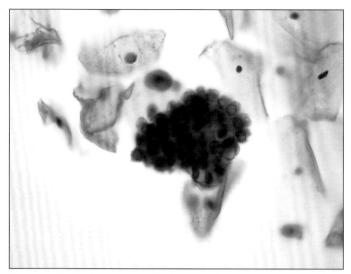

Figure 1-13. "Shed" endometrial cells. The group is three-dimensional, and the cells are generally small and have an angulated appearance. Occasional degenerative vacuoles are present in this group.

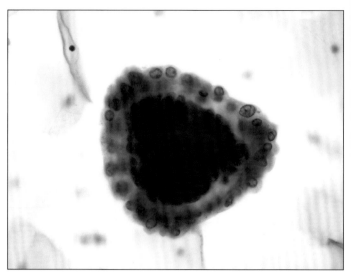

Figure 1-14. "Shed" endometrial cells showing the classic "exodus" pattern of endometrial glandular cells surrounding a core of endometrial stroma. These cell arrangements are typically present in Pap test specimens at the end of the menstrual flow period.

based preparations, shed endometrium, due to the excellent fixation of individual cells with this technique, can have a more atypical/degenerative appearance, with enlarged irregular nuclei. Such appearances can lead to overinterpretations of such cells as "atypical endometrial cells." Isolated groups of shed endometrial stromal cells may be noted, as well. These may present as hyperchromatic crowded groups showing loose cohesion. Spindled cells with elongate cytoplasm and nuclei are easily seen at the margins of the group (Figure 1-15).

Directly sampled, or abraded, endometrium can be seen in Pap specimens when the sampling device extends beyond the endocervical canal into the lower uterine segment or even into the fundus. This situation most commonly occurs in women who have had prior cervical cone biopsies and hence shortened endocervical canals. The appearance of in situ sampled endometrium will be dependent on the timing of the cycle. Proliferative endometrium will present as two-dimensional "honeycombed" crowded groups, as pseudostratified strips of cells, or even as intact tubular structures (Figure 1-16). Because these are cycling cells, mitoses may be frequent, and if the patient has anovulatory cycling, evidence of breakdown, including apoptotic bodies, may be present. This appearance can be very worrisome given the close appearance to endocervical adenocarcinoma in situ and will be discussed in greater detail in chapter 6 on glandular lesions. Nuclear size should be generally smaller than is normally present in endocervical glandular neoplasias, however, and chromatin structure should still retain a smooth "non-gritty" pattern, in distinction to the coarse granularity seen in adenocarcinoma in situ. Endometrium sampled during secretory phase will show morphology similar to normal endocervix, with prominent mucus secretion; again, nuclear size should be smaller than the normal endocervical cell, and this overall appearance does not have the worrisome look (mitoses, apoptotic bodies, pseudos-

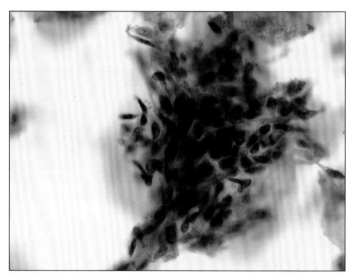

Figure 1-15. Endometrial stromal cells. The grouping is loosely aggregated, and cells present at the margins show definite spindled mesenchymal configuration.

tratification) of the proliferative phase. Because directly sampled endometrial cells are considered a normal finding, when present in women older than age 40 years, they should not be reported as would be routinely done in the Bethesda System for exfoliated benign endometrial cells.

Variations Based on Menstrual Phase, Menstrual Status, and Hormone Use

The normal cells noted above may take on various changes both in individual cell appearance and in the distribution of cell types, depending on a variety of circumstances. These circumstances may include infections, treatment effects, or trauma, which will be discussed below. More commonly, changes can be seen based on hormonal milieu changes associated with the phases of the menstrual cycle, menopausal status, and treatment with exogenous hormones.

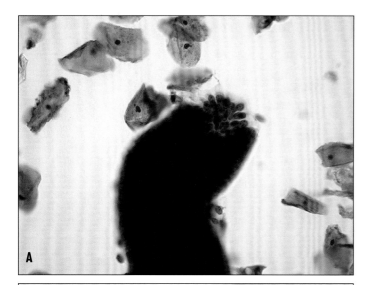

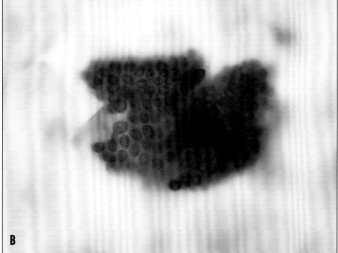

Figure 1-16. Traumatically sampled (abraded) endometrial cells. **A.** Cells displayed in an intact tubule of endometrial epithelial cells. **B.** Cells arranged in a two-dimensional honey-combed sheet indicative of direct sampling of a columnar epithelium. This arrangement is similar to that noted for endocervical cells; however, the overall cell size is significantly smaller than for endocervical cells.

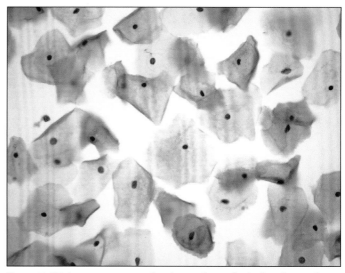

Figure 1-17. A maturation pattern of predominantly superficial cells, indicative of estrogenic effect.

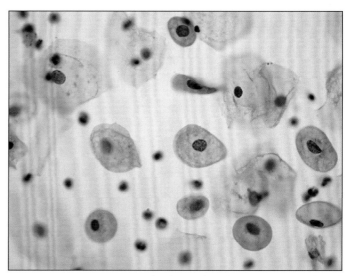

Figure 1-18. A maturation pattern of predominantly parabasal cells, indicative of lack of estrogenic effect (atrophy).

Normal endogenous estrogen stimulation of an estrogen-responsive epithelium (typically women postmenarche and premenopausal) will give a so-called mature pattern of squamous differentiation in a Pap specimen. This pattern consists of the presence of superficial and intermediate cells in variable distributions. Parabasal cells should not routinely (exception below) be noted in such hormonal states. In the past, maturation indices were routinely performed on the cells of the vaginal wall to determine if estrogenic stimulation of the squamous epithelium was present. A vaginal specimen was required, as opposed to cervical, because transformation zone sampling might normally identify metaplastic cells that could be mistaken for immature parabasal cells, the latter giving a false impression of atrophy. At present, more accurate methods to determine hormonal levels are available (blood chemical hormone analyses), and hence the cytologic method is no longer routinely utilized for hormonal assessment.

However, the general maturation appearance of the cells present, even in a cervical sample, provides important information about each specimen, including important clues to systemic health and to the identity of specimens. For instance, in postmenopausal women with no exogenous hormone use, a mature (estrogenized) pattern may indicate overexpression of endogenous estrogen (secreting tumors, obesity, etc), surreptitious use of estrogenic compounds, or even a mislabeled specimen that may belong to another patient.

A commonly used "maturation index" is the ratio of superficial to intermediate to parabasal cells. Normally only one of these types, or two "adjacent" types, should be noted in any specimen. Examples of mature and atrophic patterns, containing predominantly superficial and parabasal cells, respectively, are shown in Figures 1-17 and 1-18. Patterns composed of only intermediate cells are not good predictors of hormonal state, as this pattern can be

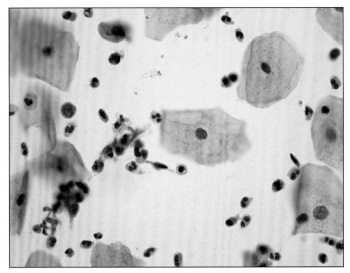

Figure 1-19. A maturation pattern composed of predominantly intermediate cells. This pattern is not predictive of any specific estrogenic status.

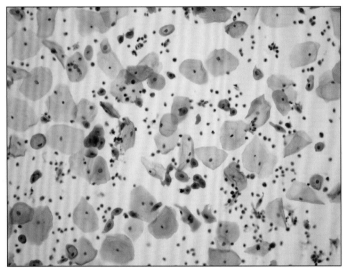

Figure 1-20. A maturation pattern composed of all three cell types: superficial, intermediate, and parabasal. This pattern is commonly noted in perimenopausal women and is thought to be associated with an epithelium showing irregular response to estrogenic stimulation.

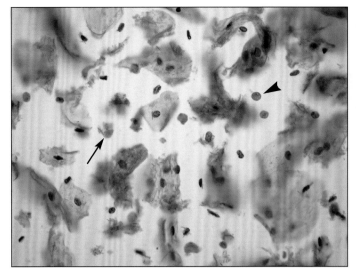

Figure 1-21. A "cytolytic" pattern, commonly noted in the luteal phase of the menstrual cycle. Squamous cells are undergoing degeneration due to lactobacilli utilizing cellular glycogen, which leads to the presence of fragments of cells (arrow) and stripped nuclei (arrowhead).

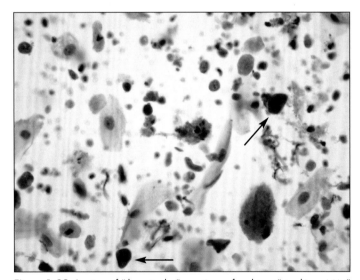

Figure 1-22. A pattern of "deep atrophy," sometimes referred to as "atrophic vaginitis." This pattern includes parabasal cells, granular debris, and amorphous blue material ("blue blobs" [arrows]).

found in estrogenized as well as nonestrogenized individuals (Figure 1-19). There is one circumstance in which significant numbers of all three cell types may be present at the same time; this occurs in the perimenopausal period in which the epithelium may be variably responsive to estrogenic stimulation. This pattern has been previously described and referred to as "early atrophy"[3] (Figure 1-20).

Squamous cells may be altered by a variety of physiologic factors. In the second half of the menstrual cycle, there is often an overgrowth of lactobacilli in the vagina, leading to dissolution of cells because the bacteria digest glycogen normally present in squamous cells. This leads to a pattern referred to as cytolysis and consists of numerous cell fragments, stripped nuclei, and amorphous cellular breakdown material in the slide background. In addition,

the intact cells remaining often are present as clumped aggregates. This pattern can lead to difficulty in smear interpretation because the Bethesda System adequacy criterion of well-preserved and presented squamous cells cannot be met, and the debris present and cell clumping leads to obscuration of nuclear detail (Figure 1-21). In deeply atrophic patients, in addition to numerous parabasal cells being present, the epithelium may show a pattern referred to as "atrophic vaginitis," in which parabasal cells undergo significant degeneration, again with a debris-laden background, many small immature cells that may become spindled, and fragments of blue breakdown material known as "blue blobs" (Figure 1-22). Use of exogenous progestational agents can cause iatro-

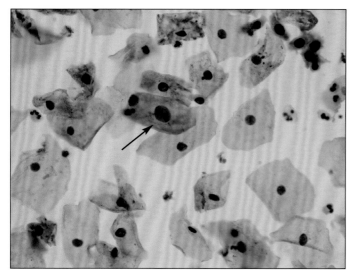

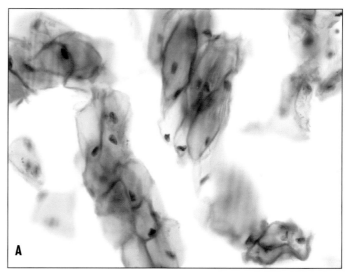

Figure 1-23. Nuclear enlargement (arrow), which may be present in squamous cells during the perimenopausal period or in circumstances of a progestational environment. These changes are sometimes referred to as "atypia of maturity" or "postmenopausal atypia." Criteria for atypical squamous cells of undetermined significance (ASC-US) (as illustrated in chapter 2) should be considered in deciding on an ultimate interpretation for such a case.

genic "atrophy" or a less-than-mature pattern in the specimen. A common finding in women using an implantable, long-acting, subcutaneous progestin for birth control is an intermediate or parabasal pattern, in which nuclei are greater in size than normal intermediate cells. In such cases, overcalling of squamous "atypia" is not uncommon, despite the finding that these women will often be HPV negative on follow-up. This "progestational" pattern is similar to that noted in peri- and postmenopausal women, in which the nuclei may be larger than normally expected. This phenomenon is called peri- or postmenopausal atypia or atypia of maturity; again, this "atypia" is not associated with the presence of HPV (Figure 1-23). In pregnant patients, squamous cells may become laden with glycogen and take on a characteristic crowded appearance, often with stellate or crescentic boat-like–shaped cells referred to as "navicular" cells (Figure 1-24).

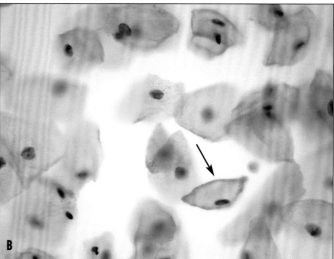

Figure 1-24. Pregnancy maturation pattern. **A.** Typical groups of angulated "navicular" cells. **B.** Isolated navicular (boat-like) cells (arrow).

References

1. Solomon D, Nayar R. *The Bethesda System for Reporting Cervical Cytology. Definitions, Criteria and Explanatory Notes.* 2nd ed. New York: Springer; 2004.
2. Boon ME, Alons-vanKordelaar JJ, Rietveld-Scheffers PE. Consequences of the introduction of combined spatula and Cytobrush sampling for cervical cytology: improvements in smear quality and detection rates. *Acta Cytol.* 1986;30:264-270.
3. Tambouret RH, Wilbur DC. The many faces of atrophy in gynecologic cytology. *Clin Lab Med.* 2003;23:659-679.

Bibliography

Bibbo M, Wilbur DC. *Comprehensive Cytopathology.* 3rd ed. London: Elsevier; 2008.

Cibas ES, Ducatman BS. *Cytology. Diagnostic Principles and Clinical Correlates.* 2nd ed. Edinburgh: Saunders; 2003.

Koss LG, Melamed MR. *Koss' Diagnostic Cytology and Its Histopathologic Basis.* 5th ed. Philadelphia, Pa: Lippincott, Williams & Wilkins; 2006.

Patten SF. *Diagnostic Cytopathology of the Uterine Cervix.* 2nd ed. Berlin: Karger; 1976.

Specimen Adequacy

George G. Birdsong, MD, Diane D. Davey, MD,
Teresa M. Darragh, MD, Paul A. Elgert, CT(ASCP),
Michael R. Henry, MD

[handwritten notes in top margin:] Bethesda Pap adequacy / satis ⟨liz = 5K sq / convent = 8-12K sq (± endocx) ⟩ / not satisf.

Background

Evaluation of specimen adequacy is considered by many to be the single most important quality assurance component of the Bethesda System. Earlier versions of Bethesda included three categories of adequacy: Satisfactory, Unsatisfactory, and a "borderline" category initially termed "Less than optimal" and then renamed "Satisfactory but limited by" in 1991. The 2001 Bethesda System eliminates the borderline category, in part, because of confusion among clinicians as to the appropriate follow-up for such findings and also due to the variability in reporting "Satisfactory but limited by" among laboratories.[1] To provide a clearer indication of adequacy, specimens are now designated as "Satisfactory" or "Unsatisfactory."

Previous criteria for determining adequacy were based on expert opinion and the few available studies in the literature. Laboratory implementation of some of these criteria was shown to be poorly reproducible.[2-4] In addition, the increasing use of liquid-based cytology necessitated developing criteria applicable to these preparations. The 2001 Bethesda adequacy criteria are based on published data to the extent possible and are tailored to conventional smears and liquid-based specimens.

Adequacy Categories

Satisfactory

Satisfactory for evaluation (*describe presence or absence of endocervical/transformation zone component and any other quality indicators, e.g., partially obscuring blood, inflammation, etc.*)

Unsatisfactory

For unsatisfactory specimens, indicate whether or not the laboratory has processed/evaluated the slide. Suggested wording:

A. Rejected specimen:
   Specimen rejected (not processed) because _____ (specimen not labeled, slide broken, etc.)

B. Fully evaluated, unsatisfactory specimen:
   Specimen processed and examined, but unsatisfactory for evaluation of epithelial abnormality because of _____ (obscuring blood, etc.)

Additional comments/recommendations, as appropriate

Explanatory Notes

For "Satisfactory" specimens, information on transformation zone sampling and other adequacy qualifiers is also included. Providing clinicians/specimen takers with regular feedback on specimen quality promotes heightened attention to specimen collection and consideration of improved sampling devices and technologies.

Any specimen with abnormal cells [atypical squamous cells of undetermined significance (ASC-US), atypical glandular cells (AGC), or worse] is by definition satisfactory for evaluation. If there is concern that the specimen is compromised, a note may be appended indicating that a more severe abnormality cannot be excluded.

Unsatisfactory specimens that are processed and evaluated require considerable time and effort. Although such specimens cannot exclude an epithelial lesion, information such as the presence of organisms, or endometrial cells in women 40 years of age or older, etc., may help direct further patient management.[5] Note that the presence of benign endometrial cells does not make an otherwise unsatisfactory specimen satisfactory.

A longitudinal study[6] found that unsatisfactory specimens that were processed and evaluated were more often from high-risk patients, and a significant number of these were followed by a squamous intraepithelial lesion (SIL)/cancer when compared to a cohort of satisfactory index specimens.

Minimum Squamous Cellularity Criteria

Conventional Smears (Figs. 2.1–2.5)

An adequate conventional specimen has an estimated minimum of approximately 8,000 to 12,000 well-preserved and well-visualized squamous epithelial cells. *Note: This minimum cell range should be estimated, and laboratories should not count individual cells in conventional smears.* This range applies only to squamous cells; endocervical cells and completely obscured cells should be excluded from the estimate as much as feasible. However, squamous metaplastic cells can be counted as squamous cells during cellularity assessment. This cellularity range should not be considered

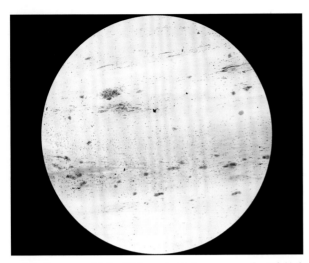

Figure 2-1. Squamous cellularity: This image depicts the appearance of a 4X field of a conventional Pap smear with approximately 75 cells. The specimen is unsatisfactory if all fields have this level, or less, of cellularity. It is to be used as a guide in assessing the squamous cellularity of a conventional smear. (Used with permission, © George Birdsong, 2003)

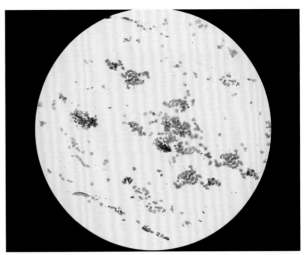

Figure 2-3. Squamous cellularity: This image depicts the appearance of a 4X field of a conventional Pap smear with approximately 500 cells. A minimum of 16 fields with similar (or greater) cellularity are needed to call this specimen adequate. (Used with permission, © George Birdsong, 2003)

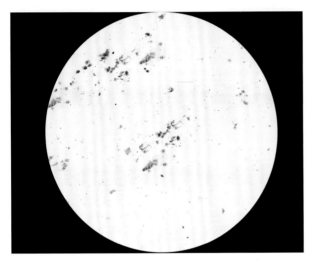

Figure 2-2. Squamous cellularity: This image depicts the appearance of a 4X field of a conventional Pap smear with approximately 150 cells. If all fields have this level of cellularity, the specimen will meet the minimum cellularity criterion, but by only a small margin. (Used with permission, © George Birdsong, 2003)

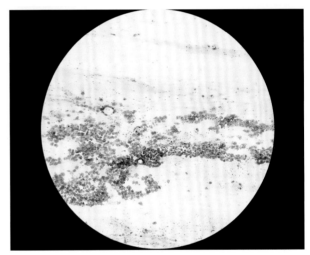

Figure 2-4. Squamous cellularity: This image depicts the appearance of a 4X field of a conventional Pap smear with approximately 1000 cells. A minimum of 8 fields with similar (or greater) cellularity are needed to call this specimen adequate. (Used with permission, © George Birdsong, 2003)

a rigid threshold (see comments below). "Reference images" of known cellularity are illustrated in Figures 2.1 to 2.5. These reference images have been computer edited to simulate the appearance of 4X fields on conventional smears. Cytologists should compare these images to specimens in question to determine if there are a sufficient number of fields with approximately equal or greater cellularity than the reference image. For instance, if an image corresponding to a 4X field with 1000 cells was used as the reference, a specimen would need to have at least eight such 4X fields to be deemed to have adequate cellularity.

Liquid-Based Preparations (Figs. 2.6–2.10)

An adequate liquid-based preparation (LBP) should have an estimated minimum of at least 5000 well-visualized/well-preserved squamous cells. Some have advocated that

LBPs with 5000 to 20,000 cells are of borderline or low squamous cellularity. In specimens with an apparent borderline or low squamous cellularity, an estimation of total cellularity can be obtained by performing representative field cell counts. A minimum of 10 microscopic fields, usually at 40X, should be assessed along a diameter that includes the center of the preparation and an average number of cells per field estimated. When there are holes or empty areas on the preparation, the percentage of the hypocellular areas should be estimated, and the fields counted should reflect this proportion. SurePath (TriPath Imaging, Inc., Burlington, NC) slides require higher cell density because of the smaller preparation diameter.

Table 2.1 provides the average number of cells per field required to achieve a minimum of 5000 cells on an LBP given a certain preparation diameter and eyepiece (ocular).

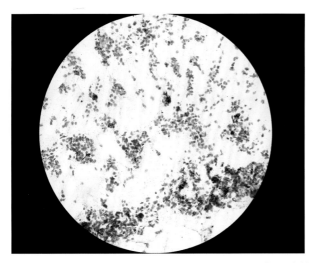

Figure 2-5. *Squamous cellularity: This image depicts the appearance of a 4X field of a conventional Pap smear with approximately 1400 cells. A minimum of 6 fields with similar (or greater) cellularity are needed to call this specimen adequate. (Used with permission, © George Birdsong, 2003)*

For individuals using oculars and preparations not shown, the formula is: number of cells required per field = 5000/(area of preparation/area of field). As of this writing, the diameters of SurePath and ThinPrep (Cytyc Corporation, Boxborough, MA) preparations are 13 and 20 millimeters (mm) respectively. The diameter of a microscopic field in millimeters is the field number of the eyepiece divided by the magnification of the objective. The area of the field is then determined by the formula used to calculate the area of a circle [pi x radius squared, πr^2]. The magnification power of the ocular does not affect this calculation. See http://www.olympusmicro.com/primer/anatomy/oculars.html for additional explanation of the pertinent optical principles.

Figures 2.6 to 2.10 show cell coverage or density in satisfactory, borderline satisfactory, and unsatisfactory LBP. These are not reference images, as they do not represent an entire microscopic field; thus, the cell density shown in the images cannot be compared directly to Table 2.1 for estimation of squamous cellularity. In some instances the cellularity on the prepared slide may not be representative of the collected sample. Slides with fewer than 5000 cells should be examined to determine if the reason for the scant cellularity is a technical problem in preparation of the slide such

as excessive blood in the specimen. When a technical problem is identified and corrected, a repeat preparation may yield adequate cellularity. However, the adequacy of each slide should be determined separately and not cumulatively. Attempts to determine cellularity cumulatively by summing the cellularity of multiple inadequate slides may be confounded by uncertainty regarding the true cellularity of the specimen (not slide), which might be substantially less than in a specimen of normal cellularity. This matter is in need of more research, and this guideline may change in the future. However, given the relatively low minimum criterion for adequate cellularity, caution is warranted in borderline cases. The report should clarify whether blood, mucus, or inflammation contributed to an unsatisfactory sample, or whether the problem was simply low squamous cellularity.

Explanatory Notes

It is recognized that strict objective criteria may not be applicable to every case. Some slides with cell clustering, atrophy, or cytolysis are technically difficult to count, and there may be clinical circumstances in which a lower cell number may be considered adequate. Laboratories should apply professional judgment and employ hierarchical review when evaluating these rare borderline adequacy slides. It should also be kept in mind that the minimum cellularity criteria described were developed for use with cervical cytology specimens. In vaginal specimens (post total hysterectomy), laboratories should exercise judgment in reporting cellularity based on the clinical and screening history. A lower cellularity may be acceptable under these circumstances. Laboratories have flexibility in determining which method for cellularity estimation is best suited for their practice setting.

The recommendation for a minimum cellularity of 5000 cells for an LBP is based on preliminary scientific evidence.[7,8] This threshold is lower than the 8,000 to 12,000 minimum cellularity for conventional smears. LBPs, by virtue of the preparation methodology, present a more random (and presumably more representative) sampling of the collected cervical material as compared to conventional smears. Although there are significant differences among various LBP procedures, there are not sufficient data to justify different minimum cellularities for the LBPs currently on the market.

Table 2.1 Guidelines for Estimating Cellularity of Liquid-Based Preparations

Prep. diameter (mm)	Area (mm²)	FN20 eyepiece/ 10X objective		FN20 eyepiece/ 40X objective		FN22 eyepiece/ 10X objective		FN22 eyepiece/ 40X objective	
		Number of fields at FN20, 10X	Number of cells/field for 5K total	Number of fields at FN20, 40X	Number of cells/field for 5K total	Number of fields at FN22, 10X	Number of cells/field for 5K total	Number of fields at FN22, 40X	Number of cells/field for 5K total
13	132.7	42.3	118.3	676	7.4	34.9	143.2	559	9.0
20	314.2	100	50.0	1600	3.1	82.6	60.5	1322	3.8

FN, field number.

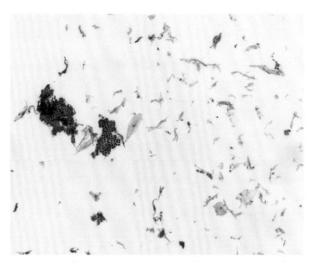

Figure 2-6. Unsatisfactory due to scant squamous cellularity. Endocervical cells are seen in a honeycomb arrangement (liquid-based preparation [LBP], ThinPrep, 10X).

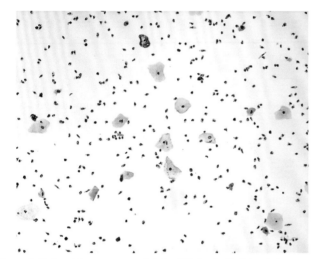

Figure 2-7. Unsatisfactory—scant cellularity (LBP, SurePath). Although this image cannot be directly compared to a microscopic field, this SurePath slide had fewer than 8 cells per 40X field. A SurePath specimen with this level of cellularity throughout the preparation would have fewer than 5000 cells.

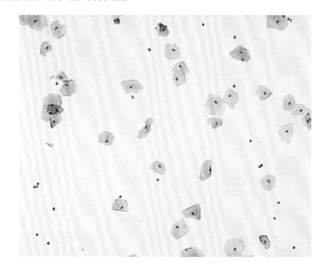

Figure 2-8. Satisfactory, but borderline squamous cellularity (LBP, SurePath). (At 40X, there were approximately 11 cells per field when 10 microscopic fields along a diameter were evaluated for squamous cellularity; this would give an estimated total cell count between 5,000 and 10,000.)

Figure 2-9. Satisfactory, but borderline squamous cellularity (LBP, ThinPrep): 10X fields of a ThinPrep specimen should have at least this level of cellularity to be considered satisfactory. (At 40X, in this ThinPrep specimen, there were approximately 4 cells per field, which would correspond to slightly over 5000 cells. Note that this level of cell density would be unsatisfactory in a SurePath LBP [see Fig. 2.7], corresponding to less than 5,000 cells because of the smaller preparation diameter.)

One preliminary study reported a higher detection rate of high-grade lesions when cellularity on LBPs exceeded 20,000.[9] However, this study did not directly investigate the possible relationship between specimen cellularity and false-negative rates, which is not necessarily the same as the relationship between specimen cellularity and the detection of high-grade lesions. Laboratories may choose to append a quality indicator comment such as "borderline or low squamous cellularity" on such specimens that meet minimal criteria for satisfactory cellularity but have only 5,000 to 20,000 cells. Patients should be managed similarly to other patients with quality indicator statements.[5]

Cellularity can be quickly and reproducibly estimated in LBPs.[7,10] Some manufacturers include estimation of LBP cellularity during training. Preliminary studies show that reference images methodology for smears is quickly learned and has better interobserver reproducibility than the previous Bethesda 10% slide coverage criterion.[11] Additional studies relating sensitivity to cell number would be useful for all preparation types. Guidelines may be revised in the future if studies demonstrate that squamous cellularity criteria different from those outlined are more appropriate.

Endocervical / Transformation Zone Component (Figs. 2.6, 2.11–2.16)

For both conventional smears and LBPs, an adequate transformation zone component requires at least 10 well-preserved endocervical or squamous metaplastic cells, singly or in clusters (Figs. 2.6, 2.11-2.15). The presence or absence of a transformation zone component is reported in the specimen adequacy section unless the woman has had a total hysterectomy. If the specimen shows a high-grade lesion or cancer, it is not necessary to report presence/

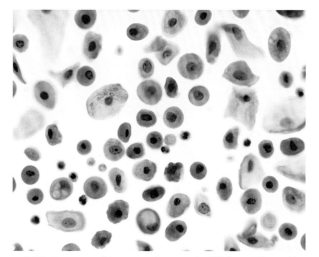

Figure 2-10. Squamous cellularity is satisfactory in this LBP from a 70-year-old woman with an atrophic cell pattern (LBP, SurePath). LBPs may show less nuclear enlargement than CPs (conventional preparations) due to fixation in the suspended state. The transformation zone component(s) may be difficult to asses in atrophy.

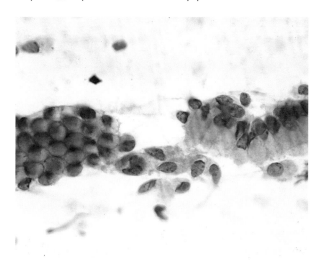

Figure 2-11. Endocervical cells (CP). Distinct cytoplasmic borders are seen in the cluster of cells on the left, giving a "honeycomb" appearance. The cell cluster on the right is seen from a side view, giving the "picket fence" appearance.

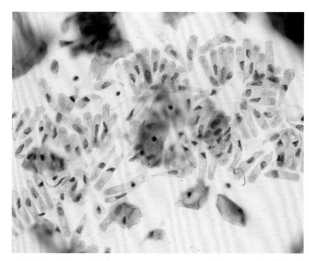

Figure 2-12. Endocervical cells (LBP). Dissociation is more frequent in liquid-based preparations than in conventional smear preparations.

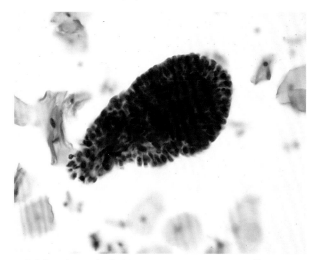

Figure 2-13. Endocervical cells (LBP). Routine screening, 27-year-old woman, NILM on follow-up. Normal endocervical cells may appear in large hyperchromatic fragments, often in the center of some LBPs. The thickness of the fragment may give the appearance of architectural disarray; however, note normal appearing cells at the periphery of the fragment. Additionally, focusing up and down through the fragment reveals normal spacing of cells, distinct cytoplasmic borders, and bland nuclear chromatin. Normal endocervical cell groups with this appearance should not be confused with dysplastic/neoplastic clusters that show more crowding (even within a single layer of cells), nuclear enlargement, nuclear membrane irregularity, and abnormal chromatin pattern.

absence of a transformation component. Degenerated cells in mucus and parabasal-type cells should not be counted in assessing transformation zone sampling. It may be difficult to distinguish parabasal-type cells from squamous metaplastic cells in specimens showing atrophy due to a variety of hormonal changes including menopause, postpartum changes, and progestational agents (Figs. 2.10, 2.16). In such cases, the laboratory may elect to make a comment about the difficulty of assessing the transformation zone component.

Explanatory Notes

Data on the importance of the endocervical/transformation zone (EC/TZ) component are conflicting. Cross-sectional studies show that SIL cells are more likely to be present on specimens in which EC/TZ cells are present.[12-14] However, retrospective cohort studies have shown that women with specimens that lack EC/TZ elements are not

more likely to have squamous lesions on follow-up than are women with EC/TZ.[15-18] Birdsong recently reviewed this subject.[19] A recent study that included colposcopic evaluation of all women with abnormal liquid-based cytology or human papillomavirus (HPV) results plus a random sample of those with negative test results failed to show an association between absent EC/TZ component and missed high-grade lesions.[20] Finally, retrospective case-control studies have failed to show an association between false-negative interpretations of specimens and lack of EC.[21,22]

The implications of the EC/TZ component could change in the future as the incidence of endocervical adenocarcinoma is increasing.[23-25] The relationship between the detection of adenocarcinoma and the presence of endocervical

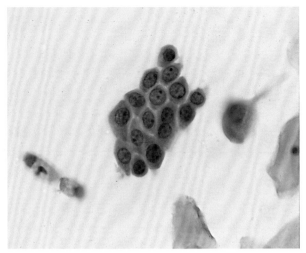

[*] **Figure 2-14.** Endocervical cells (LBP). Normal endocervical cells from the upper region of the endocervical canal can mimic squamous metaplastic cells. ([*] Bethesda Interobserver Reproducibility Project [BIRP] image.)

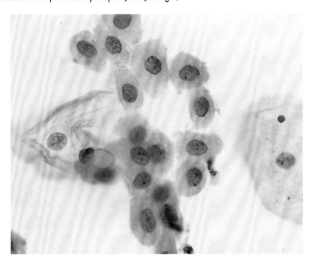

[*] **Figure 2-15.** Normal squamous metaplastic cells (LBP). Routine screening, 28-year-old woman.

cells on cervical cytology specimens is unexplored as of this writing.

Obscuring Factors (Figs. 2.17, 2.18)

Specimens with more than 75% of squamous cells obscured should be termed unsatisfactory, assuming that no abnormal cells are identified (Fig. 2.17). When 50% to 75% of the cells are obscured, a statement describing the specimen as partially obscured should follow the satisfactory term. The percentage of cells obscured, not the slide area obscured, should be evaluated, although minimal cellularity criteria

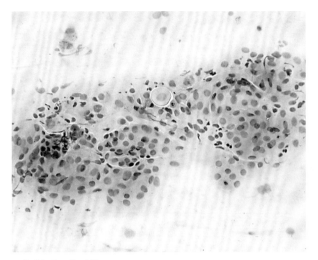

Figure 2-16. Atrophy (CP).

should also be applied. Nuclear preservation and visualization are of key importance, and changes such as cytolysis and partial obscuring of cytoplasmic detail may not necessarily interfere with specimen evaluation. Abundant cytolysis may be mentioned as a quality indicator, but most such specimens do not qualify as "unsatisfactory" unless nearly all nuclei are devoid of cytoplasm. Similar criteria apply to LBPs. In LBPs with some obscuring factors and borderline cellularity (see Figs. 2.8, 2.9), laboratories should estimate whether minimum numbers of well-visualized squamous cells are present as described above. When particular cells or areas of diagnostic interest are obscured, a report comment can be added: e.g., "air-drying of possible atypical cells" (Fig. 2.18).

Explanatory Notes

Specimens with partial obscuring factors have been shown to have fair interobserver reproducibility of adequacy assessment.[26] Although retrospective case-control studies fail to show that partial obscuring factors indicate risk for a false-negative report,[21,22] prospective studies have not been done. Reporting obscuring factors may be indicated because of patient care or quality concerns.

Management

Information on adequacy and any implications for patient follow-up may be provided optionally in an educational note. The American Society for Colposcopy and Cervical Pathology has published management guidelines for specimen adequacy and quality indicators based on the 2001 Bethesda terminology.[5]

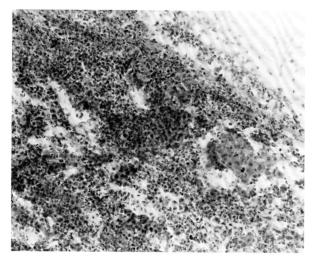

Figure 2-17. Unsatisfactory due to obscuring white blood cells (CP). If 50%–75% of the epithelial cells are covered, obscuring inflammation should be mentioned in the quality indicators section of the report (>75% obscuring is considered unsatisfactory if no abnormal cells are identified). In assessing the adequacy of a slide with respect to obscuring factors and cellularity, one should keep in mind that the minimum cellularity criteria refer to *well-visualized* cells.

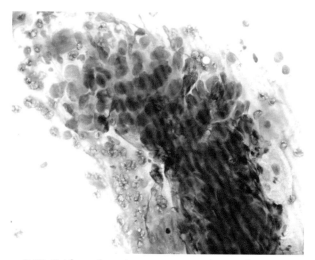

Figure 2-18. Satisfactory for evaluation; extensive air drying artifact present. Atypical squamous cells cannot exclude high grade squamous intraepithelial lesion (ASC-H) (CP). Enlarged, pale nuclei with indistinct chromatin. The nuclei are crowded and lack an orderly architectural arrangement. Note that if the interpretation is atypical cells or worse, then the specimen cannot be considered "unsatisfactory" regardless of specimen quality. Follow-up in this case was CIN 2.

Bethesda System 2001 Workshop Forum Group Moderators

Diane D. Davey, M.D., George Birdsong, M.D., Henry W. Buck, M.D., Teresa Darragh, M.D., Paul Elgert, C.T. (ASCP), Michael Henry, M.D., Heather Mitchell, M.D., Suzanne Selvaggi, M.D.

Sample Reports

Example 1

Satisfactory for evaluation; endocervical/transformation zone component present.
Interpretation:
Negative for intraepithelial lesion or malignancy.

Example 2

Satisfactory for evaluation; endocervical/transformation zone component absent/insufficient.
Interpretation:
Negative for intraepithelial lesion or malignancy.
Optional Note:
Data are conflicting regarding the significance of endocervical/transformation zone elements. A repeat cervical cytology in 12 months is generally suggested. (ASCCP Patient Management Guidelines: Am J Clin Pathol 2002;118:714-718)

Example 3

Unsatisfactory for evaluation; specimen processed and examined, but unsatisfactory for evaluation of epithelial abnormality because of obscuring inflammation.
Comment:
Trichomonas vaginalis identified.
Consider repeat cervical cytology/Pap test after treatment of *Trichomonas*.

Example 4

Interpretation:
Specimen processed and examined, but unsatisfactory for evaluation of epithelial abnormality because of insufficient squamous cellularity. Partially obscuring blood identified.
Optional:
Unsatisfactory for evaluation.
Comment:
Endometrial cells present consistent with day 5 of LMP (last menstrual period) as provided.

Example 5

Unsatisfactory for evaluation; specimen rejected because slide was received unlabeled.

References

1. Davey DD, Woodhouse S, Styer P, Stastny J, Mody D. Atypical epithelial cells and specimen adequacy: current laboratory practices of participants in the college of American pathologists interlaboratory comparison program in cervicovaginal cytology. *Arch Pathol Lab Med.* 2000;124(2):203-211.

2. Gill GW. Pap smear cellular adequacy: what does 10% coverage look like? What does it mean? *Acta Cytol.* 2000;44:873 (abstract).

3. Renshaw AA, Friedman MM, Rahemtulla A. Accuracy and reproducibility of estimating the adequacy of the squamous component of cervicovaginal smears. *Am J Clin Pathol.* 1999;111(1):38-42.

4. Valente PT, Schantz HD, Trabal JF. The determination of Papanicolaou smear adequacy using a semiquantitative method to evaluate cellularity. *Diagn Cytopathol.* 1991;7(6):576-580.

5. Davey DD, Austin RM, Birdsong G, et al. ASCCP Patient Management Guidelines: Pap test specimen adequacy and quality indicators. *J Low Genit Tract Dis.* 2002;6(3):195-199. (Also published in *Am J Clin Pathol.* 2002;118(5):714-718.)

6. Ransdell JS, Davey DD, Zaleski S. Clinicopathologic correlation of the unsatisfactory Papanicolaou smear. *Cancer (Cancer Cytopathol).* 1997;81(3):137-138.

7. Geyer JW, Carrico C, Bishop JW. Cellular constitution of Autocyte PREP cervicovaginal samples with biopsy-confirmed HSIL. *Acta Cytol.* 2000;44:505 (abstract).

8. Studeman KD, Ioffe OB, Puszkiewicz J, Sauvegeot J, Henry MR. Effect of cellularity on the sensitivity of detecting squamous lesions in liquid-based cervical cytology. *Acta Cytol.* 2003;47(4):605-610.

9. Bolick DR, Kerr J, Staley BE, et al. Effect of cellularity in the detection rates of high grade and low grade squamous intraepithelial lesions. *Acta Cytol.* 2002;46:922-923 (abstract).

10. Haroon S, Samayoa L, Witzke D, Davey D. Reproducibility of cervicovaginal ThinPrep cellularity assessment. *Diagn Cytopathol.* 2002 Jan;26(1):19-21.

11. Sheffield MV, Simsir A, Talley L, Roberson AJ, Elgert PA, Chhieng DC. Interobserver variability in assessing adequacy of the squamous component in conventional cervicovaginal smears. *Am J Clin Pathol.* 2003;119(3):367-373.

12. Martin-Hirsch P, Lilford R, Jarvis G, Kitchener HC. Efficacy of cervical-smear collection devices: a systematic review and meta-analysis. *Lancet.* 1999;354(9192):1763-1770. Erratum in: *Lancet.* 2000;355(9201):414.

13. Vooijs PG, Elias A, van der Graaf Y, Veling S. Relationship between the diagnosis of epithelial abnormalities and the composition of cervical smears. *Acta Cytol.* 1985;29(3):323-328.

14. Mintzer M, Curtis P, Resnick JC, Morrell D. The effect of the quality of Papanicolaou smears on the detection of cytologic abnormalities. *Cancer.* 1999;87(3):113-117.

15. Bos AB, van Ballegooijen M, Elske van den Akker-van Marle M, Hanselaar AG, van Oortmarssen GJ, Habbema JD. Endocervical status is not predictive of the incidence of cervical cancer in the years after negative smears. *Am J Clin Pathol.* 2001;115(6):851-855.

16. Kivlahan C, Ingram E. Papanicolaou smears without endocervical cells. Are they inadequate? *Acta Cytol.* 1986;30(3):258-260.

17. Mitchell HS. Longitudinal analysis of histologic high-grade disease after negative cervical cytology according to endocervical status. *Cancer.* 2001;93(4):237-240.

18. Mitchell H, Medley G. Longitudinal study of women with negative cervical smears according to endocervical status. *Lancet.* 1991;337(8736):265-267.

19. Birdsong GG. Pap smear adequacy: Is our understanding satisfactory...or limited? *Diagn Cytopathol.* 2001;24(2):79-81.

20. Baer A, Kiviat NB, Kulasingam S, Mao C, Kuypers J, Koutsky LA. Liquid-based Papanicolaou smears without a transformation zone component: should clinicians worry? *Obstet Gynecol.* 2002;99(6):1053-1059.

21. Mitchell H, Medley G. Differences between Papanicolaou smears with correct and incorrect diagnoses. *Cytopathology.* 1995;6(6):368-375.

22. O'Sullivan JP, A'Hern RP, Chapman PA, et al. A case-control study of true-positive versus false-negative cervical smears in women with cervical intraepithelial neoplasia (CIN) III. *Cytopathology.* 1998;9(3):155-161

23. Alfsen GC, Thoresen SO, Kristensen GB, Skovlund E, Abeler VM. Histopathologic subtyping of cervical adenocarcinoma reveals increasing incidence rates of endometrioid tumors in all age groups: a population based study with review of all nonsquamous cervical carcinomas in Norway from 1966 to 1970, 1976 to 1980, and 1986 to 1990. *Cancer.* 2000;89(6):1291-1299.

24. Stockton D, Cooper P, Lonsdale RN. Changing incidence of invasive adenocarcinoma of the uterine cervix in East Anglia. *J Med Screen.* 1997;4(1):40-43.

25. Zheng T, Holford TR, Ma Z, et al. The continuing increase in adenocarcinoma of the uterine cervix: a birth cohort phenomenon. *Int J Epidemiol.* 1996;25(2):252-258.

26. Spires SE, Banks ER, Weeks JA, Banks HW, Davey DD. Assessment of cervicovaginal smear adequacy. The Bethesda System guidelines and reproducibility. *Am J Clin Pathol.* 1994;102(3):354-359.

Human Papillomavirus: Basic Facts and Relevance to Gynecologic Cytology

Nancy A. Young, MD
David C. Wilbur, MD

Introduction

First and foremost, cervical cancer screening programs were designed and are primarily used for the detection of cervical cancer and its precursor lesions. Since virtually all cervical cancer is associated with, and at least partly caused by, the human papillomavirus (HPV),[1,2] the beginning of any discussion of cervical cancer screening should start with a basic understanding of HPV and its role in cervical carcinogenesis. HPV is one of the most extensively studied infectious organisms in medicine. It is important because some of the members of this large family of viruses play a central role in one of the most common neoplastic conditions worldwide, that being cervical cancer and its precursor lesions. Knowledge of the basic facts about the virus, its mode of transmission, and methods for viral detection is critical for the understanding of current methodologies of disease management, detection, and prevention through vaccination.

This chapter will provide the basic facts that are necessary for a full understanding of this important biologic process. The format uses a series of the most common questions and answers regarding HPV.

1. What is HPV?

HPV is a member of the papovavirus family. Its genetic material consists of an 8 Kbase circular single DNA strand, which is encapsulated by an icosahedral capsule (Figure 3-1). The HPV DNA strand contains 6 "early" genes (E genes) and a controlling regulatory region that code for the viral replication processes, and 2 "late" genes (L genes) that code for the capsule proteins (Figure 3-2). HPV requires a human host cell in which to replicate.

2. What cell in the genital tract does HPV infect?

Certain types of HPV can infect most types of epithelial cells of the anogenital tract: both squamous cells of the perineal skin, vulva, vagina, and cervix; and glandular cells of the endocervix. However, it is predominantly the metabolically active epithelial cells of the transformation zones of the cervix and anus where squamous metaplasia occurs that are the most common targets of the oncogenic actions of HPV (Figure 3-3). This feature illustrates why most cervical neoplasia arises in the transformation zones and forms the basis for the importance of sampling of these regions during the cytologic screening process.

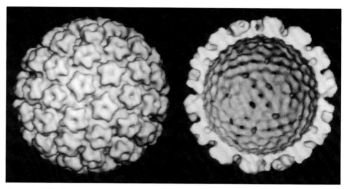

Figure 3-1. A computer reproduction of a scanning electron micrograph of the human papillomavirus. Note the icosahedral structure of the surface coat. Proteins in the coat are the immunogens utilized in the development of the currently available HPV vaccine. From: Baker TS, Newcomb WW, Olson NH, Cowsert LM, Olson C, Brown JC. Structures of bovine and human papillomaviruses: analysis by cryoelectron microscopy and three-dimensional image reconstruction. *Biophys J.* 1991;60:1445-1456. Copyright 1991 Biophysical Society. Reprinted with permission.

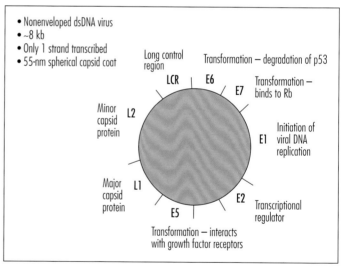

Figure 3-2. A schematic of the HPV circular genome organization. The early (E) genes control viral replication functions, and the late (L) proteins code for capsid proteins. In vegetative HPV infections, the entire genome is present, generally in an episomal form, outside of the host genome. All genes are necessary for completion of the virus life cycle and making of new virions. In true neoplastic (transformed) cells, only oncogenic portions of the genome are consistently retained and integrated into the host genome. E6 and E7 are always retained, as these are the oncogenic genes interacting with and ablating the actions of the tumor suppressor genes p53 and Rb, respectively. Integration usually disrupts the action of the E2 gene, which is responsible for viral transcription regulation; hence, E6 and E7 are transcribed in an uncontrolled fashion.

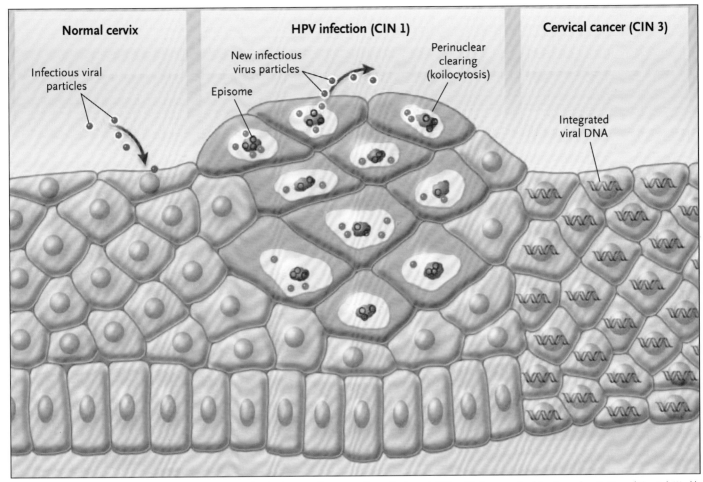

Figure 3-3. Infection of the squamous epithelium with HPV (left), development of a productive viral infection (middle), and development of a true neoplastic lesion (right). Koilocytosis is evidence of productive virion formation, whereas true neoplastic lesions do not typically complete the viral life cycle and hence do not show koilocytosis.

From: Goodman A, Wilbur DC. Case records of the Massachusetts General Hospital. Weekly clinicopathological exercises. Case 32-2003. A 37-year-old woman with atypical squamous cells on a Papanicolaou smear. *N Engl J Med.* 2003;349:1555-1564. Copyright © 2003 Massachusetts Medical Society. All rights reserved. Reprinted with permission.

3. How is HPV transmitted?

Genital HPV infection is considered to be almost exclusively sexually transmitted. There is some evidence to suggest that a small number of genital infections may be due to nonsexual contact via fomites (inanimate carriers). However, the virus has difficulty surviving for long periods of time outside of its normal host environment; hence, fomite transmission is generally thought to be a very minor pathway in comparison with the usual sexual route.

4. How many women are infected?

This figure depends on the age and population studied. Generally, younger women have higher prevalence rates. These rates may be as high as 30% in the late teens and early twenties, fall through the reproductive years to as low as 5%, and then may rise again in the late forties and fifties, sometimes to as high as 10% to 20%. The reasons for this second rise are uncertain. Two possibilities have been suggested: (1) increased number of new sexual partners in this age group or (2) alterations in immune surveillance

status, allowing persistent subclinical infections to become detectable.

In a meta-analysis study of more than 150,000 women with normal cytology reported from 78 separate studies, the overall prevalence of detectable HPV worldwide was 10.4%. This background prevalence varied by continent, with Africa having the highest prevalence at 22.9%; followed by Central, South, and North America at 20.5%, 14.3%, and 13.8%, respectively; Asia overall at 8.3% (China/South Korea at 18.5%); and Europe overall at 6.6% (Russia and Eastern Europe at 29.1%)[3] (Figure 3-4).

5. Does an HPV infection imply the presence of clinical disease?

Not always. Most women with detectable HPV will have either no manifestation of cervical disease (squamous intraepithelial lesion [SIL] or cancer) or will manifest only a low-grade squamous intraepithelial lesion (LSIL), which generally represents an acute infection rather than a neoplastic state. Such infections generally will clear after several months to years (see question 9).

Worldwide High-Risk HPV Prevalence in Cytologically Normal Women		
Africa		22.9%
	Eastern Africa	35.4%
	Northern Africa	21.5%
	Southern Africa	15.5%
	Western Africa	16.5%
The Americas		15.5%
	Central America	20.5%
	South America	14.3%
	North America	13.8%
Europe		6.6%
	Eastern Europe	29.1%
	Northern Europe	8.0%
	Southern Europe	5.7%
	Western Europe	6.1%
Asia		8.3%
	Eastern Asia	18.5%
	Japan and Taiwan	7.5%
	Southeast Asia	6.2%
	India	6.6%
Total		10.4%

Figure 3-4. Data from a meta-analysis of 78 separate studies on high-risk HPV prevalence in cytologically benign women worldwide. The overall average is 10.4%. Underdeveloped areas show increased prevalence as compared with developed countries, which have higher levels of cervical cancer screening. Source: de Sanjose et al.[3]

6. What is the difference between "low-risk" and "high-risk" HPV types?

Low-risk HPV types are virtually never associated with high-grade cervical cancer precursors and invasive carcinomas. High-risk types are the only viruses that cause lesions that are true precursors of invasive carcinoma (both squamous and endocervical). Basically, the difference has to do with how effective the oncogenic portions of their genomes are at transforming normal cells into malignant ones; low-risk HPVs have little transforming potential. This biologic difference is the reason that clinical testing for low-risk types is considered to be of no management value and the reason that all management guidelines include testing for high-risk types only. It is important to remember that most low-grade lesions are still associated with high-risk viral types (as high as 85% to 90%); therefore, low-grade disease does not imply low-risk virus.[4]

7. What are the specific disease associations of HPV types?

Specific HPV types have been shown to be more commonly associated with different morphologic lesions. HPV type 16 is more commonly associated with squamous cancers, and HPV type 18 is more commonly associated with endocervical adenocarcinoma and neuroendocrine (small cell) carcinoma. HPV types 6 and 11 are the most common low-risk types and are most commonly associated with benign

Clinical Lesion	HPV Types
Common warts	2, 4
Plantar warts	1
Condyloma acuminatum	6, 11
Laryngeal papillomatosis	11, 6
LSIL	All mucosotropic types
HSIL and squamous cancer	16, 18, 31, 33, 35, 39, 45, 51, 51+
Other anogenital cancer	16

Figure 3-5. The types of virus most commonly associated with various morphologic entities. As noted, condylomatous lesions of the external genitalia are typical associated with low-risk viral types 6 and 11. Low-grade cervical lesions are most commonly associated with high-risk types but can also be associated with low-risk types. High-grade lesions are virtually always associated with high-risk viral types.

genital warts (condyloma) (Figure 3-5). In addition, there are HPV type subdivisions, referred to as HPV type variants. These subdivisions are based on intratype genetic variability in portions of the viral genome. Variants differ by less than 2% in the genetic sequence, whereas division into types requires greater than a 10% difference.

Variant HPVs are clustered along geographic lines, meaning that humans evolving in one geographic population (eg, European, Asian, North American) will have slightly different genetic makeup in their HPV 16 than will those derived from other geographic locations. These differences most likely arise from host-virus interactions over time, with geographic "matching" of the HPV variant into the most advantageous situation (presumably for propagation and survival) based on host factors such as population-specific HLA types and other genetic factors.[5] The differences between variants has been implicated (by as yet incompletely understood factors) as a potential factor in differences in morphogenesis of cancers of the cervix (eg, squamous versus glandular).[6]

8. What is the most prevalent HPV type?

HPV type 16 is the most prevalent high-risk viral type in all populations studied and can comprise as many as 40% of the infections. Its associated family members, types 18, 45, 31, 33, 35, 52, and 58, are the next most frequent types. Types 16 and 18 account for 71% of all cervical cancers worldwide. Together with types 16 and 18, the six additional most common types mentioned account for 87% of all cervical cancers.[7]

9. What is the biologic difference between low-grade and high-grade cervical lesions?

Low-grade squamous intraepithelial lesion (LSIL) is the cytologic correlate of lesions that, on histology, are classified as cervical intraepithelial neoplasia grade 1 (CIN I).

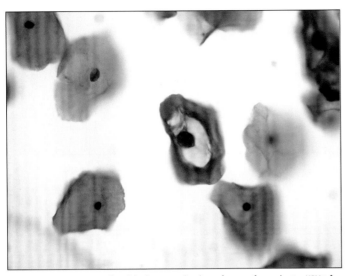

Figure 3-6. Squamous cell with koilocytosis, the classic feature of a productive HPV infection (low-grade squamous intraepithelial lesion [LSIL]).

These lesions are generally associated with replicative infections of HPV where the viral DNA is present as an episome outside the host cell DNA. These productive infections allow completion of the viral life cycle and the production of whole infectious virions capable of infecting other cells. The koilocyte, the classic morphologic feature of LSIL (Figure 3-6), is a cell filled with complete virions ready to spill out. Low-grade lesions typically run a benign course and resolve—similar to cutaneous HPVs associated with common warts of the skin. Studies have shown that if followed for a 3-year period, LSIL will clear to normal, with nondetectable HPV in greater than 90% of cases.[8]

High-grade squamous intraepithelial lesion (HSIL) and cancer may contain only the oncogenic portions of the HPV genome. These genes are most commonly integrated into the host's DNA in specific ways that allow uncontrolled expression and cellular replication, so-called cellular transformation. Some true high-grade lesions can retain these oncogenic genes in an episomal form, and therefore integration is not universal. In either case, because a functional complete genome is not present, these are not replicative infections and no intact virions are produced; hence, koilocytosis is not a feature of these lesions. These changes are generally considered to represent true neoplastic precursors.

One of the important issues to remember is that not all HSIL lesions are truly biologic high grade, with a potential for invasion. A spectrum of "moderate dysplasia" (CIN II) may represent either low-grade or high-grade disease processes but would, under the Bethesda System classification scheme, fall into HSIL. This situation occurs because it is not possible on a morphologic basis to discriminate between the CIN II cases that represent low-grade versus high-grade disease; hence, the Bethesda System consensus decision was to err on the side of safety in this categorization in order not to miss true high-grade disease processes (maximization of cytologic sensitivity at the expense of

specificity for true high-grade disease). It should be noted that other classification schemes in use distinguish CIN II from CIN III lesions cytologically primarily because of this issue and the more conservative management differences that are associated.

10. What are the oncogenic genes of HPV and what do they do?

In virtually all biologic high-grade neoplasias and cancer, two HPV genes are always conserved. These are the E6 and E7 genes. The E6 gene acts by interfering with the host p53 tumor suppressor gene function, and the E7 gene acts by interfering with the host retinoblastoma (Rb) tumor suppressor gene function. Hence, both host tumor suppressor genes are "disabled," leading to an increased propensity for cellular neoplastic transformation. In neoplastic lesions, breakage of the HPV circular DNA during insertion into the host genome occurs in the region of the E2 gene, thus disrupting the regulation of the expression of the E6 and E7 genes, which leads to uncontrolled transcription. E6 and E7 gene actions disable the ability to repair DNA mutations prior to DNA replication (aberrant S-phase initiation), leading to accumulations of somatic mutations in infected cells (Figure 3-3).

11. What are the methods for detecting HPV?

Hybrid Capture® 2 (hc2), "the Digene® test" (Qiagen, Gaithersberg, Maryland), is the most commonly utilized method for the detection of HPV DNA. It has been the method of choice in a large number of clinical studies (most notably the National Cancer Institute's ASCUS-LSIL Triage Study [ALTS]), and it forms the basis for the most current management schemes, including the 2006 guidelines from the American Society for Colposcopy and Cervical Pathology (ASCCP).[9] The test detects high-risk virus in a sensitive manner but lacks specificity for clinical disease, meaning that not all patients testing positive for HPV have SIL (dysplasia) or cancer. It is relatively inexpensive and easy to perform. It operates on the principle of the detection of HPV DNA by hybridization with a whole genomic RNA probe. Hybrids formed are then detected in a chemiluminescent assay, which is semiquantitative for the amount of HPV DNA in the overall sample. At the time of this writing, hc2, using either The ThinPrep® Pap Test (Hologic Inc, Bedford, Massachusetts) or Standard Transport Medium (Qiagen) collection methods, is the only test for HPV detection cleared by the US Food and Drug Administration (FDA).

Another signal amplification technology for the detection of HPV is the Third Wave Invader® technology, which utilizes a proprietary isothermal process to enhance the signal. Early studies have shown greater sensitivity of HPV detection compared to Hybrid Capture 2, and this method has the advantage of an included internal control (human anti-actin) to ensure that an adequate specimen has been obtained.[10] At the time of this writing, a clinical trial for FDA approval of the HPV Invader technology has been initiated.

In situ hybridization (ISH) is a method that has been utilized in research laboratories for a long time, but which has only recently been commercialized into a proprietary laboratory test (INFORM®; Ventana Medical Systems Inc, Tucson, Arizona). It is performed directly on cellular specimens, and therefore direct visualization of infected cells and correlation with a morphologic abnormality is possible. Preliminary studies comparing this method with the hc2 method suggested that ISH may not be as sensitive as hc2 for the detection of HPV but may be more specific for the detection of disease, meaning that cells infected, but producing no cytologic manifestations, may not be positive with this test.[11] However, additional studies have indicated that the sensitivity may not be as high as originally hoped, and thus further study is required to verify ISH's operating characteristics.[12] The Ventana test is performed on its automated Benchmark staining system and hence is a very simple test (Figure 3-7). This test has not been cleared by the FDA for routine clinical use, and, as such, like the Third Wave method, laboratories using this test for HPV DNA detection are required to perform appropriate analytic and clinical validation studies prior to use.[13]

Polymerase chain reaction (PCR) is the standard reference method for the detection of the presence of HPV and has the added advantage of allowing specific viral typing or, in the case of real-time PCR techniques, can also provide assessments of viral load. It is highly sensitive for the detection of the presence of HPV DNA but shares the lack of specificity for disease detection that is observed with hc2. The assay is commercially available (Amplicor HPV, Roche Diagnostics, Switzerland). At the time of this writing, no FDA clearance has been given for PCR-based detection of HPV, and hence appropriate analytic and clinical validation studies are required in any laboratory prior to clinical use.

With immunocytochemistry, antibodies are available for the detection of HPV viral capsid antigen. Because these antibodies detect only the viral coats of intact virions, they are not clinically useful for screening for biologic high-grade disease and are not in general use in any of the clinical triage protocols. New markers for proliferation antigens combined with aberrant cell cycle antigens are promising in their ability to detect high-grade disease with reasonable sensitivity and specificity.[14,15] Again, as an "in situ" assay, the ability to visualize the underlying cellular morphology may be useful in fine-tuning interpretation.

12. Are there other diseases associated with HPV and what are they?

Anal Cancer. The anus resembles the cervix in that both have a transformation zone, connecting glandular to squamous epithelium, which is susceptible to HPV infection with a high risk of neoplastic transformation.[16] Non-keratinizing squamous cell carcinoma of the anus is more strongly associated with HPV than the keratinizing type. Overall, approximately 90% of anal cancers are attributable to HPV. The risk of anal cancer has been associated with

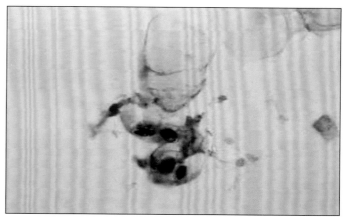

Figure 3-7. Positive staining for HPV DNA in an in-situ hybridization reaction. The nucleus of the cell is dark blue compared to the surrounding negative (pink) nuclei.

the number of sex partners of the opposite sex, homosexual contact (for men), other sexually transmitted infections, and receptive anal intercourse. In addition to HPV, constant irritation and chronic inflammatory changes may also play a role in cancer development. As in the case of cervical cancer, HIV infection is also strongly associated with an increased risk of anal cancer, which may in part be due to the suppressed immune system.

Penile Cancer. Penile cancer is similar to vulvar cancer in that HPV is related only to certain histologic subtypes.[17] Little is known about the natural history of penile HPV infection (acquisition, clearance, or persistence). The overall prevalence of HPV in penile cancers ranges from 15% to 71% in the largest published studies.[18] HPV-related lesions can be commonly observed on all parts of the penis as whitening following the application of acetic acid. Sometimes the lesions may appear precancerous microscopically; however, given the low risk of transformation to cancer, they are not true surrogates for cancer.[16]

Recurrent Respiratory Papillomatosis (RRP). In the United States, approximately 600 infants are diagnosed with RRP annually. It is associated with low-risk HPV types 6 and 11. It is hypothesized that these infants acquire HPV infection during passage through a heavily infected birth canal. The disease is manifested as rapidly growing exophytic lesions in the upper airway, most often in the larynx, causing severe respiratory and speech impairment. Repeated excision is often needed for management of airway obstruction, which can be life threatening. Severity of the disease has been linked primarily to cases with HPV type 11 infections. Host genetic and immune factors are thought to be associated with the development of this disorder, as many infants are infected with HPV 6 and/or 11 at birth, but only a small number are affected with RRP. Rare cases of progression to invasive squamous cell carcinoma have been reported.[19]

Other Non-anogenital HPV-associated Malignancies. HPV has been associated with malignancies involving the aerodigestive tract, including oropharyngeal carcinoma, lung cancer, and esophageal cancer. Recent evidence has linked HPV types 16 and 18 to lung cancer among non-smoking females in Taiwan,[20] HPV type 18 to esophageal cancer among Greek men and women,[21] and HPV type 16 to schistosomiasis-associated bladder cancer.[22] Multiple studies have also linked HPV to oropharyngeal squamous cell carcinoma among individuals who neither smoke nor abuse alcohol.[23-27]

References

1. Walboomers JM, Jacobs MV, Manos MM, et al. Human papillomavirus is a necessary cause of invasive cervical cancer worldwide. *J Pathol*. 1999;189:12-19.

2. Schiffman M, Castle PE, Jeronimo J, Rodriguez AC, Wacholder S. Human papillomavirus and cervical cancer. *Lancet*. 2007;370:890-907.

3. de Sanjose S, Diaz M, Castellsague X, et al. Worldwide prevalence and genotype distribution of cervical human papillomavirus DNA in women with normal cytology: a meta-analysis. *Lancet Infect Dis*. 2007;7:453-459.

4. Stoler MH. Testing for human papillomavirus: data driven implications for cervical neoplasia management. *Clin Lab Med*. 2003;23(3):569-583.

5. Schiffman M, Herrero R, DeSalle R, et al. The carcinogenicity of human papillomavirus types reflects viral evolution. *Virology*. 2005;337:76-84.

6. Sichero L, Villa LL. Epidemiological and functional implications of molecular variants of human papillomavirus. *Braz J Med Biol Res*. 2006;39:707-717.

7. Muñoz N, Bosch FX, Castellsagué X, et al. Against which human papillomavirus types shall we vaccinate and screen?: the international perspective. *Int J Cancer*. 2004;111:278-285.

8. Moscicki AB, Shiboski S, Hills NK, et al. Regression of low-grade squamous intra-epithelial lesions in young women. *Lancet*. 2004;364:1678-1683.

9. Wright TC Jr, Massad LS, Dunton CJ, Spitzer M, Wilkinson EJ, Solomon D; for the 2006 ASCCP-Sponsored Consensus Conference. 2006 consensus guidelines for the management of women with abnormal cervical screening tests. *J Low Genit Tract Dis*. 2007;11:201-222.

10. Schutzbank TE, Jarvis C, Kahmann N, et al. Detection of high-risk human papillomavirus DNA with commercial Invader technology-based analyte specific reagents following automated extraction of DNA from cervical brushings in ThinPrep media. *J Clin Microbiol*. 2007;45(12):4067-4069. Epub 2007 Oct 24.

11. Qureshi MN, Rudelli RD, Tubbs RR, Biscotti CV, Layfield LJ. Role of HPV DNA testing in predicting cervical intraepithelial lesions: comparison of HC HPV and ISH HPV. *Diagn Cytopathol*. 2003;29:149-155.

12. Hesselink AT, van den Brule AJ, Brink AA, et al. Comparison of hybrid capture 2 with in situ hybridization for the detection of high-risk human papillomavirus in liquid-based cervical samples. *Cancer*. 2004;102:11-18.

13. Stoler MH, Castle PE, Solomon D, Schiffman M. The expanded use of HPV testing in gynecologic practice per ASCCP-guided management requires the use of well-validated assays. *Am J Clin Pathol*. 2007;127:1-3.

14. Homer P, Heinz D, Singh M. Validation of a novel immunocytochemical assay for topoisomerase II-alpha and minichromosome maintenance protein 2 expression in cervical cytology. *Cancer*. 2006;108:324-330.

15. Guo M, Hu L, Baliga M, He Z, Hughson MD. The predictive value of p16(INK4a) and hybrid capture 2 human papillomavirus testing for high-grade cervical intraepithelial neoplasia. *Am J Clin Pathol*. 2004;122:894-901.

16. Schiffman M, Kjaer SK. Chapter 2: natural history of anogenital human papillomavirus infection and neoplasia. *J Natl Cancer Inst Monogr*. 2003;31:14-19.

17. Bezerra AL, Lopes A, Landman G, Alencar GN, Torloni H, Villa LL. Clinicopathologic features and human papillomavirus DNA prevalence of warty and squamous cell carcinoma of the penis. *Am J Surg Pathol*. 2001;25:673-678.

18. Rubin MA, Kleter B, Zhou M, et al. Detection and typing of human papillomavirus DNA in penile carcinoma: evidence for multiple independent pathways of penile carcinogenesis. *Am J Pathol*. 2001;159:1211-1218.

19. Lee JH, Smith RJ. Recurrent respiratory papillomatosis: pathogenesis and treatment. *Curr Opin Otolaryngol Head Neck Surg*. 2005;13:354-359.

20. Lin TS, Lee H, Chen RA, et al. An association of DNMT3b protein expression with P16INK4a promoter hypermethylation in non-smoking female lung cancer with human papillomavirus infection. *Cancer Lett*. 2005;226:77-84.

21. Lyronis ID, Baritaki S, Bizakis I, Tsardi M, Spandidos DA. Evaluation of the prevalence of human papillomavirus and Epstein-Barr virus in esophageal squamous cell carcinomas. *Int J Biol Markers*. 2005;20:5-10.

22. Yang H, Yang K, Khafagi A, et al. Sensitive detection of human papillomavirus in cervical, head/neck, and schistosomiasis-associated bladder malignancies. *Proc Natl Acad Sci USA*. 2005;102:7683-7688.

23. Elamin F, Steingrimsdottir H, Wanakulasuriya S, Johnson N, Tavassoli M. Prevalence of human papillomavirus infection in premalignant and malignant lesions of the oral cavity in U.K. subjects: a novel method of detection. *Oral Oncol*. 1998;34:191-197.

24. Scully C. Oral squamous cell carcinoma: from an hypothesis about a virus, to concern about possible sexual transmission. *Oral Oncol*. 2002;38:227-234.

25. Miller CS, Johnstone BM. Human papillomavirus as a risk factor for oral squamous cell carcinoma: a meta-analysis, 1982-1997. *Oral Surg Oral Med Oral Pathol Oral Radiol Endod*. 2001;91:622-635.

26. Mork J, Lie AK, Glattre E, et al. Human papillomavirus infection as a risk factor for squamous-cell carcinoma of the head and neck. *N Engl J Med*. 2001;344:1125-1131.

27. D'Souza G, Kreimer AR, Viscidi R, et al. Case-control study of human papillomavirus and oropharyngeal cancer. *N Engl J Med*. 2007;356:1944-1956.

Benign Changes and Mimics of Malignant and Premalignant Epithelial Lesions

Camilla J. Cobb, MD

[handwritten annotations: inflam rxn △ / ↑v3 nuc / fine nuc / bi nuc / nucleoli // degen △ clumpy chromatin]

General Features

The recognition of benign changes, organisms, and artifacts in cervical/vaginal cytologic samples is important for all cytology practitioners. Many benign conditions observed in Pap slides are notorious for their ability to mimic malignant and premalignant epithelial lesions. Awareness of these entities and recognition of their unique cytomorphology are important to avoid misdiagnosis and, especially, overdiagnosis. The observation of various organisms may be useful in the treatment of diseases related to their presence. Recognition of various artifacts is also important for proper interpretation. The cytomorphology of common and uncommon benign conditions is discussed in this chapter, with emphasis on the features that are most useful in distinguishing them from malignant and premalignant epithelial lesions.

[handwritten annotation: neoplasia = ↑v3 nuc (x3 intmed)]

Benign Inflammatory Conditions

Figure 4-1. Reactive and inflammatory epithelial cell changes.

Inflammatory epithelial cell changes include nonspecific reactive features such as nuclear enlargement, prominent nucleoli, fine and evenly distributed chromatin, binucleation and multinucleation, and smooth nuclear borders (A through D). These changes may be seen in either squamous or endocervical cells. A benign finding that may be confused with low-grade squamous intraepithelial lesion (LSIL) is that of small perinuclear vacuoles, which are distinguished from koilocytes by their small diameter, lack of a sharp "cookie-cutter" edge, and absence of associated dysplastic nuclear changes (see Figure 7-17). These shallow vacuoles can also be found with specific infections, such as *Candida* and *Trichomonas* (E and F). Degenerative change (eg, dark clumpy or smudgy chromatin, karyopyknosis, karyorrhexis) is common in association with these processes (H). Distinction from dysplasia is sometimes difficult. However, dysplasia is associated with greater nuclear enlargement (greater than three times the size of a normal intermediate nucleus); darker, more coarsely granular, irregularly distributed chromatin; and frequent irregularity of the nuclear borders (I). Background inflammation is predominantly acute in nature, but remember that an acute inflammatory background can be seen with dysplasia as well.

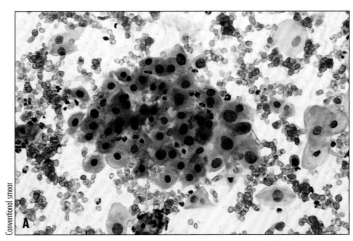

Conventional smear

A

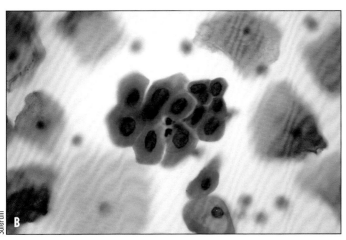

SurePath

B

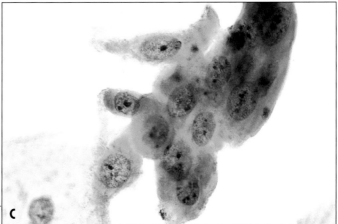

ThinPrep

C

Figure 4-1 continued.

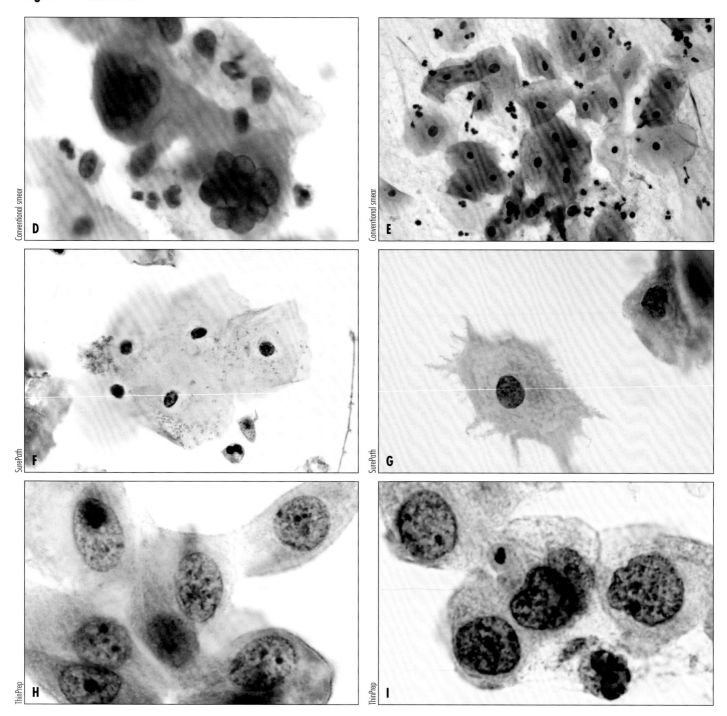

Figure 4-2. Parabasal and squamous metaplastic cells.

These two cell types are morphologically similar, and their presence in Pap specimens reflects sampling from a relatively thin, immature, squamous mucosal surface predisposed to conditions (eg, infection, irritation, erosion, ulceration) that lead to reactive/reparative and degenerative changes. Parabasal-like cells often dominate during the postpartum and postmenopausal periods and are also seen in some cyclic women taking Depo-Provera or other progestational drugs (C). These cells reflect the lack of maturation of the squamous epithelium due to low estrogen levels. Squamous metaplasia occurs at the transformation zone of cyclic women and may yield large numbers of immature squamous cells. Reactive/reparative change (prominent nucleoli, mild hyperchromasia, nuclear enlargement, mitotic activity) and degenerative changes (dark clumpy or smudgy chromatin) in these small squamous cells are sometimes confused with dysplasia or carcinoma (E and H). Cytologic features that support an accurate benign interpretation include nuclear uniformity, smooth nuclear borders, polarity in cell groups, and finely granular and evenly distributed chromatin (see Figure 7-19). In conventional Pap smears, these cells most often appear in two-dimensional sheets (D), but they can form more rounded groups in liquid-based preparations (F).

benign metaplasia = smooth nuclear borders

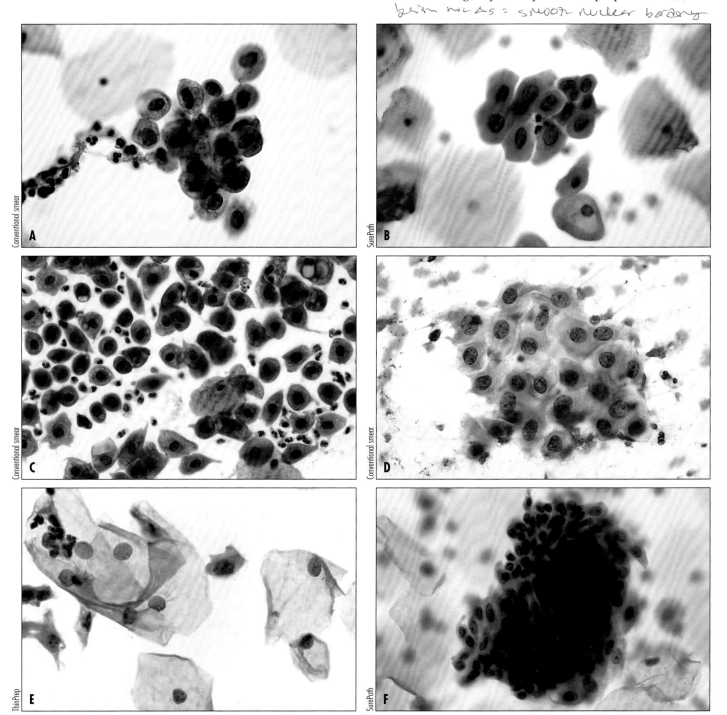

Figure 4-3. Anucleated squamous cells.

Anucleated squamous cells (ANSC) are indicative of super-ficial epithelial keratosis and, when present in small numbers, may represent contamination from skin and can be ignored, as this does not represent a significant clinical finding (A). ANSC, especially in larger numbers, may represent keratosis involving the cervix or vagina, where the cause is chronic irritation due to an infection or uterine prolapse. ANSC may also overlie squamous intraepithelial lesions and even, on occasion, squamous cell carcinoma (B). Therefore, careful review of the slide for an underlying epithelial lesion is warranted whenever abundant ANSC are present, especially when in large plaque-like aggregates (C).

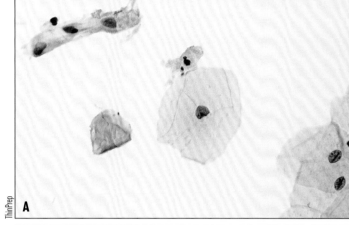

ThinPrep   A

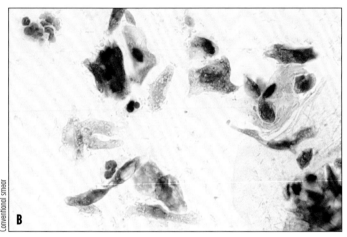

Conventional smear   B

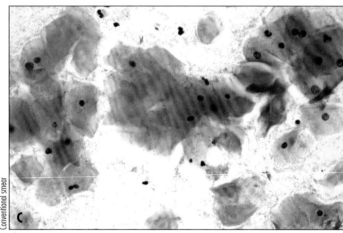

Conventional smear   C

Figure 4-4. Atrophic vaginitis.

Atrophic vaginitis (AV) is usually observed in post-menopausal women or, uncommonly, in postpartum patients. Pap slides with AV show variable inflammation, marked background necrosis (simulating a tumor diathe-sis), and degeneration of the small, parabasal squamous cells. "Blue blobs," which are degenerating parabasal cells, resemble large, abnormal, bare nuclei (B, arrow). These findings can be confused with malignancy, especially when the atrophic changes include background necrosis or a degenerative pseudo-parakeratotic change (F, G, and H). Close examination of the viable cells and noting the absence of significant atypia in these cells help to avoid overinterpretation. In benign atrophy, there is most often a spectrum of atrophy ranging from obvious benign changes to the more atypical groups. Occasionally a diagnosis of atypical squamous cells of undetermined significance (ASC-US) or atypical squamous cells, cannot exclude high-grade squamous intraepithelial lesion (ASC-H) is warrant-ed (see Figure 5-8), in which case follow-up testing for high-risk human papillomavirus (HPV) and/or col-poscopy would be warranted, according to the latest American Society for Colposcopy and Cervical Pathology (ASCCP) guidelines.

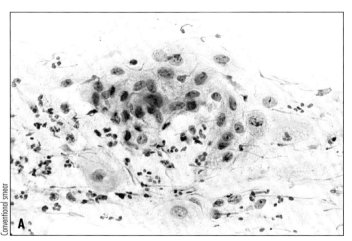

Conventional smear   A

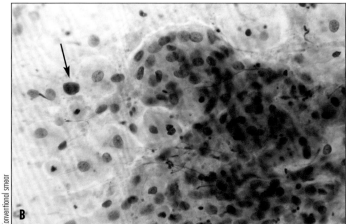

Conventional smear   B

Figure 4-4 continued.

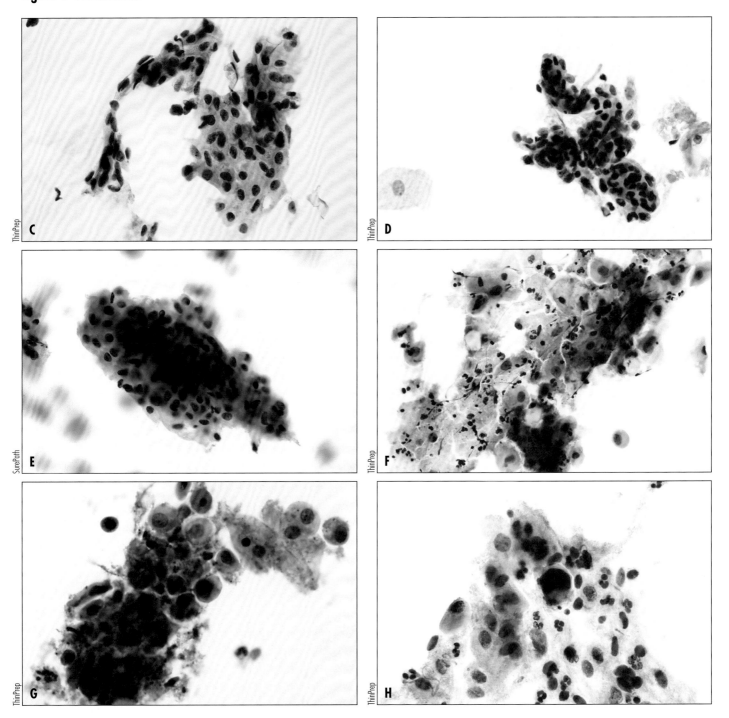

Figure 4-5. Degenerative changes in benign cells.

Degenerative changes include cytoplasmic and nuclear vacuolization, cellular and nuclear enlargement, chromatin clumping, karyopyknosis (very dense chromatin that lacks detail), karyorrhexis (the breaking up of nuclear chromatin following rupture of the nuclear membrane), and karyolysis (dissolution of the nuclear chromatin) (A, B, and C). The degenerative finding that is perhaps most worrisome for cancer or dysplasia is chromatin clumping. However, degenerative chromatin clumps are more smoothly contoured and regular in size, shape, and distribution than are those found in dysplasia or carcinoma (D and E). Exercise caution when evaluating for dysplasia or malignancy in groups of cells showing obvious degenerative changes.

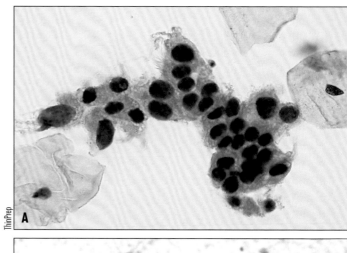

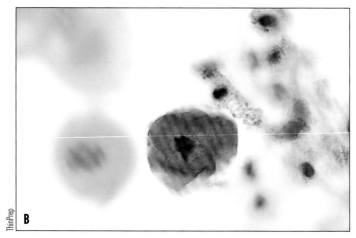

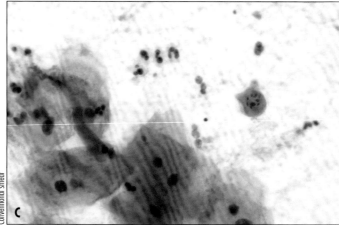

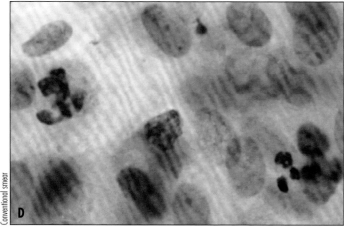

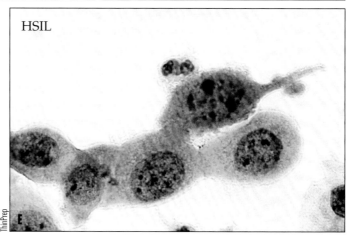

Figure 4-6. Chronic follicular cervicitis. = germinal center of chlon.

Chronic follicular (ie, germinal center) cervicitis (CFC) is limited to the cervical submucosa. Therefore, Pap slides may show evidence of CFC only when there is erosion or ulceration of the overlying mucosa or if the mucosa is very thin, as in markedly atrophic squamous conditions. CFC is characterized by focal collections of polymorphous lymphocytes with scattered intermixed tingible body macrophages. The differential diagnosis can include HSIL, small cell carcinoma and lymphoma/leukemia. Most helpful for interpretation is the appreciation of the characteristic dark, clumped chromatin of the small mature lymphocytes and the recognition of the larger, phagocytic tingible body macrophages (A, arrow). In HSIL, the chromatin is not as coarsely granular, and cells are overall larger and more pleomorphic, with some cells showing obvious squamous differentiation. In HSIL, abnormal epithelial clusters are also usually present elsewhere on the slide. Pap slides involved with a small cell malignancy (eg, primary or metastatic small cell carcinoma, leukemia/lymphoma) are typically dominated by the malignant cells and show a tumor diathesis and significant nuclear abnormalities. In contrast, CFC is a focal and minor component of the slide and is not associated with necrosis or a diathesis. When lymphoma or leukemia presents in Pap slides, there is usually a history of such, as primary lymphoma of the cervicovaginal area is extremely rare. With regard to CFC, there are differences between conventional smears and liquid-based preparations. In conventional smears, CFC presents as dispersed cells in localized areas (A and B), whereas in liquid-based preparations, the cells of CFC usually form loose clusters, with scattered isolated small lymphocytes present in the slide background (C, D, and E).

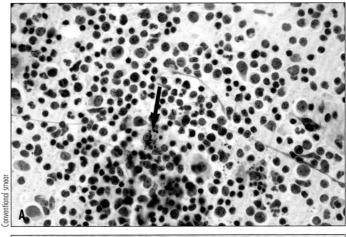

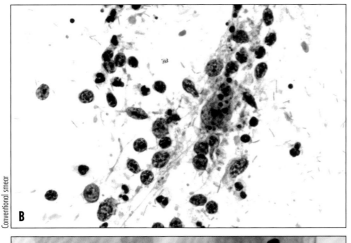

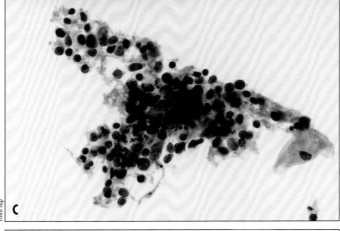

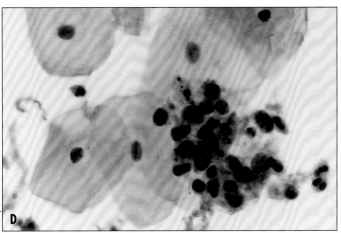

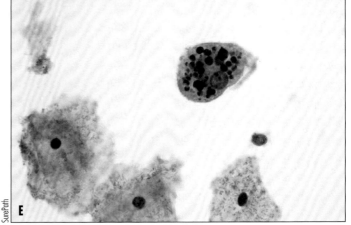

Figure 4-7. Parakeratotic cells.

Parakeratotic (PK) cells are tiny versions of superficial squamous cells, but with dense, glassy cytoplasm that stains pink, blue, or orange (A and B). Most often PK cells replace surface squamous cells in response to chronic irritation of a benign nature (eg, infection, uterine prolapse). PK may present as single cells, small plaques or sheets, or as a keratin pearl (C). Typical PK, with round to oval pyknotic nuclei and low nuclear to cytoplasmic (N:C) ratios, is considered to be a benign finding. Infrequently, benign-appearing PK cells overlie squamous dysplasia or invasive squamous cell carcinoma, in which case the Pap slide typically contains other obvious abnormal squamous cells representative of these lesions. The finding of PK cells always warrants a careful search for more abnormal cells. Atypical PK will demonstrate more nuclear variability and dyskeratotic changes, as described in chapter 5, and should be diagnosed as an epithelial abnormality (D). These atypical PK cells are one of the most common manifestations of HPV cytopathic change.

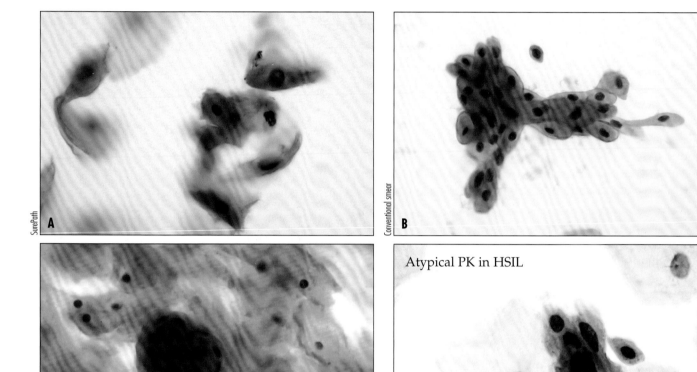

Figure 4-8. Repair.

Reparative changes are characterized by orderly sheets of squamous or glandular (and sometimes stromal) cells that are oriented, or stream, in one direction (like a "school of fish"). Cytoplasm is increased in amount and is usually more dense than in nonreparative cells. Cytoplasm at the margins of the groups tends to extend in pseudopods, indicating normal cohesion with the cells adjacent to those that were sampled. This cytoplasm is often drawn-out in a "taffy-pull" configuration. The nucleoli in repair are prominent, round, and may be multiple. Nuclear chromatin may be pale or slightly hyperchromatic but is fine and even in distribution. Nuclei may vary in size but tend to be oval to elongate. Nuclear contours are smooth. Occasionally, normal mitoses are noted. Inflammatory cells, most commonly neutrophils, are typically intermixed within the groups. The differential diagnosis of repair often includes adenocarcinoma and nonkeratinizing squamous cell carcinoma, which are distinguished by loss of polarity in the groups of cells, cell dyshesion, nuclear hyperchromasia with irregular chromatin distribution, nuclear pleomorphism, nuclear membrane irregularity, and prominent irregular nucleoli.

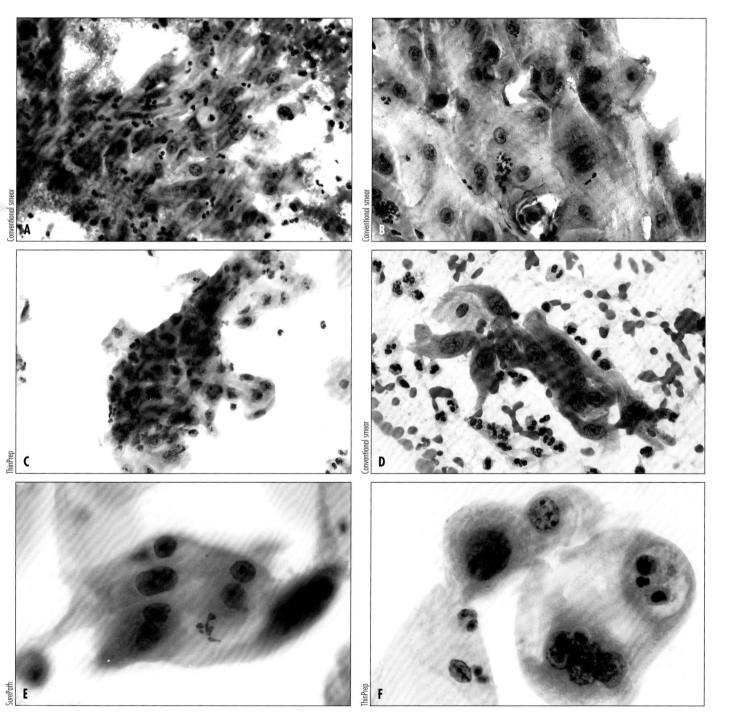

Figure 4-9. Reserve cells.

Reserve cells are small immature cells that have the potential to mature into squamous or glandular cells. Reserve cells proliferate under endocervical glandular cells either at the native squamo-columnar junction or in the transformation zone. On histology, reserve cells make up one to several layers of small immature epithelial cells beneath a row of endocervical glandular cells. Although a rare finding in Pap slides, when present, reserve cells are arranged in cohesive groups of small bland, uniform cells with slightly hyperchromatic nuclei and scant, delicate, blue-staining cytoplasm. The major differential diagnostic consideration is with HSIL or ASC-H. The small size of reserve cells, their rarity, and the uniformity of the cells should allow a proper interpretation.

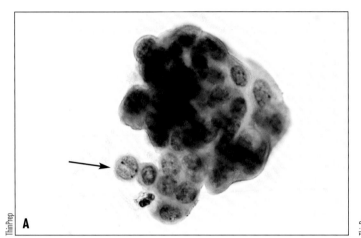

A

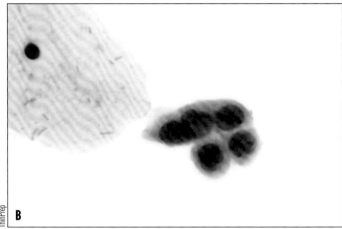

B

Organisms

branching filaments
back of IUD of
ch. endometr?y

Figure 4-10. Actinomyces.

Actinomyces species are <u>branching</u> filamentous bacteria that are almost always associated with the presence of chronic endometritis, usually caused by an intrauterine device (IUD) (approximately 25% of patients with IUDs will have *Actinomyces* present in their Pap specimens). In cervical samples, the filaments of *Actinomyces* are densely clustered and generally associated with a heavy concentration of small companion bacteria. The dense clustering results in a central, poorly stained area. The companion bacteria can impart a fuzzy appearance to the bacterial cluster and can largely obscure the *Actinomyces* (D). By focusing up and down, the filamentous *Actinomyces* organisms can be seen radiating from the edges of the bacterial clusters. *Actinomyces* may be associated with nonspecific inflammatory changes in the epithelial cells, or the specimen may be otherwise unremarkable.

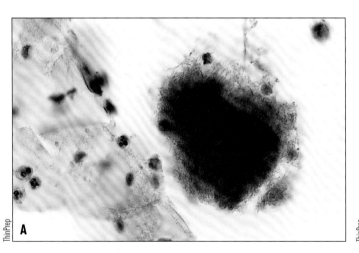

A

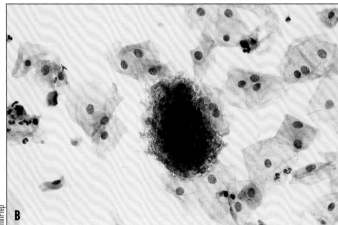

B

Figure 4-10 continued.

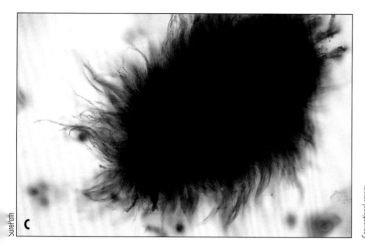

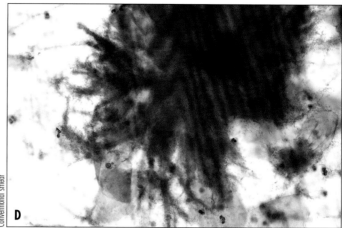

Figure 4-11. Amoeba.

Two types of amoebic trophozoites can be found in Pap slides, *Entamoeba histolytica* and *Endameba gingivalis*, which have similar morphology. Trophozoites are usually 15 to 30 μm in diameter and have a single nucleus with a distinctive small central karysome. The nuclear chromatin is evenly distributed along the periphery of the nucleus. In *E histolytica*, the finely granular endoplasm may contain ingested red blood cells. *E histolytica* (A) resides in the intestine and enters the female genital tract via local transmission. *E gingivalis* (B) lives in/on the teeth, gums, and sometimes tonsils of nearly all adult humans, and transmission to the female genital tract is thought to be through oral-genital contact. Rarely, other types of amoeba may present in cervical samples as a contaminant from the preparation or staining of the specimen. In this circumstance, no associated inflammation or cell changes are noted within the specimen. The amoeba illustrated in C was found to be present in the water used in the staining process.

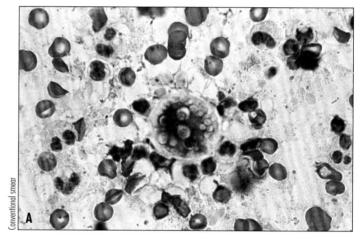

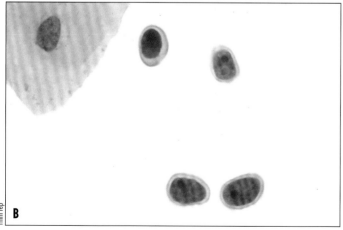

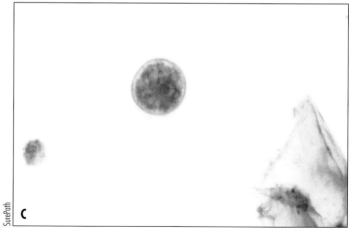

Figure 4-12. Bacterial vaginosis.

Bacterial vaginosis (BV) in Pap slides is characterized by numerous coccobacilli that cover mature squamous cells (clue cells) and are clumped and loosely arranged in the background. In conventional preparations, the coccobacilli are diffusely spread throughout the smear (A). In liquid samples, the background coccobacilli are more clumped, with loose clusters of bacteria as well as the diagnostic clue cells (B and C). The associated inflammatory infiltrate, usually comprising neutrophils, can range from minimal to obscuring. Epithelial cells may show inflammatory and reactive/reparative changes (D). Several types of microorganisms are associated with BV, including *Gardnerella vaginalis* as well as a variety of anaerobic bacteria. BV is associated with an increase in the vaginal Ph, with replacement of the normal population of lactobacilli. It is important to remember that the presence of increased numbers of coccobacilli is not necessarily an indication of the clinical manifestation of BV. In light of this, the recommended Bethesda System interpretation is "shift in flora suggestive of bacterial vaginosis."

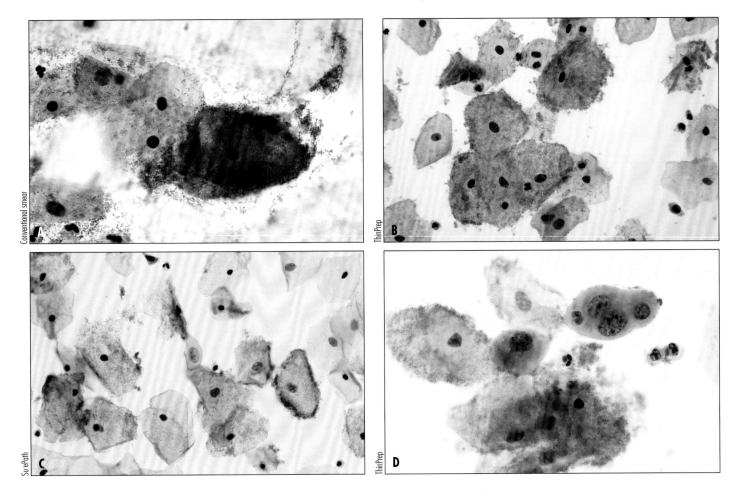

Figure 4-13. Candida species. = pseudohyphae / yeast ~~OOOO~~ skewered dsq.

The most common fungal organism present in cervical/vaginal specimens is *Candida* species (albicans or glabrata). Budding yeast and/or pseudohypheal forms can be seen, often in the background of inflammation. In liquid-based specimens, a classic low-power finding is a long row of mature squamous cells that appear "skewered" by pseudohyphae (A). If only small yeast forms are present, the organism is likely *Candida glabrata* (C). These small yeast forms are often hidden among the cells and are easily missed. Epithelial changes observed with infection by *Candida* species include inflammatory changes, such as keratotic change (ie, anucleated squamous cells,

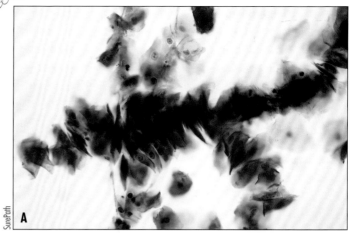

A — SurePath

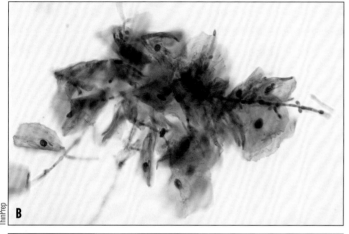

B — ThinPrep

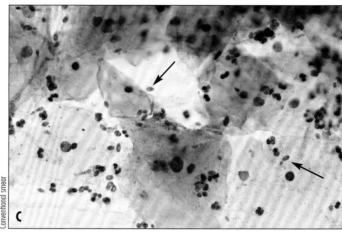

C — Conventional smear

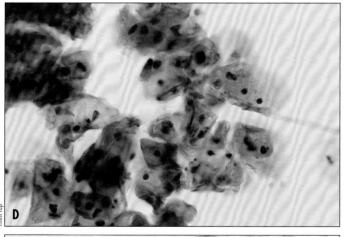

D — ThinPrep

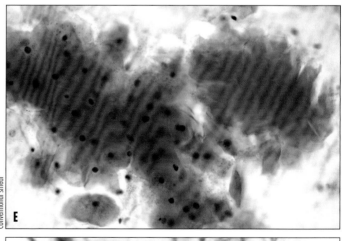

E — Conventional smear

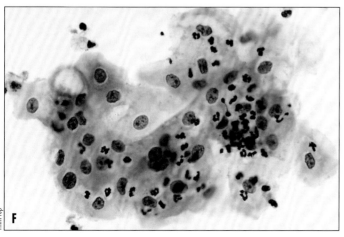

F — ThinPrep

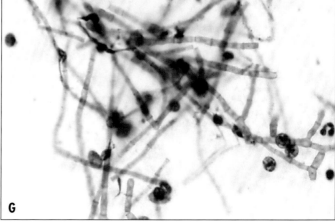

G — Conventional smear

Figure 4-13 continued.

orangeophilia, and dense eosinophilia), and a "moth-eaten" appearance of the cytoplasm (D, E, and F). Other cells may show evidence of edema manifesting as small perinuclear halos. ASC-US or LSIL is frequently in the differential diagnosis when these changes are noted. True epithelial abnormalities show greater nuclear hyperchro-

masia and enlargement (see Figure 7-6). Care must be taken to diagnose only true *Candida* fungal elements. If only pseudohyphae are present, the differential also includes *Geotrichum* and may also include various fibers and other artifacts (G, H, and I). The finding of diagnostic well-formed pseudohyphae and/or spores is needed to make a correct interpretation of *Candida* species.

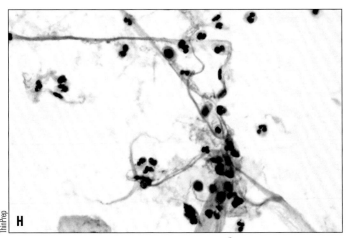

ThinPrep

H

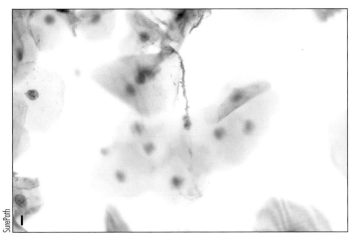

SurePath

I

Figure 4-14. Cytomegalovirus.

The cytopathic changes associated with cytomegalovirus (CMV) infection affect the ectocervical squamous and endocervical glandular cells, and include cellular and nuclear enlargement and large intranuclear viral inclusions having a prominent halo. Small cytoplasmic inclusions can also be present in CMV, in contrast to herpes simplex, where inclusions are only intranuclear (C). The large CMV-infected cells are sometimes confused with bizarre tumor cells. Causing further confusion is the fact that along with other debilitating states, malignancy can predispose to infection by CMV. Indeed, malignancy and CMV can coexist and be observed in the same specimen.

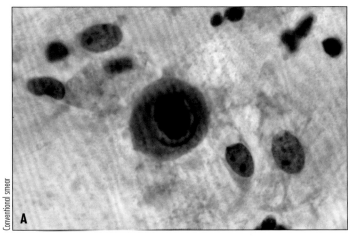

Conventional smear

A

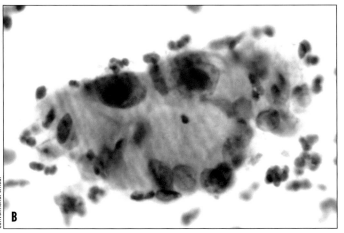

Conventional smear

B

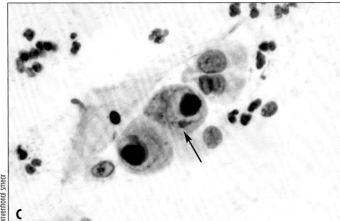

Conventional smear

C

HSV = N inclution
nuclear/Margination/Multinuc

Figure 4-15. Herpes simplex.

Herpes simplex, a DNA virus, causes cytopathic changes in mature squamous cells that include multinucleation, nuclear molding, margination of chromatin (the "3 M's"), nuclear enlargement, and ground-glass nuclei, all of which result in a slightly hyperchromatic, homogenous nuclear appearance, which can mimic LSIL. Careful evaluation for the classic cytopathic effects noted above helps prevent misinterpretation. The diagnosis of herpes is most obvious if the cytopathic effects also include the characteristic large intranuclear inclusion with a surrounding halo (A).

Classically, herpes causes epithelial ulceration, necrosis, and regeneration, which sometimes overshadow the cytopathic viral changes and can simulate invasive carcinoma. Both a careful search for viral changes and noting the absence of significant epithelial pleomorphism help to avoid a false-positive diagnosis. Nonspecific reactive changes may be seen in the background of herpes or as an initial presentation (F). Care must be taken only to diagnose herpes when definitive viral changes are present. Liquid-based specimens can lead to increased numbers of isolated herpetic cells, which, when mononuclear, can lead to misinterpretation as HSIL (D).

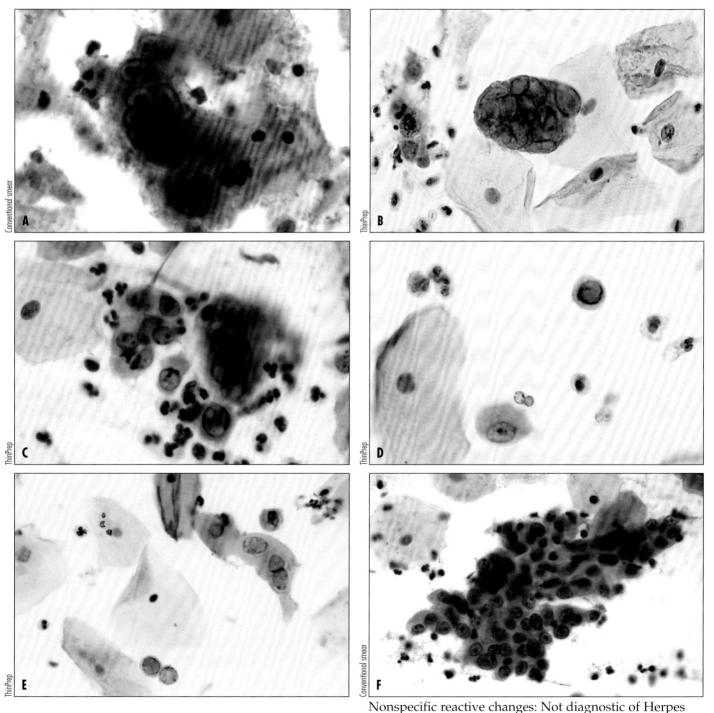

Nonspecific reactive changes: Not diagnostic of Herpes

Figure 4-16. Leptothrix (with discussion on Trichomonas).

Leptothrix is similar morphologically to *Actinomyces* species, except that in Pap slides, *Leptothrix* is nonbranching, is much less-densely clustered, and is not associated with "companion" bacteria. Clinically, *Leptothrix* is not in itself a pathogen, but diagnostically it is of interest because its presence is often associated with *Trichomonas vaginalis*. *Leptothrix* may be the first finding noted in such cases and should always prompt further investigation for the presence of *Trichomonas* ("if you find the spaghetti, look for the meatballs!"). *Leptothrix* does not cause any epithelial cell changes and, by itself, does not need to be reported.

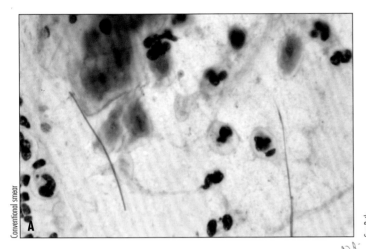

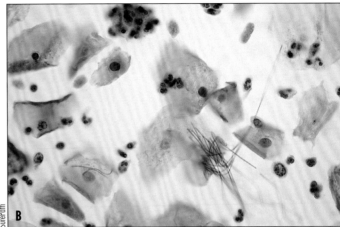

Figure 4-17. Molluscum contagiosum. *= poxvirus / eos- cyto inclusion*

Molluscum contagiosum is a poxvirus that causes human skin and squamous mucosal infections that are sometimes sexually transmitted and involve the genital tract. The lesions present as smooth umbilicated papules (3 to 6 mm) and are sometimes sampled incidentally in Pap slides. On histology, the raised cup-shaped lesions show large (up to 35 μm), homogenous, eosinophilic intracytoplasmic viral inclusions (molluscum bodies) that push the nucleus of the mature squamous cell to the periphery. Rarely, these dense, red or polychromatic molluscum bodies may be seen in Pap slides, either intracellularly or extracellularly (A).

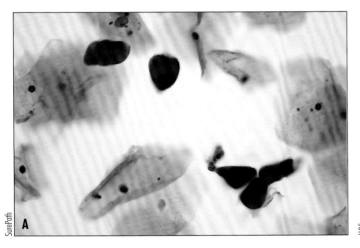

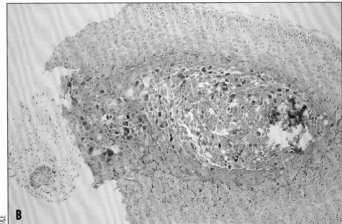

Figure 4-18. Pinworm (Enterobius vermicularis).

Pinworms (*Enterobius vermicularis*) are parasitic round worms that infect the large intestine and deposit eggs perianally, causing intense anal and vaginal pruritis. The infection is highly contagious and typically affects many or all members of a family. The parasite ova are thick-shelled, 50 to 60 µm by 20 to 30 µm, and ovoid, with one flat surface.

Occasionally, pinworm ova present in Pap slides, where they are easily distinguished from normal and abnormal epithelial cells, but they may be dismissed as an insignificant contaminant (eg, food) if not recognized. Recognition of pinworm ova in Pap slides is important because this may be the initial indication of possible infection in the patient and other members of her family.

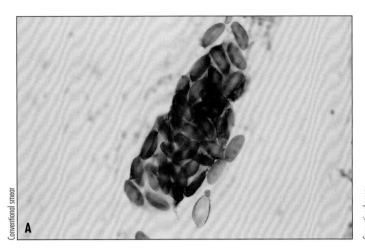

A — Conventional smear

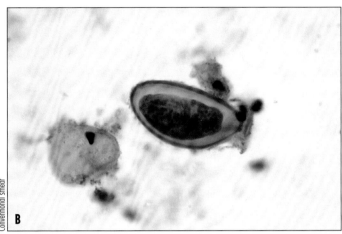

B — Conventional smear

Trich. = parasite
motile x3 Flagella

Figure 4-19. Trichomonas vaginalis.

Trichomonas vaginalis (TV) is the most common sexually transmitted, parasitic infection in the vagina. TV is a flagellate protozoan parasite with an eccentric nucleus and three flagella. In Pap specimens, the organisms are pear-shaped and blue-gray, with a distinctive elliptical nucleus, and frequently contain red cytoplasmic granules. They generally range in size from 15 to 30 microns. While the flagella are almost never present on conventional smears, in liquid-based preparations the flagella may be distinct (A). TV organisms are usually isolated but, especially in liquid-based specimens, can form aggregates, sometime referred to as "Trich parties" (C). *Trichomonas* infection

shows inflammatory epithelial cell changes, as described previously, and small perinuclear halos are a common finding, which may be the first clue to the presence of TV when the slide is viewed at low magnification ("Trich change") (D). Mild nuclear hyperchromasia, slight nuclear enlargement, and pseudokeratinization are also often present (E). Other findings that are frequently observed include a tumor-like granular diathesis, *Leptothrix*, and neutrophils arranged in round clusters ("poly-balls") (F). At times, the reactive changes can mimic an epithelial lesion. However, as in other reactive conditions, the nuclei found in dysplasia and carcinomas are larger and darker, and display more chromatin and nuclear membrane irregularity.

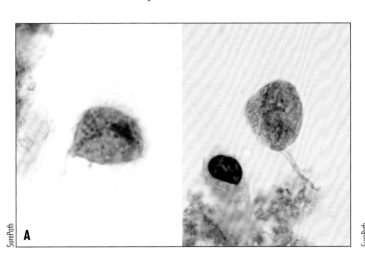

A — SurePath

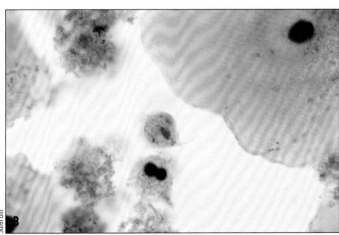

B — SurePath

Figure 4-19 continued.

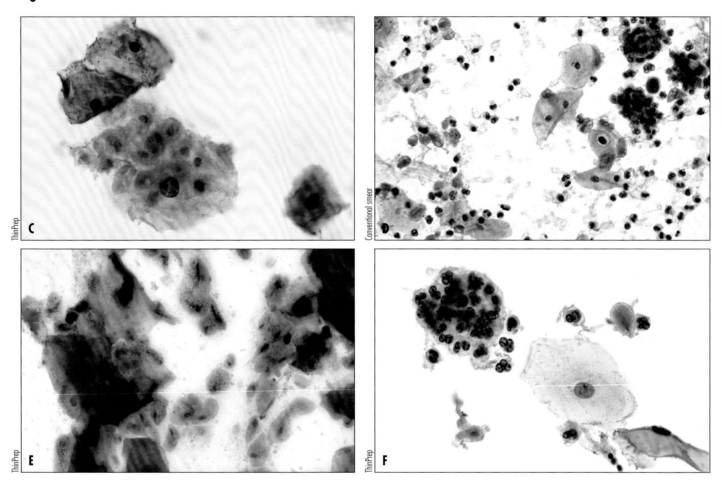

Pregnancy-Related Changes

Figure 4-20. Arias Stella change.

Arias Stella change is a benign, reactive, progestational effect observed in either endocervical or endometrial glandular cells. These changes are usually associated with pregnancy but may also be seen following progestigen therapy in older women. The cellular changes are related to increased levels of both estrogens and progestins and reflect nuclear polysomy, with no evidence of aneuploidy. The changes are often quite focal and regress when the hor-

monal stimulus returns to normal levels. Characteristic changes observed on Pap slides include single and clustered cells showing cellular and nuclear enlargement, with prominent nucleoli, isolated large and bizarre cells, and variable degenerative changes. A characteristic change that may be seen is the presence of intranuclear holes (E, arrow). These features can simulate adenocarcinomas, especially clear cell adenocarcinoma (F). To avoid overinterpretation, obtaining history is important, along with noting any associated cells having clearly reactive changes and the absence of viable, definitively malignant cells.

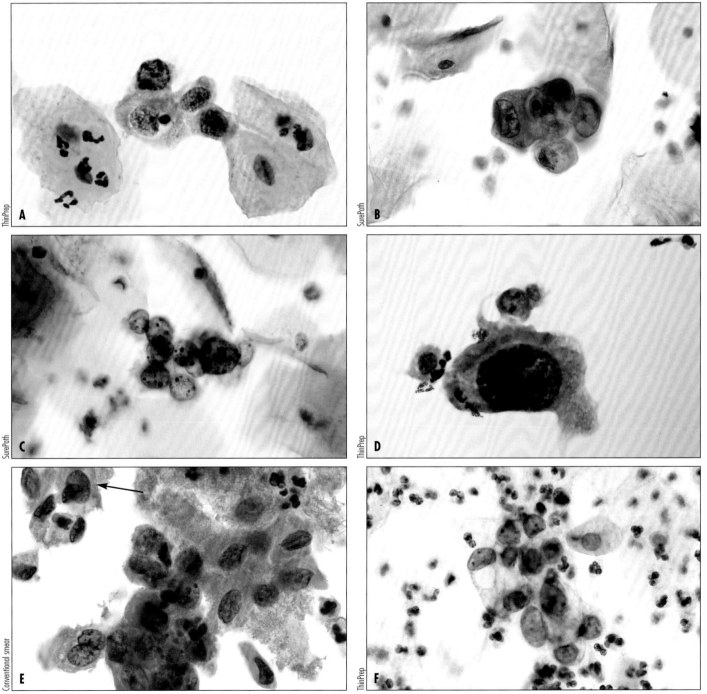

Clear cell adenocarcinoma

Figure 4-21. Decidual change.

Decidual change involving the cervical stroma is common in pregnant and postpartum patients. With ulceration or erosion of the overlying mucosa, decidual cells can be found in Pap slides following spontaneous exfoliation or direct sampling. Decidual cells are about the size of mature squamous cells, are loosely clustered or isolated, and have defined cell borders and large reactive-appearing nuclei (ie, pale, finely granular, and evenly distributed chromatin; smooth nuclear borders; and prominent nucleoli). Decidual cells are most often misinterpreted as benign reactive squamous cells but, when abundant or showing degenerative changes, may be mistaken for LSIL. Awareness of a history of pregnancy or recent delivery, in which reactive or decidual cells would be expected, helps to prevent an overinterpretation of SIL or carcinoma.

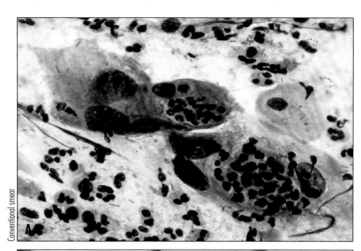

Conventional smear

A

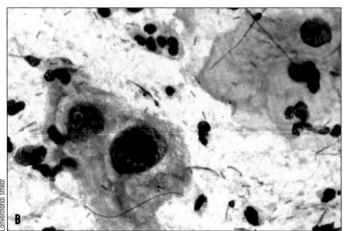

Conventional smear

B

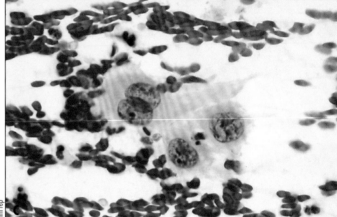

ThinPrep

C

Figure 4-22. Trophoblastic cells.

Cytotrophoblasts. Placental cytotrophoblasts may exfoliate into the cervicovaginal area during pregnancy, but their morphologic overlap with other cell types found in Pap slides usually precludes specific identification. Cytotrophoblasts most closely resemble reactive squamous cells (A and B) and are very rarely misinterpreted as dysplastic or malignant.

Syncytial Trophoblasts. The multinucleated placental syncytial trophoblasts are occasionally seen in Pap slides during pregnancy, following delivery, or post abortion. Syncytial trophoblasts are one of several types of multinucleated giant cells that can present in Pap slides. Syncytial trophoblasts are distinguished by tapering of the dense defined cytoplasm at one end (this is where the cell was attached to the placenta) and nuclei that tend to bunch towards the center of the cell and that have dark coarse chromatin (C and D). Most often there will be over 50 nuclei in each cell. The distinctive nuclear and cytoplasmic features represent degenerative changes.

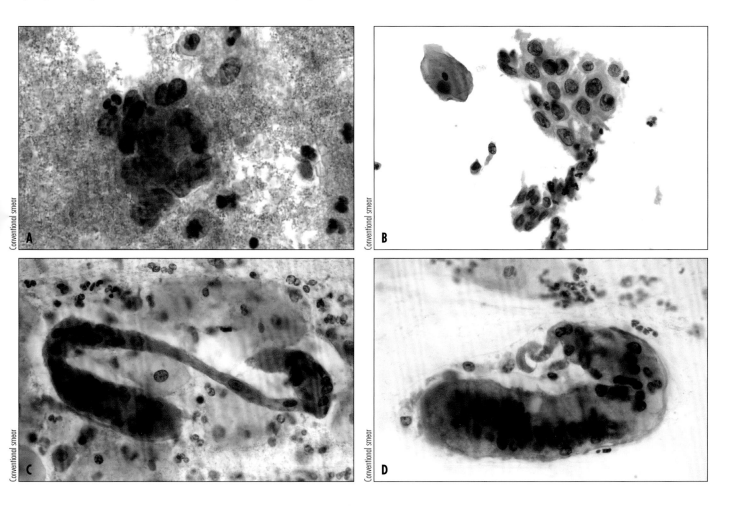

Benign Glandular Changes

Figure 4-23. Microglandular hyperplasia.

Microglandular hyperplasia (MGH) is associated with a progestigenic effect usually observed in patients who are pregnant, taking progestins for perimenopausal bleeding, or taking oral contraceptives. Histologically, MGH is characterized by hyperplastic, endocervical, glandular epithelium, with extensive perinuclear vacuolization. The cells of

MGH are relatively fragile, exfoliate in large loose clusters, and readily degenerate. Cytologically, the degenerated glandular cells can mimic HSIL, with variably shaped, dark, smudged to pyknotic nuclei and granular orangeophilic cytoplasm, interspersed with nuclear and cytoplasmic debris. These changes usually comprise a minor component of the Pap slide. Clinical correlation and the finding of viable bland-appearing glandular cells, along with the absence viable dysplastic cells in association, helps prevent a false-positive interpretation.

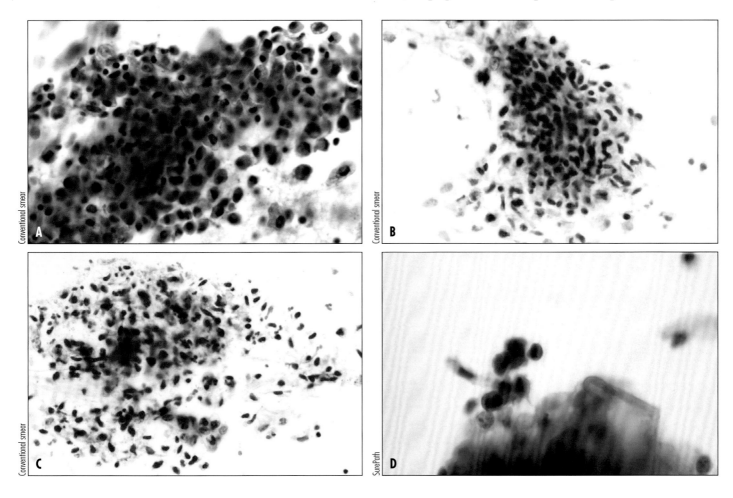

Figure 4-24. Endocervical cells.

Endocervical cells present as sheets or strips of uniform columnar cells with basally situated nuclei and tall, pale, frothy cytoplasm when viewed from the side (A and B). When viewed on end, the cells have a honeycombed appearance (C, D, and F). In liquid-based preparations, the cells tend to form rounded groups of uniform cells, and the columnar shape is best appreciated in cells at the edges of the group (E). Multinucleation in endocervical cells is a very common, nonspecific, benign reactive change (G and H). In Pap slides, these multinucleated cells are easily recognized when they are well preserved and associated with normal endocervical cells. However, there is a tendency for these cells to round up and lose their columnar shape. This is especially true in liquid-base preparations, in which case

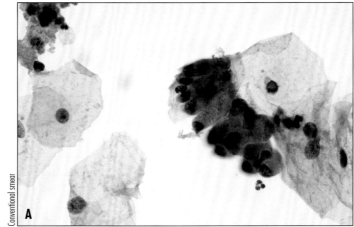

Figure 4-24 continued.

they could be confused with multinucleated histiocytes or even with the multinucleated cells associated with Herpes simplex infection (H). Problems arise when the nuclei of some of these rounded cells start to degenerate, darken, swell, and fuse, appearing as one large dysplastic nucleus. To avoid overinterpretation, it is important to note the association with normal benign endocervical cells, and that the degenerated nuclei of the multinucleated cells appear dark and smudged, with lack of normal chromatin detail. In uncertain cases, an interpretation of AGC or ASC-US may be reasonable (see Figure 6-4, A through D).

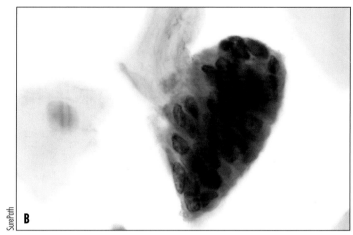

SurePath **B**

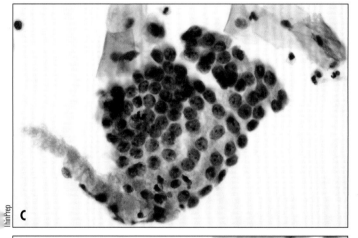

ThinPrep **C**

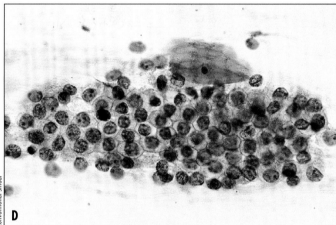

Conventional smear **D**

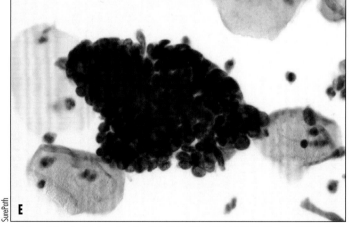

SurePath **E**

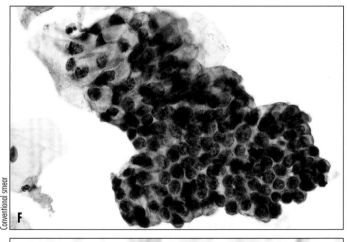

Conventional smear **F**

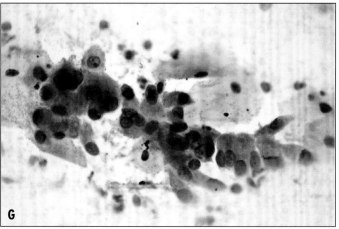

Conventional smear **G**

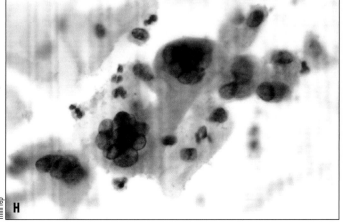

ThinPrep **H**

Figure 4-25. Endometrial exodus.

The term "exodus" is given to a distinctive arrangement of benign, spontaneously exfoliated endometrial stromal and glandular cells that usually presents in Pap slides around days 6 to 10 of the menstrual cycle. Its presence is indicative of shed endometrium, most commonly of menstrual type. The endometrial cells of exodus are arranged in three-dimensional, double-contoured groups, with central small, dark endometrial stromal cells rimmed by larger, paler endometrial glandular cells (A and B). Usually, exodus is readily identified, especially when observed during the first half of the menstrual cycle, where it is essentially a normal finding. However, the exodus pattern can be seen with abnormal shedding in anovulatory cycling and other

conditions. As such, reporting of cells identified in this pattern will depend on the particular history of each patient.

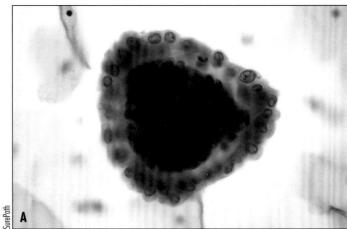

A

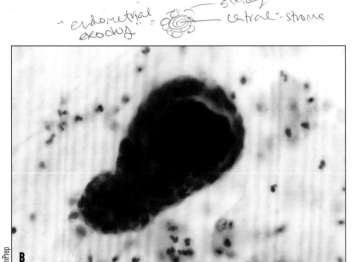

B

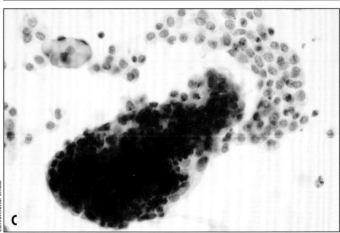

C

Figure 4-26. Endometrial glandular cells.

Endometrial glandular (EMG) cells are the smallest epithelial cells normally found in Pap slides. Most are derived from spontaneously exfoliated cells from the endometrium, which then travel through the endocervical canal to the cervicovaginal area. As a result, EMG cells usually present in Pap slides as small, shrunken cells in three-dimensional

groups, with degenerative nuclear (dark, clumpy, smudged chromatin) and cytoplasmic (frayed or absent, ill-defined, vacuolar) changes. EMG cells in Pap slides can be confused with other "hyperchromatic crowded groups" of cells, including HSIL and squamous and adenocarcinoma carcinoma (see Figure 7-9). HSIL cells are generally much larger, and the groups appear less three-dimensional and, instead, may present in loose clusters and as single cells. In addition,

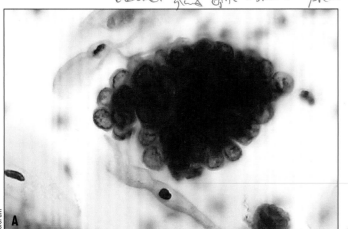

A

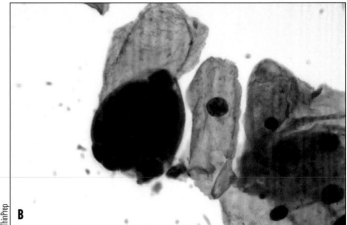

B

Figure 4-26 continued.

the cytoplasm in HSIL is more dense and well defined compared to the delicate ill-defined cytoplasm of EMG cells. EMG cells might also be confused with microinvasive or invasive squamous carcinoma, especially the small cell variant. In a cyclic-age woman, squamous cell carcinoma is much more likely than endometrial carcinoma, but a biopsy would be needed for precise clarification of the process. Benign EMG cells are found in greatest numbers on Pap slides when the sample is taken during the menses, at which time EMG cells are larger, reactive appearing, and present on a bloody, necrotic-appearing background, which could simulate a diathesis. For this reason, Pap testing should be done at mid-cycle. To avoid overinterpretation, knowledge of the menstrual history is always important. The finding of EMG cells—even when benign appearing—in a Pap slide from a postmenopausal woman may indicate the presence of endometrial pathology, which can range from benign processes, such as endometrial polyp, to endometrial neoplasia, and a biopsy is warranted for diagnosis. According to the Bethesda System of reporting, the finding of benign-appearing EMG cells in women older than 40 years should be reported, as the risk of endometrial neoplasia increases with age.

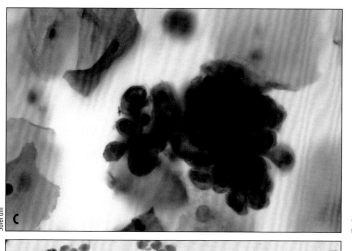

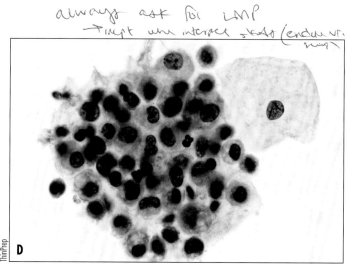

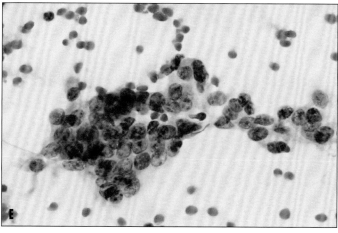

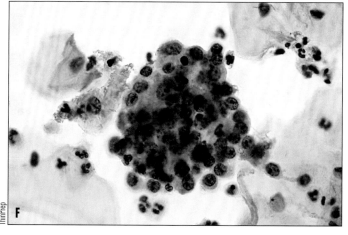

Figure 4-27. Endometrium from the lower uterine segment.

Cells from the lower uterine segment (LUS) occur in Pap slides as a result of direct sampling and present as two-dimensional sheets or tissue fragments containing orderly, compactly arranged, small uniform cells with high N:C ratios and dark, uniform, oval to elongated nuclei. Gland openings, tubular arrangements, and palisading are also frequently observed. These cells can be seen in Pap slides from any patient when the sampling brush is extended high enough into the endocervical canal. However, Pap testing done following a recent loop electrosurgical excision (LEEP) or conization procedure yields the greatest amount of LUS material. LUS cells are in the differential diagnosis of "hyperchromatic crowded groups" (see Figure 7-9). Confusion with HSIL is greatest when LUS cells present in small cell groups. In larger cell groups, the glandular origin of LUS cells is more obvious, but confusion with a significant glandular lesion is possible (see Figure 6-7, A through D). Recognition of the maintenance of polarity, the lack of cellular atypia, the overall small cellular size, and the presence of attached endometrial stromal fragments are most helpful in distinguishing LUS cell groups from

epithelial lesions. Knowledge of a recent cervical LEEP or conization may also be very useful. Because LUS cells are usually directly sampled during Pap testing, they may be seen at any time during the menstrual cycle. However, in distinction to EMG cells, they should not be reported as "endometrial cells present in a woman over 40" when observed in Pap slides from women older than 40 years, because they do not have significance for endometrial pathology.

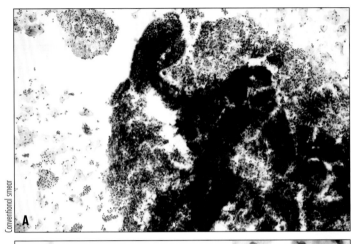

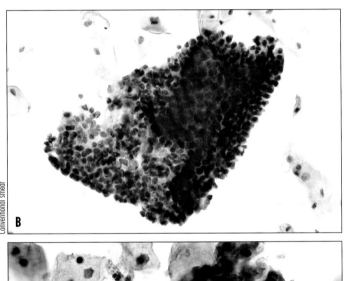

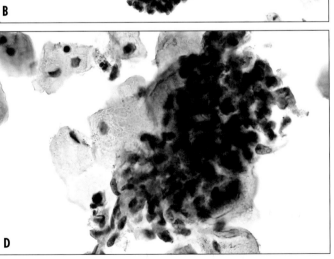

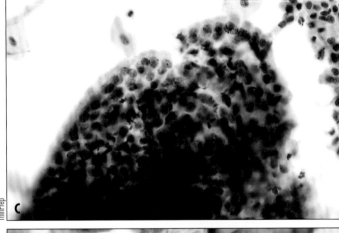

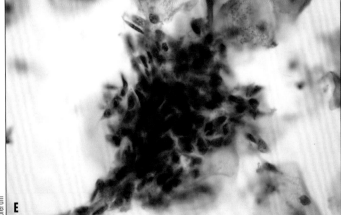

Figure 4-28. Endometrial stromal cells.

Two types of endometrial stromal (EMS) cells are recognized: the smaller, dark, oval to elongated cells from the deep stroma (A and B); and the larger, pale, histiocytic-like cells (C through F) from the superficial stroma. Like endoglandular (EMG) cells, EMS cells are normally observed during the first half of the menstrual cycle but can also be seen in patients with endometrial lesions, including hyperplasia and carcinoma. Unlike EMG cells, which usually present in tight three-dimensional groups, EMS cells are usually arranged in loosely cohesive, two-dimensional cell groups. Like EMG cells, EMS cells can show variable degenerative changes. In many cases, distinction between endometrial glandular and stromal cells is not possible. In this circumstance, reporting of "endometrial cells, not otherwise specified" when required, is appropriate. Confusion with HSIL is most likely when EMS cells show marked degenerative change, including shrunken cells, nuclear pyknosis, and cytoplasmic mummification, which can suggest keratinization (F). The absence of atypia in the viable cells in these EMS cell groups and correlation with the menstrual history help to avoid overinterpretation.

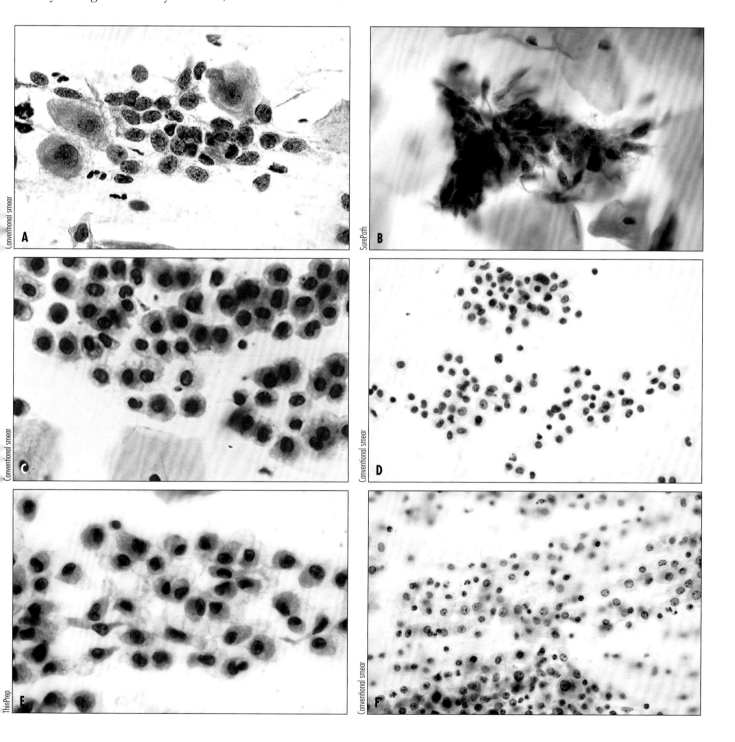

Figure 4-29. Endometriosis.

Endometriosis can involve the cervix and vagina, especially following excisional procedures, such as a LEEP. The cells from endometriosis in these sites are occasionally sampled during the Pap test. Cells that spontaneously exfoliate from these sites present on Pap slides, as do other endometrial cell groups (A). Because of the location, direct sampling is also possible, in which case the cells may appear larger and better preserved, in a fashion similar to that described previously for directly-sampled endometrium (B). Figure C is a biopsy from the same patient as B. The additional finding of hemosiderin-laden macrophages and/or stromal spindle cells in a cyclic woman would also suggest endometriosis.

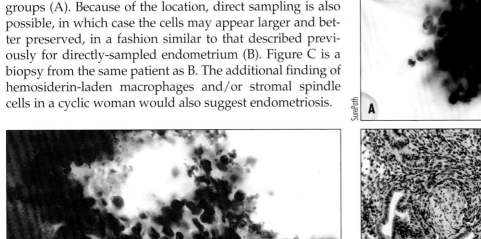

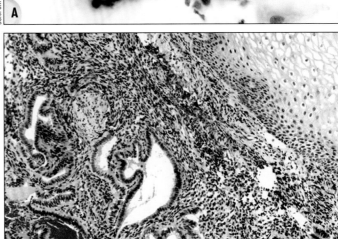

Figure 4-30. Changes associated with intrauterine device.

Intrauterine device (IUD)-associated changes in Pap slides are widely recognized and characterized by small clusters of rounded cells (squamous metaplastic and/or glandular cells), with individual cells showing large vacuoles that push the bland uniform nucleus towards the edge of the cluster ("bubble-gum vacuoles") (A, B, and C). While this cell arrangement is a characteristic IUD-associated finding, it is not specific and can be seen in women without a history of IUD placement. A less-commonly recognized IUD-associated change is the presence in the Pap slide of a few,

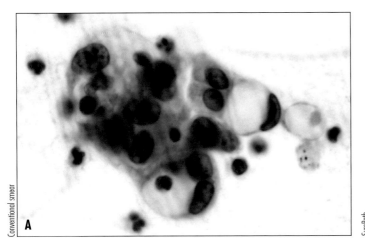

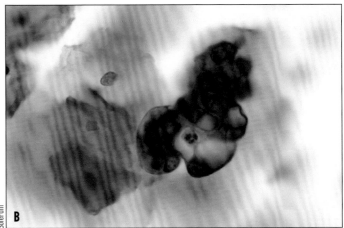

IUD ∝ metap / bubble gum vacuoles
& actinomyces

Figure 4-30 continued.

small, scattered isolated cells with dark, but smudged, nuclei and smooth nuclear borders that mimic HSIL (D, E, and F). All of these cellular changes are thought to represent degenerated high-endocervical-canal and/or endometrial cells that exfoliate spontaneously in response to the presence of the IUD and the string that extends into the endocervical canal. In contrast, the cells of HSIL are more abundant, variable in overall size and shape, and show coarse granular chromatin, nuclear membrane irregularity, and variation in nuclear size and shape. Careful examination of the slide for other viable dysplastic cells and noting a history of either abnormal Pap slides or IUD placement are helpful for the differential diagnosis. The presence of *Actinomyces* on the slide is an important clue to the presence of an IUD, as it can be seen in association in about 25% of cases. Unfortunately, history of an IUD is not always given by the patient or known by the specimen taker; hence the changes noted previously may allow the cytologist to report the potential presence of an IUD to the clinician.

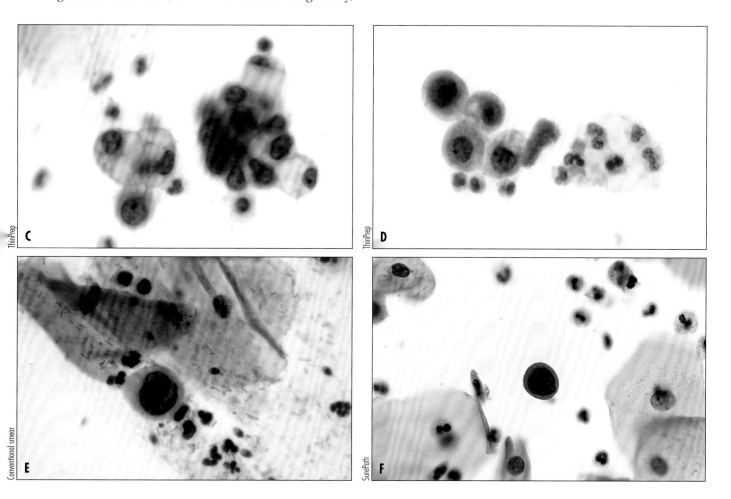

Figure 4-31. Endocervical and endometrial polyps.

Benign endocervical (A, B, and C) and endometrial polyps (D, E, and F) that present at the cervical os are prone to erosion and ulceration. This, in turn, leads to degenerative, reparative, and squamous metaplastic changes in the native glandular epithelium, which can mimic neoplasia. In addition, cell groups sampled from the polyp surface may also show macronucleoli, mitoses, hyperchromasia, cellular crowding, and a slight loss of polarity. Overinterpretation is avoided by noting that the abnormal cells are usually limited to only a few, cohesive, two-dimensional cell groups showing smooth nuclear borders and finely granular, evenly distributed chromatin. A diagnosis of ASC-US or AGC may be warranted in some cases and may lead to the initial discovery of the polyp (see Figure 6-4, C and D, and Figure 6-8, C).

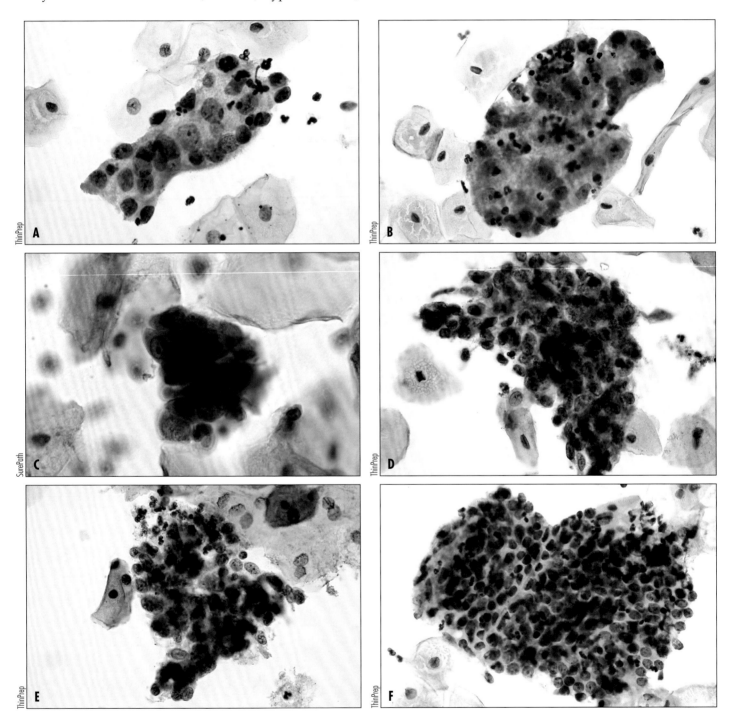

Figure 4-32. Tubal metaplasia.

The tubal metaplastic epithelium of endocervical glands is similar to fallopian tube mucosa, which is pseudostratified and comprises several cell types, including ciliated columnar, nonciliated secretory, and intercalated cells. In Pap slides, these cells may appear as crowded groups (due to pseudostatification) (D and E) and may be mildly pleomorphic (due to the multiple cell types) (F), which can render them difficult to differentiate from neoplastic and preneoplastic glandular cell groups. The most important distinguishing feature in crowded cell groups is the finding of cilia and/or terminal bars, which essentially rules out the possibility of malignancy for the group in which they appear (A, B, and C). Cilia and terminal bars should be sought in all groups of atypical glandular cells. Nuclear features are otherwise most helpful. Tubal metaplastic nuclei tend to be round to slightly oval compared to the more-elongated nuclei of low-grade endocervical adenocarcinoma, including adenocarcinoma in situ. In addition, the nuclei of tubal metaplasia show evenly distributed, finely granular chromatin—sometimes even "washed-out"—in distinction to the coarsely granular, dense chromatin of endocervical neoplasia. Hyperchromasia and increased N:C ratios can be found in both tubal metaplasia and adenocarcinoma, so these characteristics are not helpful in distinguishing between the two processes. In difficult cases, an interpretation of AGC is warranted and should prompt an appropriate clinical investigation (see Figure 6-5, A through D).

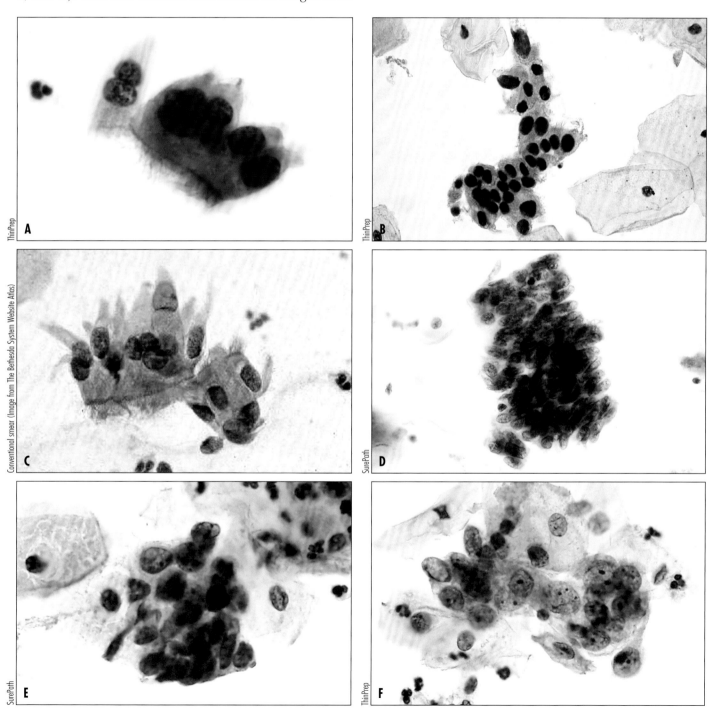

55

Iatrogenic, Metabolic, Systemic

Figure 4-33. Chemotherapy/radiation.

Chemotherapy. The morphologic effects of systemically administered chemotherapeutic agents (eg, Busulfan, Imuran) can be observed in all types of subsequently examined cytologic specimens. Like radiation therapy, the effects of chemotherapy occur at the molecular level, and the associated morphologic changes can persist indefinitely. Initially, the site of the malignancy shows obvious tumor necrosis and degeneration. In Pap slides, characteristic chemotherapeutic changes overlap with dysplasia and carcinoma and include nuclear enlargement, hyperchromasia, irregular nuclear borders, and, sometimes, prominent nucleoli. However, the chromatin is often smudged with chemotherapy effect (A and B). Many of the radiation-induced changes described below can also be seen after chemotherapy. The treatment history for malignancy is most important for the differential cytodiagnosis, and with a positive history of treatment, extreme caution is required when evaluating for recurrent or new malignancy.

Radiation. Radiation therapy produces atypical to bizarre cell changes that, in Pap slides, are most prominently featured in squamous cells. Radiation-induced epithelial cell changes include cytomegaly with normal N:C ratios; delicate, wispy, polychromatic (ie, pink and blue or two-tone staining) cytoplasm; degenerative vacuoles in the cytoplasm and nuclei; smooth or wrinkled nuclear contours; and dark, granular, evenly distributed chromatin or dark, smudged nuclei (C through F). The cytoplasmic vacuoles may contain inflammatory cells. The background contains various inflammatory cells, including multinucleated histiocytes, and the latter can on occasion dominate the smear. Very similar epithelial cell changes can be seen with folate deficiency, and the cytologic differential diagnosis also includes chemotherapy effect, LSIL, and carcinoma. The latter two entities are distinguished by nuclear enlargement leading to an increase in the N:C ratio; dark, irregularly distributed, coarsely granular chromatin; denser, well-defined cytoplasm; and frequent koilocytotic change in LSIL. Keratinization, if present, would fit with dysplasia or carcinoma and is not a typical radiation-induced change. When correlated with the clinical history, recognition of radiation change is usually straightforward. Since radiation causes cell damage at the molecular level, the cytomorphologic effects can last indefinitely. Therefore, it is important that any past history of radiation therapy be provided with the Pap test sample.

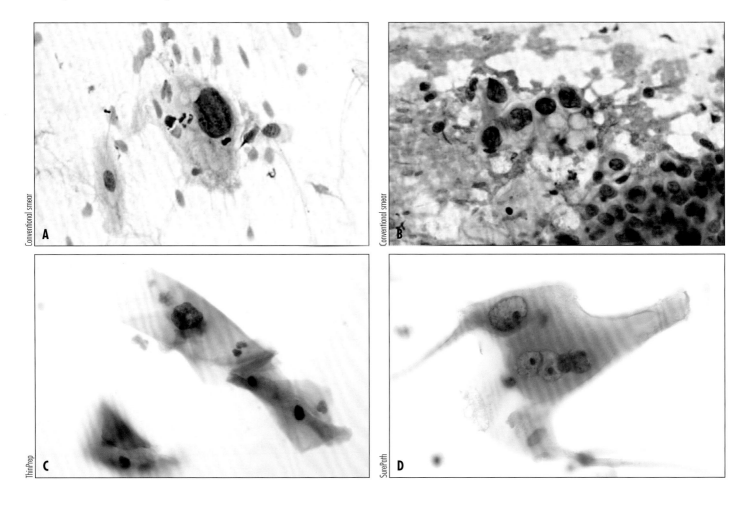

A — Conventional smear
B — Conventional smear
C — ThinPrep
D — SurePath

Figure 4-33 continued.

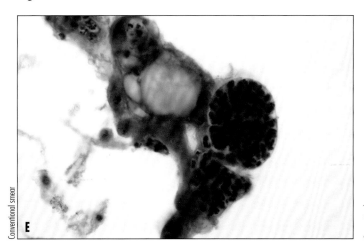

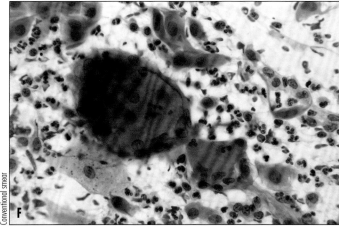

Figure 4-34. Depo-Provera.

When prescribed as a contraceptive therapy, Depo-Provera can cause a decreased estrogenic effect in the cervicovaginal squamous mucosa. The time it takes to develop this change and the extent of this change vary widely among patients, and hormonal patterns can range from normal to intermediate cell dominant to atrophy. Artifacts (eg, air-drying on conventional preparations) and reactive/reparative changes in large numbers of immature-appearing cells on such slides from cyclic age women can potentially be overinterpreted as ASC-US or SIL. Awareness of this potential effect of Depo-Provera on the cervicovaginal mucosa and utilization of strict criteria in the cytological assessment help avoid pitfalls in cytologic interpretation.

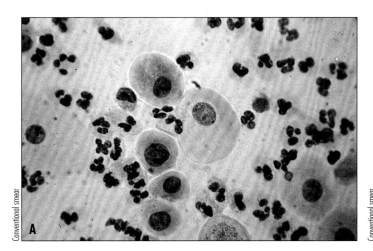

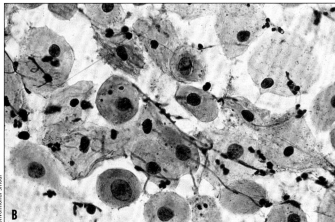

Figure 4-35. Fistula: Colon cells and food.

Colonic contents can drain through a recto-vaginal fistula into the cervicovaginal area and be subsequently sampled during Pap testing. The resulting Pap slide will typically contain some or all of the following: degenerating colonic mucosa cells (A), vegetable cells, and golden-brown granular fecal debris. This pattern may suggest invasive carcinoma, and often these patients will have a history of regional malignancy with surgery and/or radiation. Colonic mucosa cells pose the greatest challenge, because they are much larger than glandular cells normally found in the cervical-vaginal area and, in this setting, show marked degenerative change that could be misinterpreted as cancer (B). If a history of recto-vaginal fistula is provided, an accurate interpretation is likely. Otherwise, the recognition of vegetable cells (C and D) or fecal material is important and should trigger an investigation of the clinical history. Recto-vaginal fistulas also occur in patients with colonic carcinoma that invades into the cervix or vagina. In this circumstance, the background may show similar changes of inflammation and necrosis, but malignant columnar cells indicative of colonic adenocarcinoma can also be present in the Pap slide (E). Goblet cells simulating colonic mucosa may also be seen in the intestinal variant of adenocarcinoma in situ (F).

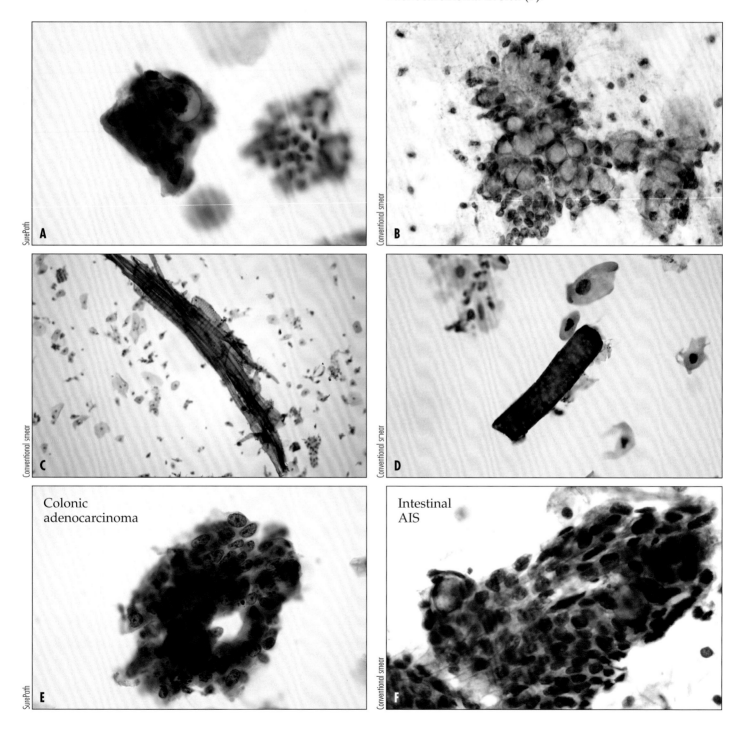

Figure 4-36. Folate and vitamin B$_{12}$ deficiency.

Folate deficiency (as may occur in patients who are pregnant, postmenopausal, or taking oral contraceptives) and vitamin B$_{12}$ deficiency are associated with cytologic epithelial changes similar to those observed in radiation therapy, ie, nuclear and cellular enlargement, vacuolar change, and polychromasia. The differential diagnosis for these vitamin deficiencies also includes LSIL, with the helpful differential features as described previously for radiation therapy. Folate and vitamin B$_{12}$ both function as coenzymes in DNA synthesis.

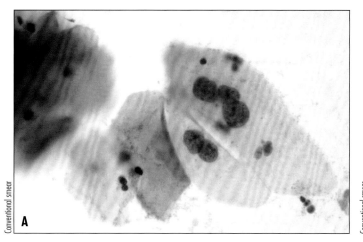
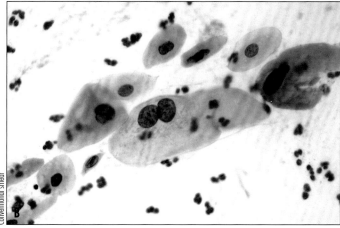

Figure 4-37. Pemphigus.

Pemphigus is an autoimmune disorder associated with blistering of both the skin and other squamous mucosal surfaces. Cervicovaginal lesions secondary to pemphigus are sometimes sampled during Pap testing. Characteristic findings on Pap slides include loosely clustered, metaplastic squamous cells with spidery and bridging cytoplasmic extensions (acantholysis) and very prominent bullet- or rectangular-shaped nucleoli. Cells from pemphigus otherwise look reactive/reparative and are usually interpreted as such, because the chromatin is pale, fine, and even; the nuclear borders are smooth; there is no pleomorphism; and the lesional cells comprise a minor component of the slide. Clinical correlation is supportive of the reactive cytologic features.

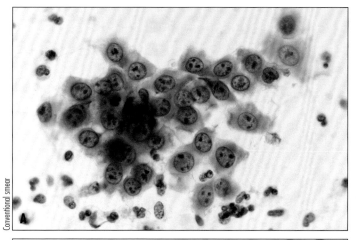
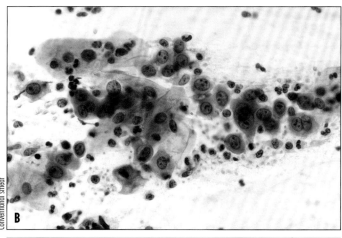
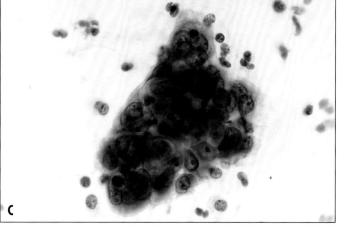
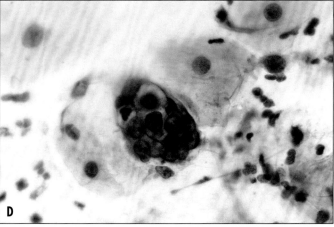

Noncervical Cells and Artifacts

Figure 4-38. Air-drying artifact.

Air-dried cells in Pap slides are almost exclusively confined to conventional smeared specimens. Cells having air-drying artifacts appear larger than normal and have pale, faded, ill-defined cytoplasm, and pale or slightly darker, washed out, smudged nuclei compared to their preserved counterparts. Benign air-dried cells have normal N:C ratios, uniform cell and nuclear size and shape, and smooth nuclear contours (A). When these cells comprise a minor component of the Pap slide, they can usually be disregarded. By contrast, dysplastic or malignant air-dried cells exhibit high N:C ratios, variation in cell and nuclear size and shape, and irregular nuclear contours (B). When these cells are observed in Pap slides, a careful search for non-dried abnormal cells is important. Even if none are found, a diagnosis of ASC-US or a request for a repeat Pap test should be considered. Pap slides with significant air-drying artifact (>75% of the smear,

per the Bethesda System of reporting) and no abnormal cells identified (ASC-US and above) should be reported as "unsatisfactory." Although air-drying artifact is most often present on conventional preparations, similar features may sometimes be seen at the edge of a ThinPrep sample (C).

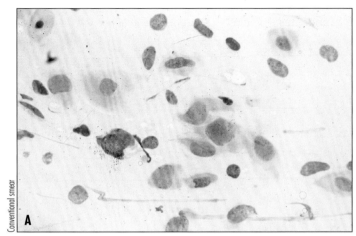

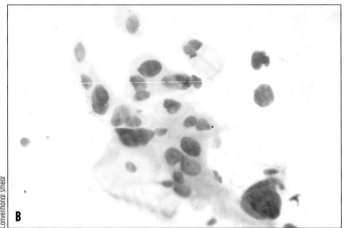

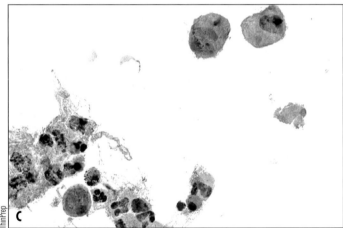

Figure 4-39. Alternaria.

Alternaria is a ubiquitous plant fungus and an occasional contaminant in cytologic preparations, where its large (7 to 10 by 23 to 34 µm), brown, horizontally and vertically sep-

tate and snowshoe-shaped conidia (or spores) render it readily recognizable. *Alternaria* is a rare cause of infection in humans, and affected patients are typically immunocompromised.

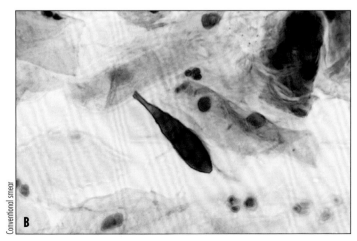

Figure 4-40. Bare nuclei.

Bare nuclei on Pap slides are usually of endocervical or parabasal cell origin, and recognition is aided by their close association with nearby viable intact cells with similar features. Bare nuclei often show degenerative changes, including dark smudged nuclei, and can be confused with lymphocytes, organisms such as *Trichomonas vaginalis*, and rarely a small cell neoplasm. Occasionally, bare nuclei derived from HSIL may be seen. In this circumstance, which is more commonly noted on liquid-based specimens, nuclei will generally be hyperchromatic and may show coarsely granular chromatin and nuclear outline irregularities. When bare nuclei with features suggesting dysplasia are noted, a close search for intact HSIL cells should be performed. Bare nuclei can also be present in cytolytic specimens from the luteal phase of the menstrual cycle. In this circumstance, the typical dissolution of cytoplasm and the background bacteria should be present and will allow a correct interpretation.

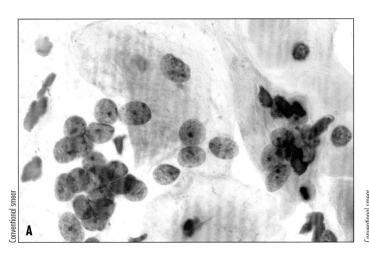

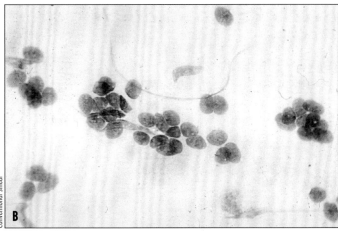

Figure 4-41. Cockleburs.

A cocklebur is a spoke-like arrangement of yellowish crystalloid material surrounded by mixed inflammatory cells, including histiocytes. Once thought to contain predominantly hematoidin, cockleburs contain mostly glycoproteins and calcium. Cockleburs are found infrequently in Pap slides and are most often observed during pregnancy. This interesting artifact has no known clinical significance, and their presence in Pap slides need not be reported.

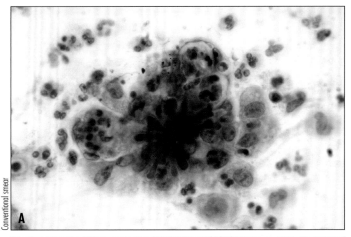

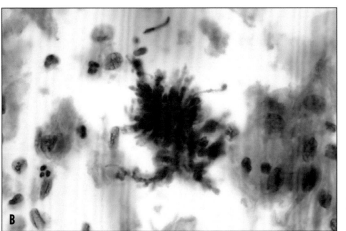

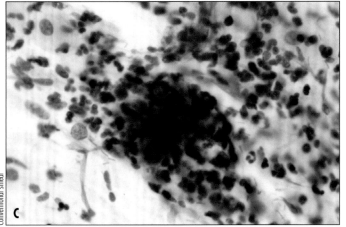

Figure 4-42. Cornflaking.

Cornflaking, a very common artifact of coverslipping, is readily recognized by most cytologists. It occurs when mounting media starts to evaporate prior to placing the coverslip on the stained slide. At the point on the cell surface where evaporation occurs, air bubbles can become trapped between the coverslip and the surface of the cells. Usually, mature squamous cells are involved. When viewed with the light microscope, the air bubbles appear as coarse, dark brown, refractile granules that cover much of the surface of the cells—thus the resemblance to corn flakes. At high magnification, the air bubbles are seen slightly above the plane of the cell surface. When extensive, cornflaking can significantly obscure epithelial cells, in which case recoverslipping is required for better evaluation of the smear.

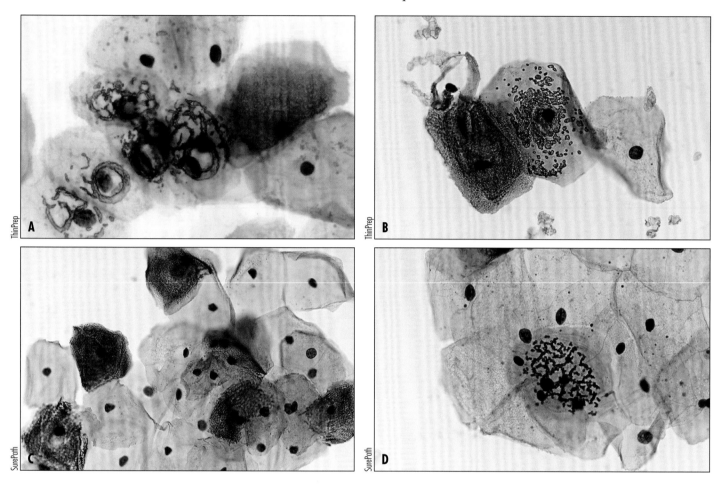

Figure 4-43. Ferning.

Ferning is observed in conventional Pap preparations obtained near mid-cycle (ie, at ovulation), when cervical mucus is relatively thin. Ferning is the formation of a palm-leaf pattern by the crystallized cervical mucus as it dries on a smear. Ferning was historically used as a test to determine the date of ovulation.

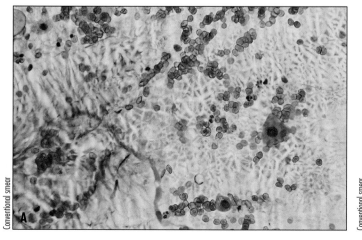

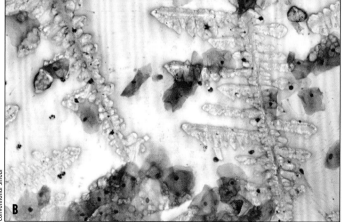

Figure 4-44. Fibers.

The origins of various fibers and threads in Pap slides include clothing, menstrual pads, tampons, and other foreign objects (eg, wooden spatulas, cotton swabs) introduced into the vagina. Fibers of foreign materials are usually readily recognized but on occasion can be confused with *Candida* or other fungi.

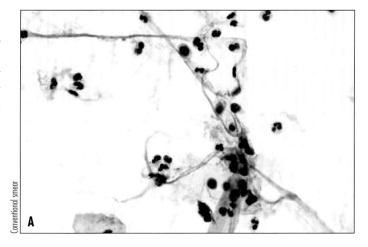

Conventional smear

A

Figure 4-45. Fibrocytes/fibroblasts.

Spindle cells of fibroblastic origin may be seen in post-abortion or post-delivery patients, when granulation tissue from the healing wound is present. If the cells are fibroblastic or reactive, confusion with a well-differentiated squamous cell carcinoma (which is often associated with spindled squamous cells) is possible. Reactive fibroblastic cells have a dense granular cytoplasm, as opposed to the glassy keratinized cytoplasm of squamous cells. The paucity of spindle cells and the absence of diagnostic malignant and keratinized cells should prevent overinterpretation.

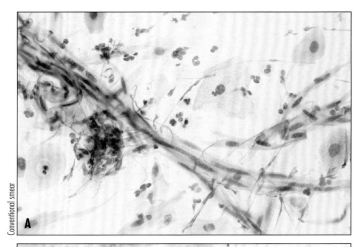

Conventional smear

A

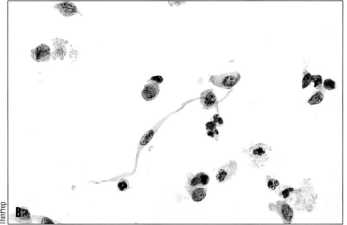

ThinPrep

B

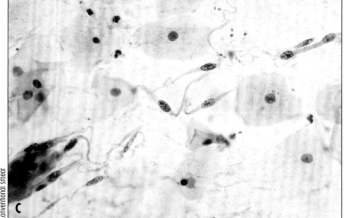

Conventional smear

C

Figure 4-46. Geotrichum.

Geotrichum (A, B, and C) is a rarely pathogenic fungus that has hyphal forms similar to *Candida* species (D), but without spore or yeast formation. *Geotrichum* forms septate true hyphae that are 3 to 6 µm in diameter. The fungi are widespread and can be found on the skin, in food products such as cereals and dairy, and in textiles, soil, and water. There are no reports of clinically significant vaginal infections, and these organisms do not need to be reported.

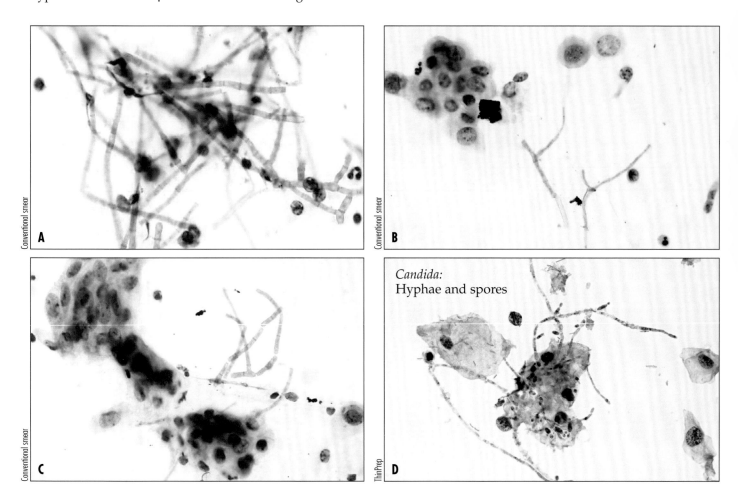

Figure 4-47. Glycogen.

Glycogen is a normal component found in the cytoplasm of squamous cells, especially intermediate cells. Normal vaginal flora (ie, lactobacilli, aka Doderline bacilli) feed on the intracellular glycogen, which leads to cytolysis and lactic acid production. This, in turn, helps to maintain an acid Ph, which supports the normal bacterial flora (A). Because glycogen is most abundant in the intermediate squamous cell, cytolysis is most often observed in Pap slides when these cells predominate, as during the luteal phase of the menstrual cycle or pregnancy. Intracellular glycogen imparts a yellow or golden color to the perinuclear cytoplasm, often with no obvious change in cytoplasmic consistency. When the color is very pale, the perinuclear cytoplasm appears empty and can be confused with the perinuclear HPV koilocytic cavity (B, arrow). However, the latter is distinguished by an empty sharp-edged cavity and an associated large dark (ie, dysplastic) nucleus. Sometimes intracellular glycogen is more distinct and clumpy and may appear to crack like dried clay. During pregnancy, intermediate cells accumulate an abundant amount of glycogen, which stains deeply and imparts a rigid, slightly elongated or boat-shaped configuration to the cell. These distinctive cells are called navicular cells, and they can also be seen in Pap slides from postmenopausal women.

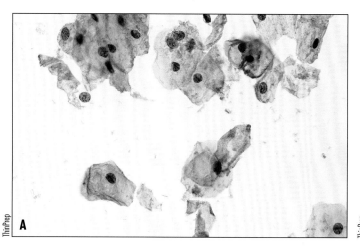
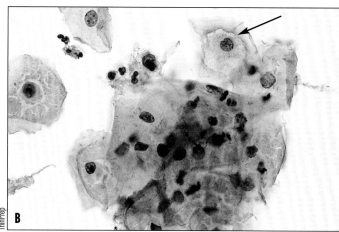

Figure 4-48. Lubricant.

The background blue material in the illustration represents lubricant used to insert the speculum for the pelvic examination (A). It usually does not cause problems in interpretation but may dilute the sample for Pap testing and thus can be the cause of an unsatisfactory Pap slide. Rarely, lubricant can plug the filter in a ThinPrep sample, resulting in a scantly cellular or unsatisfactory preparation (B).

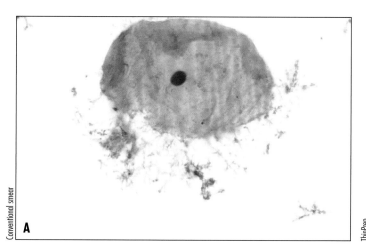
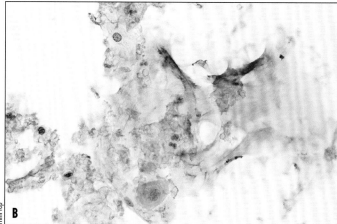

Figure 4-49. Multinucleated histiocytes.

Multinucleated histiocytes are fairly common in Pap slides, especially those from postmenopausal women. This finding is of no clinical import and does not need to be reported. These cells are also common in post-radiation slides, where they are sometimes the dominant cell type present. They are often associated with mononuclear histiocytes. Very rarely, giant cells may be seen in the background of a tuberculous infection. Multinucleated histiocytes should be differentiated from syncytial trophoblasts, as described previously (see Figure 4-22). Multinucleated histiocytes will be smaller and have fewer nuclei than syncytial trophoblasts.

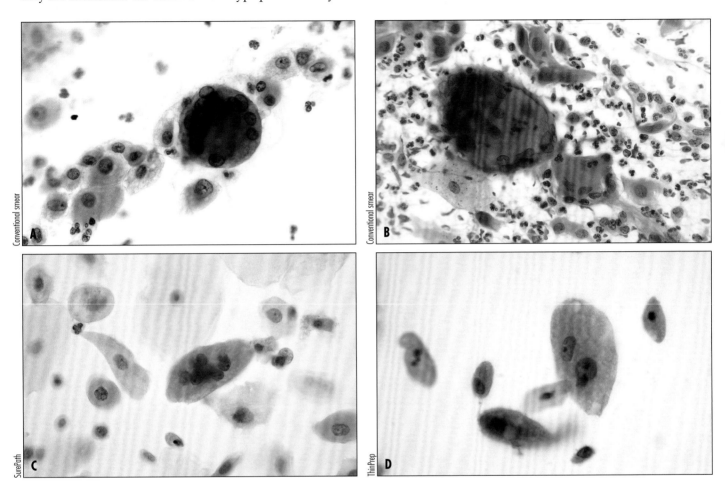

Figure 4-50. Pencil cells.

Pencil cells are thin, elongated endocervical cells thought to be caused by a hypertonic milieu, with resulting shrinkage of the endocervical cells. Pencil cells may be seen in Pap slides taken subsequent to the application of Lugol's iodine solution (A). Another potential cause of these cells is the elongation caused by the electrical loop cautery device used in LEEP procedures. Endocervical samples taken immediately after such procedures may show considerable artifactual change (B and C). Pencil cells may be confused with other benign cells, such as rolled mature squamous cells or benign mesenchymal cells (smooth muscle cells or fibrocytes), but their blandness and uniformity usually preclude confusion with a neoplastic or preneoplastic process.

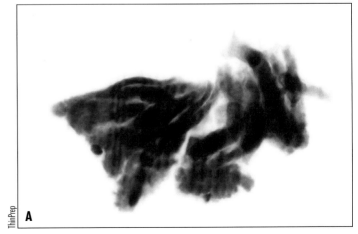

Figure 4-50 continued.

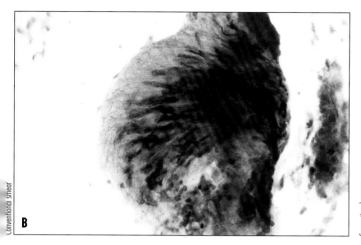

B

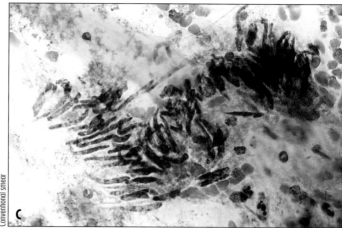

C

Figure 4-51. Pollen.

Pollen is a large vegetable cell, and on Pap slides it can rarely be confused with a keratinized squamous cell. Pollen varies in size but is generally about the size of a mature squamous cell. Unlike epithelial cells, the central region of the pollen cell does not contain a nucleus and is homogenous and dense orange—thus the superficial resemblance to keratinized squamous cells (A, B, and C). Another helpful finding is the presence of the variably shaped, rigid cell wall that is one of the characteristics of plant cells. Although pollen is variable in size and shape, the presence of a cell wall and the lack of a nucleus are consistent features. Talc may be confused with pollen but presents as refractile small granules without cellular features (D).

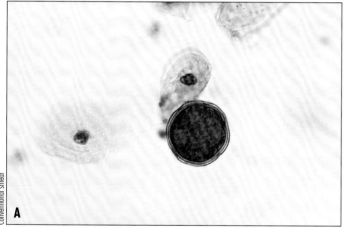

A

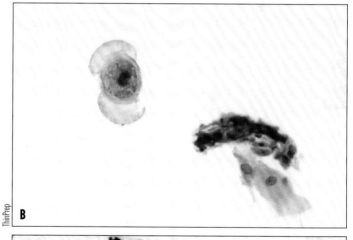

B

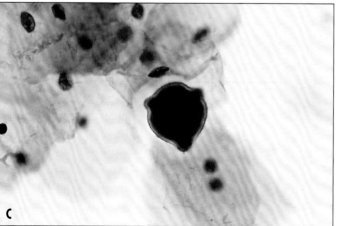

C

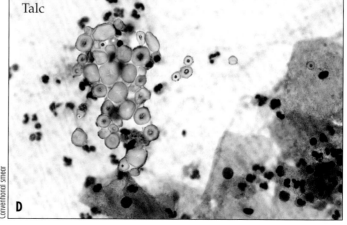

Talc

D

Figure 4-52. Smooth muscle cells.

Smooth muscle (SM) cells are rarely observed in Pap slides but may, on occasion, present post abortion or exfoliate from a submucosal leiomyoma that has undergone erosion of the overlying mucosa. SM cells present singly or in small clusters and have defined cytoplasmic borders that taper at the two ends. The nuclei are also smoothly contoured, with tapered ends. The nuclear chromatin is pale, finely granular, and evenly distributed. Nucleoli are small and uniform. There may be considerable reactive changes if the cells are derived from an ulcerated submucosal leiomyoma (B and D). Rolled-up mature squamous cells are commonly present on Pap slides and are sometimes misinterpreted as SM cells. Invasive squamous cell carcinoma frequently contains abnormal spindled squamous cells, and careful cytologic review of nuclear features is very important to evaluate for squamous cell carcinoma whenever spindled cells are seen in Pap slides. Malignant spindled squamous cells typically have enlarged, elongated, dark, or pyknotic nuclei, and the cytoplasm is often densely keratinized.

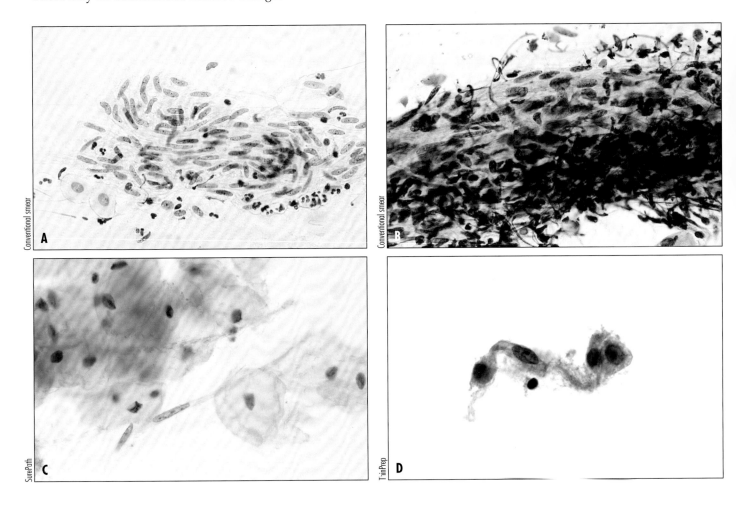

Squamous Epithelial Abnormalities

Michael R. Henry, MD

Atypical Squamous Cells of Undetermined Significance

The concept of atypical squamous cells of undetermined significance (ASC-US) as a diagnostic category for cervical cytology reflects the reality of the limitations of light microscopy in classifying cytologic changes. Under ideal circumstances, all lesions would have classic appearances and fall quite nicely into their respective categories. In reality, the cellular changes seen in a cervical/vaginal sample represent a broad and continuous spectrum of change. Often there will be cells demonstrating overlapping criteria or small numbers of abnormal cells, which makes an exact diagnosis problematic. These equivocal findings lead to the necessity for an indeterminate diagnostic category such as ASC-US. Because of these limitations, the initial version of the Bethesda System invented the term "atypical squamous cells of undetermined significance" (ASCUS). This diagnostic category was to be used for cellular abnormalities that were more than those attributable to reactive changes but that quantitatively or qualitatively fell short of squamous intraepithelial lesion (SIL).[1] The term "of undetermined significance" was used because the cellular changes in the ASCUS category might reflect either an exuberant benign change or alternatively a potentially serious lesion.[2] It was also suggested that qualifying terms, such as "probably reactive" or "suggestive of LSIL" (low-grade SIL), be added to the diagnosis of ASCUS in order to more accurately define the risk of having true disease.

Over the ensuing decade, the term ASCUS became well accepted in the clinical community, and studies have shown that the use of ASCUS as a diagnostic category significantly improves the clinical usefulness of the Pap test. Pitman et al demonstrated that the elimination of ASCUS as a diagnostic category (a series of ASCUS cases were reclassified as either benign or SIL) resulted in a significant decrease in the sensitivity of the Pap test from 100% to 41% for high-grade squamous intraepithelial lesion or worse (HSIL+), with no associated increase in the specificity of the test.[3] While the relative risk for HSIL+ is low for a patient with ASC-US (less than 10%),[4,5] ASCUS is by far the most commonly diagnosed Pap abnormality leading to a true abnormality found on subsequent work up. Kinney et al[4] clearly demonstrated the importance of minimally abnormal Pap tests in a prospective study of over 46,000 women. In that study, the authors showed that the most common initial cytologic diagnosis in women with histologically-proven HSIL+ was ASCUS, with 38.8% of these

HSIL+ cases having ASCUS as the initiating event. They also noted that while a cytologic diagnosis of high-grade intraepithelial lesion was very specific, only 31.4% of biopsy-proven HSIL+ was diagnosed as HSIL on the initial Pap test.

With the support of similar data, the 2001 Bethesda System consensus conference retained the general category of atypical squamous cells (ASC), with minor modification of the terminology and definition. The qualifiers of "probably reactive" and "suggestive of LSIL" were eliminated because they were found to have no real clinical significance. Instead, two more specific categories of ASC were adopted: (1) atypical squamous cells of undetermined significance (ASC-US) and (2) atypical squamous cells, cannot exclude HSIL (ASC-H).[6] ASC-US is defined as "cytologic changes suggestive of an LSIL that are quantitatively or qualitatively insufficient for a definitive diagnosis." ASC-H is defined as "cytologic changes suggestive of a HSIL that are quantitatively or qualitatively insufficient for a definitive diagnosis." It is important to note that both the clinical significance and clinical management vary considerably between the two entities. For example, the recommended management for ASC-H is colposcopic examination. On the other hand, ASC-US may be initially managed with either reflex testing for high-risk human papillomavirus (HPV), follow-up with cervical cytology at 6 and 12 months, or immediate colposcopic examination. The 2006 American Society for Colposcopy and Cervical Pathology (ASCCP) guidelines recommend, as the preferred method of triage to colposcopic examination, offering reflex HPV testing (if using liquid-based cytology or obtaining co-collected HPV samples) for women older than age 20 years who have an initial diagnosis of ASC-US.[7]

It is important to remember that ASC is not a single diagnostic entity but encompasses a spectrum of cellular changes and reflects a variety of pathologic processes. Thus, ASC should always be considered a diagnosis of exclusion, and it should never be used if a more specific result is possible.

Conceptually, ASC-US can be divided into two subcategories, both of which show changes suggestive but not diagnostic of LSIL. First there are cases where some, but not all, of the diagnostic features of HPV infection are present (Figure 5-1). For example, a hallmark of HPV infection is the perinuclear halo or koilocytosis. However, if this change is present in small numbers or with relatively normal nuclear morphology, a definitive diagnosis of LSIL may not be possible, and the correct interpretation would be ASC-US. Cytoplasmic vacuolization or ill-defined perinuclear halos may be reactive in nature and, if possible, should be placed into a benign category (see Figures 7-6 and 7-16). Another atypical cellular change often associated with HPV infection is atypical or pleomorphic parakeratosis. These cells are small keratinizing squamous cells with atypical features, such as variable nuclear size and shape or elongated, sometimes snakelike, nuclei and dense eosinophilic cytoplasm. While these cells are not of themselves diagnostic of SIL, they are certainly suggestive of possible HPV cytopathic effect (see "Low-Grade Squamous Intraepithelial Lesions" below) (Figure 5-1, E through G). Again, these changes need to be differentiated from benign parakeratosis, often described as miniature superficial squamous cells with round, regular, pyknotic nuclei (see Figure 7-19).

Secondly, there are cases with nuclear abnormalities that approach those of LSIL (Figure 5-2). These nuclei are enlarged two to three times the size of a normal intermediate cell. There may be mild variation in size and shape, slight hyperchromasia, and occasional binucleation. These changes are seen in mature squamous cells with mature cytoplasm and low nuclear to cytoplasmic (N:C) ratios. These changes should not be confused with benign nuclear enlargement, which may be seen in the perimenopausal age group. This perimenopausal nuclear enlargement consists of mature squamous cells with large nuclei (two to three times normal), with a concomitant increase in cytoplasmic size and no nuclear hyperchromasia or membrane wrinkling, and with a finely granular chromatin structure. This change and other benign ASC-US mimics are illustrated in chapter 7 (see Figure 7-6).

Atypical Squamous Cells, Cannot Exclude HSIL

Most commonly, ASC-H is represented by changes in immature squamous metaplastic cells or reserve cells, which fall between benign cellular changes and HSIL. These cells have immature cytoplasm and larger nuclei than normal metaplastic cells. There is an increase in the N:C ratio along with some degree of anisonucleosis, nuclear membrane irregularity, and mild hyperchromasia. However, the changes seen fall short of the criteria needed for a diagnosis of HSIL (Figure 5-3). At other times, cells with the cytologic features of HSIL may be present on the slide, but there are not enough cells to confidently make the diagnosis. In many cases, these cells are seen as scattered single cells that are easily missed during the screening process and may be a cause of false-negative cases (Figure 5-4).[8,9] Cells suggestive of HSIL may also be seen in hyperchromatic crowded groups, where the density of the cells makes evaluation of the nuclei difficult and therefore precludes a definitive diagnosis (Figure 5-5).

Another variant of ASC-H consists of cellular clusters with features of both repair (a benign cellular change) and an epithelial abnormality, often suggesting the possibility of invasive carcinoma (Figure 5-6). The cells in question are typically immature squamous or glandular cells with

prominent nucleoli. In a benign reparative process, the cells are present in flat, cohesive, syncytial sheets, with streaming of the cells (see Figure 4-8 and Figure 7-21). An atypical reparative process will contain groups of cells with piled up nuclei, more anisonucleosis, and uneven chromatin distribution, or loosely cohesive groups with occasional single cells. Numerous single cells or tumor diathesis is not present. Most often these changes represent an exuberant reactive or reparative process. Because the differential diagnosis includes invasive carcinoma, these cases should be included in the generic category of ASC-H, with a suggestion that the features are suggestive of carcinoma in order that appropriate clinical follow-up will be obtained.[7] Pleomorphic parakeratosis may also fall into this category when the abnormal cells suggest the possibility of keratinizing dysplasia (HSIL) or even keratinizing squamous cell carcinoma (Figure 5-7).

The spectrum of change seen in atrophy is broad and may include cells that are difficult to distinguish from an epithelial cell abnormality. The differential diagnosis of the immature cells present in atrophy may include LSIL, HSIL, or even carcinoma. Thus, atypical cellular changes in atrophy may be included in either ASC-US or ASC-H (depending on the severity of the abnormality). Atypical findings in atrophy may include nuclear enlargement with concomitant hyperchromasia, marked irregularity in the nuclear membranes, irregular chromatin distribution, hyperchromatic crowded groups, or the presence of pleomorphic spindle or tadpole cells (Figure 5-8).

Low-Grade Squamous Intraepithelial Lesion

At the first Bethesda consensus conference, the terms low-grade squamous intraepithelial lesion (LSIL) and high-grade squamous intraepithelial lesion (HSIL) were devised to cover the preinvasive squamous lesions seen in cytologic samples. The term squamous intraepithelial lesion (SIL) is a cytologically specific concept; cervical intraepithelial neoplasia (CIN) is a histological term. While the cytologic features of SIL correlate with histological features, SIL should be reserved for cytologic samples. The 2001 Bethesda System confirmed the use of these terms as clinically relevant. This support is based on the strong biological justification for a two-tiered diagnostic terminology in which the dividing line is placed between the histologic entities of mild dysplasia (CIN I) and moderate dysplasia (CIN II).[10] Both LSIL and HSIL encompass the spectrum of squamous precursors leading to carcinoma of the cervix.

LSIL on Pap tests is characterized by cells with the diagnostic features of mild dysplasia or the definitive changes associated with HPV infection—so-called HPV cytopathic effect. The category is inclusive of the older diagnostic classes of mild dysplasia as well as the previously utilized terms of HPV infection, such as "koilocytic atypia." The cells of LSIL may be seen as single cells or as sheets of dysplastic cells, with or without HPV cytopathic effect. The hallmark of this HPV-associated change is the perinuclear cytoplasmic halo known as koilocytosis. A diagnostic koilocyte has a well-defined, optically clear, perinuclear halo, with a dense peripheral rim of cytoplasm and nuclear abnormalities (Figure 5-9). In preparations with the features of "classic" nonkeratinizing (or mild) dysplasia, LSIL is characterized by mature squamous cells with large nuclei, ranging from four to six times the size of a normal intermediate nucleus. The nuclei also demonstrate hyperchromasia, irregular nuclear membranes, and frequent binucleation. The chromatin is typically finely granular and evenly distributed. Nucleoli are infrequent (Figure 5-10). The nuclear changes of LSIL may consist of enlargement, nuclear membrane wrinkling, hyperchromasia, binucleation and multinucleation, and often some degenerative changes, such as chromatin smudging or pyknosis, resulting in changes described as "raisinoid" (Figure 5-11). Most often, slides with LSIL will demonstrate a combination of the above features, with both "classic" mild dysplasia and HPV cytopathic change.

In liquid-based cervical samples, the cytologic criteria for LSIL are essentially the same as for conventional smears, although in some cases there is a tendency towards nuclear normo- or even hypochromasia.

High-Grade Squamous Intraepithelial Lesion

The category of HSIL encompasses the histologic categories of moderate and severe dysplasias and carcinoma in situ (CIN II-III). The cytologic features of HSIL are characterized by cells with immature cytoplasm, abnormal nuclear features, and an increased N:C ratio.

The nuclei of HSIL are smaller than those of LSIL, especially in the more severe lesions. The nuclear size typically ranges from two to five times the size of an intermediate cell nucleus. Of importance, the cytoplasmic area is always decreased, yielding a marked increase in the N:C ratio. The nuclei are hyperchromatic with a fine to coarsely granular, evenly distributed chromatin pattern. The nuclear membranes are often wrinkled, and there is typically a significant degree of anisonucleosis. Nucleoli are generally absent (Figure 5-12).

The two most important differences between LSIL and HSIL are the immaturity of the cytoplasm and the high N:C ratio in cases of HSIL. The cells of HSIL are present singly, in sheets, and, at the high end of the spectrum, may be seen in syncytial-like aggregates (Figures 5-13 and 5-14). Some sampling devices will often pull aggregates of HSIL off from the surface or from endocervical glands, yielding three-dimensional clusters or hyperchromatic crowded groups of abnormal immature cells (Figure 5-15).

Keratinizing dysplasia is a variant of HSIL. Unlike the immature cells of classic HSIL, this variant consists of cells with a glassy keratinizing (often pleomorphic) cytoplasm. These cells may take on a caudate or tadpole shape. The N:C ratio is very high, and the nuclear membranes are irregular. The chromatin is typically very dense and may be opaque (Figure 5-16). These cells are placed in the HSIL category because the biopsy is most often CIN II+ and these features are similar to those of invasive keratinizing

carcinoma. Indeed, the only difference between keratinizing dysplasia and keratinizing invasive carcinoma is the presence of a tumor diathesis and/or nucleoli and subtle chromatin irregularity (clearing), which may be present in invasive carcinoma (see Figure 7-19).

Unlike LSIL, there are sometimes significant variations in the diagnostic criteria for HSIL in liquid-based samples.[11] While the morphologic changes are generally similar for both preparations, HSIL cells from the liquid-based samples may appear to be somewhat smaller than their counterparts in conventional smears. This is especially true in the cells derived from the highest grade lesions, such as carcinoma in situ, and is especially marked in ThinPrep specimens. Cells from HSIL can be found singly and in groups. Syncytial aggregates noted in association with carcinoma in situ are clearly identified on liquid-based cytology preparations but may mimic glandular groups, due to smoother contoured borders and smaller nuclei.[12] Challenges occur when only a few high-grade cells are present in the background of the slide. These cells are often small and may approximate the size of a small histiocyte. In the clean background encountered on liquid-based preparations, these small cells are easily missed on routine screening (Figure 5-17). The increased N:C ratios seen in moderate and severe dysplasias are evident on liquid-based preparations. Irregular nuclear contours are clearly displayed and may even be accentuated in liquid-based preparations. Fine to coarse nuclear granularity of the chromatin pattern is preserved. Hyperchromasia may be somewhat decreased in liquid-based preparations and should be considered to be a lesser criterion (Figure 5-18).

Squamous Cell Carcinoma

Squamous cell carcinoma (SCC) comes in two common morphologic variants: keratinizing and nonkeratinizing. While the Bethesda System does not subdivide SCC into these categories, the cytologic features are somewhat different. Nonkeratinizing SCC features cells with immature cytoplasm, high N:C ratios, and nuclei with prominent nucleoli, irregular chromatin distribution, and irregular nuclear membranes (Figure 5-19). These cells may be seen in loose or syncytial groups or as isolated cells (Figure 5-20). Associated features may include a tumor diathesis composed of necrotic debris, old blood, and inflammation.

Keratinizing SCC displays all of the cellular characteristics of keratinizing HSIL, with the addition of variable numbers of cells demonstrating nucleoli or the addition of a tumor diathesis. Features include marked cellular variation with tadpole, spindle, and caudate shapes; dense eosinophilic cytoplasm; and markedly hyperchromatic, often opaque, nuclei with high N:C ratios. Cells may be present singly or in loose or even thick groups (Figure 5-21).

A definitive interpretation of SCC is often difficult to make on cervical/vaginal preparations, especially in women without a clinical history of cervical cancer or other suggestive physical findings. In these cases, the Bethesda System recommends the use of "HSIL with features suggestive of invasive carcinoma." As mentioned above, often the only difference between keratinizing HSIL and keratinizing SCC is the presence of a tumor diathesis and nucleoli. To complicate matters, because of the frequent exophytic growth pattern, a diathesis may not be present in some cases of invasive carcinoma, and the dense nuclear features make nucleoli difficult to identify. Thus, a careful search should be made for more immature cells with less nuclear opacity to identify the presence of nucleoli. A mixture of keratinizing cells and the markedly atypical cells associated with nonkeratinizing SCC is another clue to the presence of invasive carcinoma.

The presence of a tumor diathesis suggests an invasive carcinoma. This finding is still noted on liquid samples but may be somewhat patchier. It has been described as "clinging" diathesis because it seems to cling to abnormal cells and often coagulates into aggregates of debris, in distinction to the diffuse diathesis in smeared specimens (Figure 5-22). The presence of background blood and inflammation in women with SCC often makes the smears difficult to evaluate. This material may plug the filters used for ThinPrep preparations, yielding scantly cellular smears.[13] At times the diagnostic cells are hidden in this obscuring material and may be missed during screening. Look for numerous pleomorphic, pyknotic cells that are caught up in necrotic debris. It is always important to thoroughly examine bloody and inflamed smears for the presence of these hidden malignant cells, even—or especially—when they are otherwise technically unsatisfactory.

Figure 5-1. ASC-US with changes suggestive of LSIL (HPV cytopathic effect).

The changes seen in these images suggest the possibility of HPV cytopathic effect and LSIL. The atypical cells present with varying degrees of dyskeratotic and koilocytic change. In some cases, while the individual cells (as in C) strongly suggest an HPV infection, the limited number of atypical cells present on the entire slide may preclude a diagnosis of LSIL. The sheets of cells in A and B show variably sized nuclei with focal binucleation. In A there is a suggestion of halo formation, but definite koilocytosis is not seen. The two atypical cells in C show halo formation, but the nuclei are small and do not demonstrate the quantitative nuclear changes sufficient for LSIL. The nuclei in D are larger, irregular, and hyperchromatic but fall short of the features of LSIL. Atypical keratin pearls are seen in E and F, with irregular nuclei rather than the round nuclei that would be associated with a benign pearl. Two types of atypical parakeratosis are seen in G and H. The cells in G are probably derived from surface cells. The more atypical cells in H have increased N:C ratios, variably-sized large nuclei, and irregular membranes. These cells are on the borderline between ASC-US and cells suggesting keratinizing dysplasia (ASC-H).

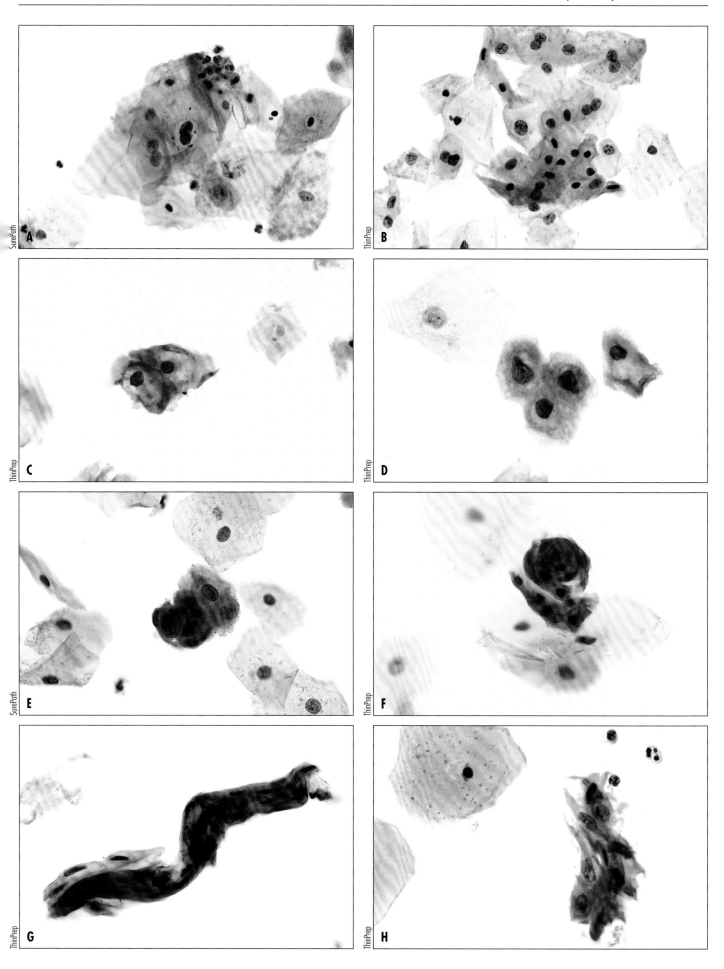

Figure 5-2. ASC-US with features suggestive of LSIL (mild dysplasia).

These images illustrate ASC-US nuclear changes suggestive of LSIL. The common feature is the abnormal nuclear enlargement without concomitant HPV cytopathic change, although there is a suggestion of a halo noted in D. All of the nuclei demonstrate variable degrees of hyperchromasia and nuclear membrane irregularity, which is most pronounced in C. The abnormal cells are for the most part mature squamous cells with abundant cytoplasm. The age of the patient must be taken into consideration in these cases because scattered cells with large nuclei, abundant cytoplasm, and no evidence of HPV change (such as in A and B) may be a normal component in a sample from a perimenopausal patient. Immature cytoplasm is seen in G, but the low N:C ratios are suggestive of LSIL instead of HSIL. Repair-like features are noted in H, but the lack of prominent nucleoli and cytoplasmic streaming combined with nuclear size variation suggests the possibility of LSIL.

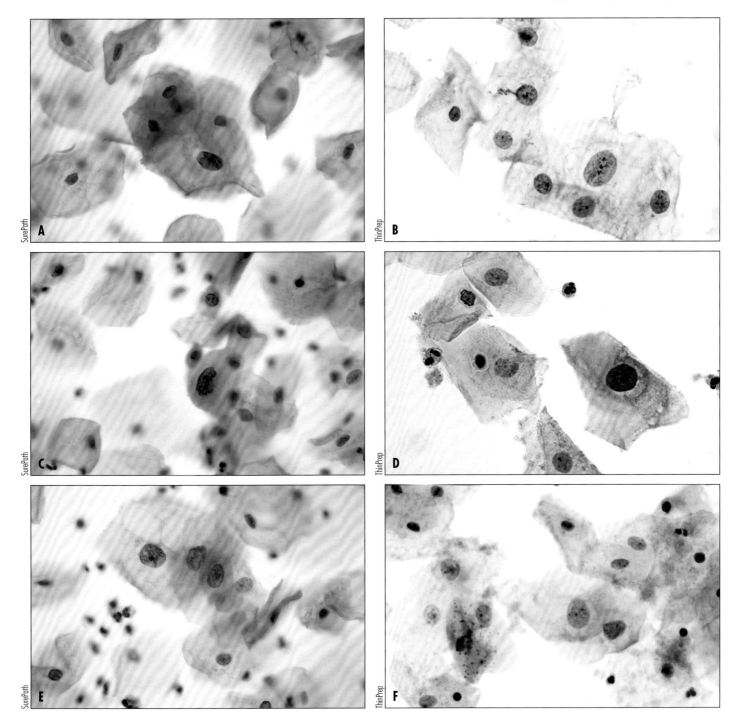

Figure 5-2 continued.

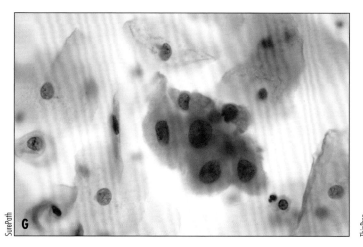

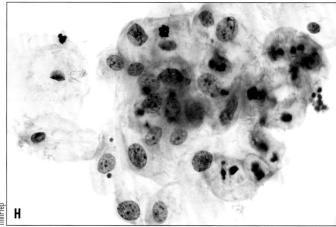

Figure 5-3. ASC-H: Immature squamous metaplasia.

The cells seen in these images have immature cytoplasm with features of immature squamous metaplasia. However, the nuclei show variation in nuclear size, with some nuclear membrane irregularities. This size variation combined with increased N:C ratios seen within groups or sheets of cells is an important criterion, suggesting the possibility of HSIL, rather than a benign process. The immature cells seen in A and B have large nuclei with slightly increased N:C ratios, suggesting moderate dysplasia. In B, the two abnormal cells at the bottom of the image can be compared to the benign squamous metaplastic cells seen on the left of the image. In C and D, there are loose sheets of smaller immature cells with increased N:C ratios, variability in nuclear size, and mild hyperchromasia, suggesting the possibility of severe dysplasia. Note that in C these nuclei are about the same size as a normal intermediate nucleus.

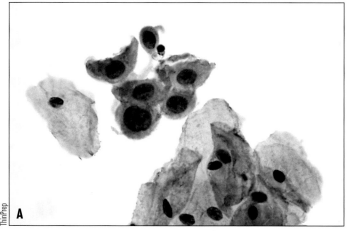

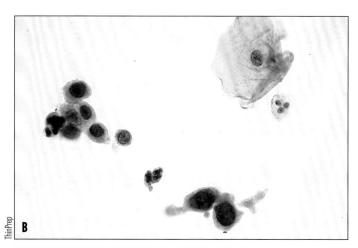

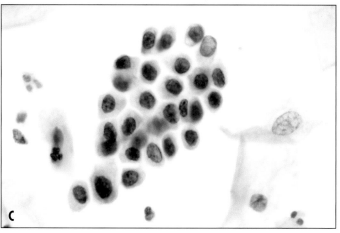

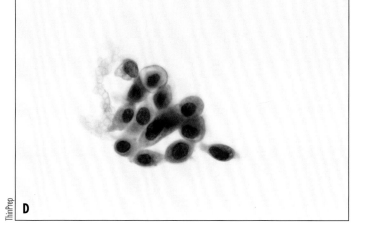

Figure 5-4. ASC-H: Scattered single cell pattern.

These are single atypical cells with moderately sized hyperchromatic nuclei, very irregular nuclear membranes, and scant cytoplasm. This pattern may not meet the quantitative criteria for a definitive diagnosis of HSIL. As presented in A, these cells individually have features consistent with HSIL (severe dysplasia/carcinoma in situ); however, if only a few of these cells are present on the slide, a conclusive interpretation of HSIL may not be possible. In C and D, the cells have increased N:C ratios, slight hyperchromasia, and nuclear membrane wrinkling suggestive but not diagnostic of HSIL. These single cells are usually dispersed and hide "in plain sight" in the white (or blank) areas of liquid-based specimens. Alternatively, they may lie on top of other cells, also making identification difficult (B). The differential diagnostic consideration is often degenerative changes, which may be seen in single small cells, as noted in chapter 7 (see Figure 7-8).

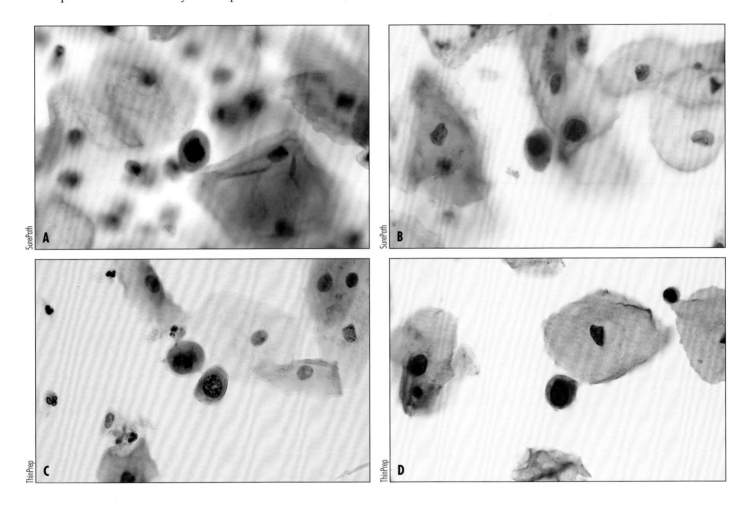

Figure 5-5. ASC-H: Hyperchromatic crowded groups.

Immature small cells arranged in crowded three-dimensional groups with hyperchromasia and nuclear size variation is suggestive of HSIL. These thick groups are often difficult to evaluate. All the cellular groups seen here are composed of small cells with scant cytoplasm and hyperchromatic nuclei with somewhat coarse chromatin. There is some nuclear size variation (anisonucleosis), and, when visible, the nuclear membranes are slightly wrinkled with occasional notches. Apoptotic bodies (arrow in D) and mitoses may be present in these groups and are more indicative of HSIL. Often the differential is between glandular groups of reactive endocervical or endometrial cells. The horizontal arrangement of the cells around the periphery of the groups confirms the squamous nature of the cells.

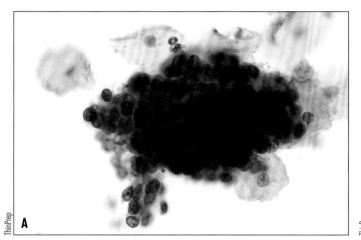

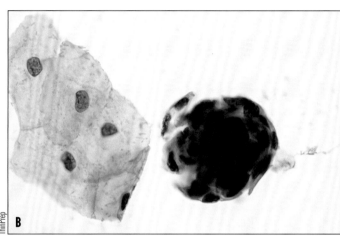

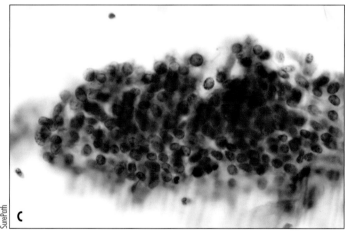

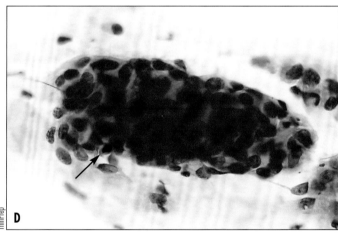

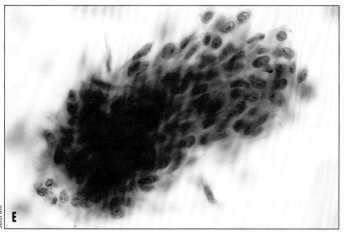

Figure 5-6. ASC-H: Atypical repair.

Atypical reparative cells may suggest the possibility of invasive carcinoma. Although conceptually these cells may fall within the category of ASC-H, in reality an interpretation should be made that alerts the clinician to the possibility of cancer. An immediate colposcopic examination should be recommended. The cells present in A and B show thick sheets with scant cytoplasm, variably sized nuclei with focal irregular chromatin distribution, and multiple prominent nucleoli. There are no single cells, mitoses, or tumor diathesis. As in the more common variants of ASC-H, the features fall short of the qualitative or quantitative criteria needed for an interpretation of squamous cell carcinoma. While these groups may represent a benign reactive process, invasive carcinoma or dysplasia with reactive changes secondary to inflammation cannot be excluded.

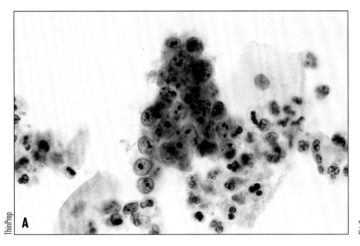

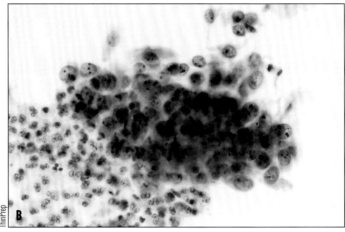

Figure 5-7. ASC-H: Pleomorphic parakeratosis suggestive of keratinizing dysplasia.

Dyskeratotic cells with irregular hyperchromatic nuclei and high N:C ratios may be seen in both keratinizing dysplasia (HSIL) and keratinizing squamous cell carcinoma. However, a benign degenerative process may also shed similar cells. Because of the possibility of HSIL+ in these cases, it is best to place cases with these types of cells into the general category of ASC-H. Both of these images demonstrate abnormal cells with dense eosinophilic cytoplasm. A cluster of cells with more typical immature cytoplasm and irregular nuclei suggestive of HSIL is also noted in A, reflecting the common finding of the mixture of cells that may be seen in cases of keratinizing dysplasia. Similar cells with cyanophilic cytoplasm are noted in B.

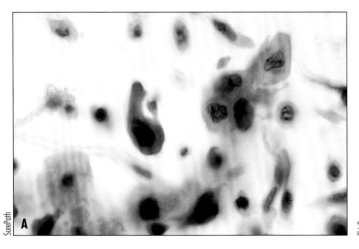

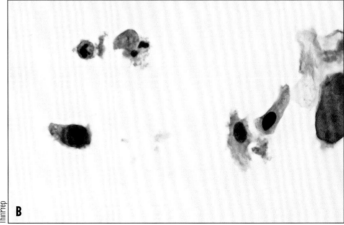

Figure 5-8. ASC-H: Atypical squamous cells in atrophy.

Atypical changes seen in atrophy are variable. Degenerative changes can lead to apparent dyskeratotic cells with tadpole shapes, suggesting the possibility of keratinizing dysplasia or even carcinoma, as shown in A. Cells noted in B are more typical for atrophy but show increased nuclear variability and increased size. Interestingly, the cells presented in A reverted to normal with a trial of estrogen. In case B, the follow-up revealed squamous cell carcinoma.

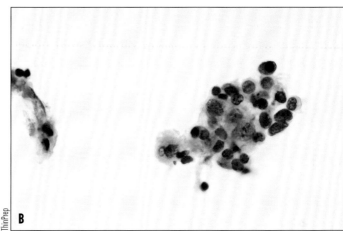

Figure 5-9. LSIL: Cellular morphology of HPV cytopathic effect.

The hallmark of HPV cytopathic effect (LSIL) is the koilocyte. A koilocyte is a cell with a large, optically clear, perinuclear halo; a peripheral rim of condensed cytoplasm; and some degree of nuclear change. The rim of the halo is most often irregular, with sharply demarcated borders. The nuclei are enlarged, hyperchromatic, irregular, and may have coarse chromatin. Degenerative changes of pyknosis or smudging of the chromatin is common. Binucleation or multinucleation is also common but not diagnostic of LSIL. The diagnostic cells may be isolated, as in B, or present as sheets or plaques of cells, as noted in C, G, and H. Most often the halo is large, but occasionally it may be contracted around the nucleus, as seen in F.

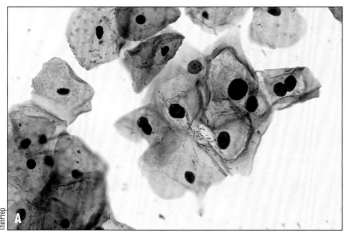

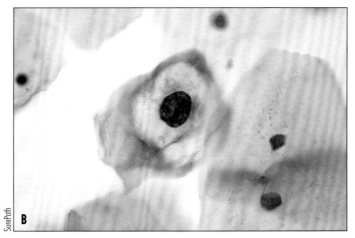

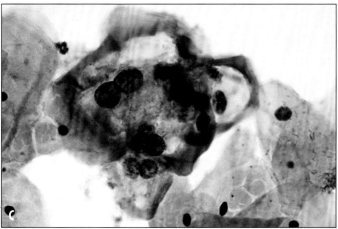

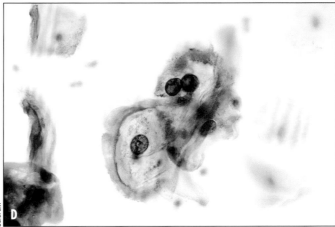

Figure 5-9 continued.

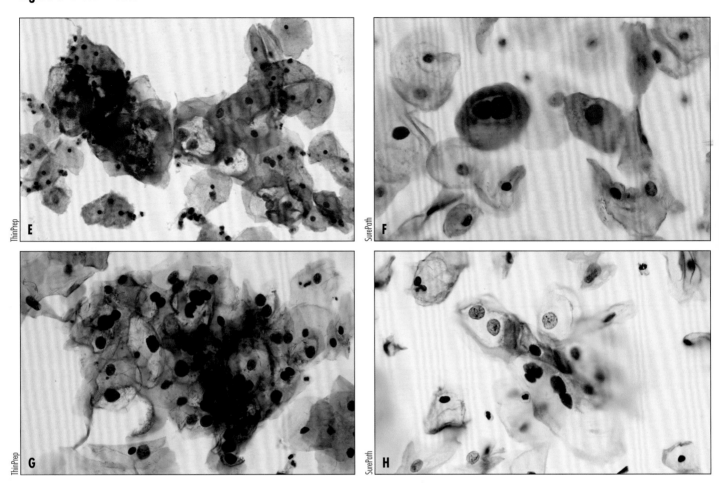

Figure 5-10. LSIL: Cellular morphology of mild dysplasia.

Classic mild dysplasia is the other major cellular finding in LSIL. The majority of the slides will contain cells with both HPV cytopathic effect and more pronounced nuclear features of dysplasia, but occasionally slides will only show one of these features. The hallmark of mild dysplasia is an enlarged nucleus, often as much as six to eight times the area of a normal intermediate nucleus. The largest dys-plastic nuclei are seen in LSIL. The cellular cytoplasm is mature and the N:C ratio is low. Other features include multinucleation (C and G), hyperchromasia (A and E), nuclear membrane irregularity (B and H), and anisonucle-osis (E, G, and H). In general, the chromatin is dense and compact, and nucleoli should be rare. Hyperchromasia varies, especially in liquid-based samples, from normo-chromatic (F) to densely dark (E).

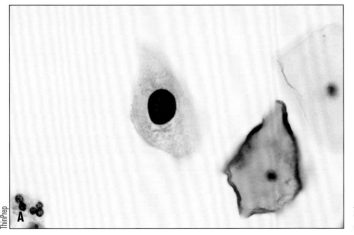

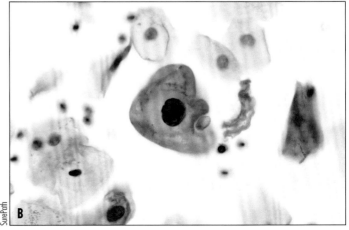

Figure 5-10 continued.

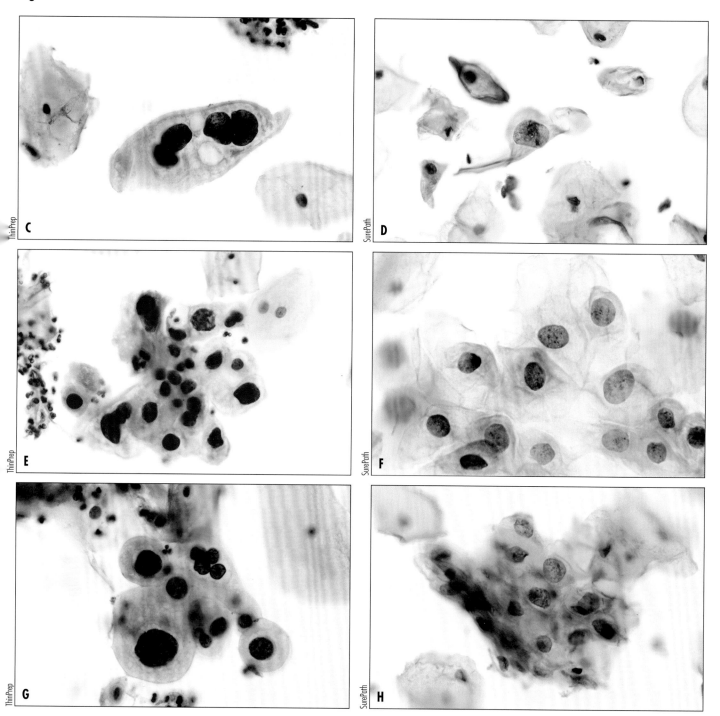

Figure 5-11. LSIL: Nuclear morphology.

As mentioned in Figure 5-10, the hallmark of the nuclei of LSIL is the large size (as much as six to eight times the size of an intermediate nucleus). The nuclei also have variably irregular nuclear membranes with occasional angulation (B and D). The chromatin is evenly distributed and ranges from coarse (A) to finely granular (B). Prominent nucleoli should not be present, but occasional chromocenters are noted (A and C). The LSIL nuclei noted in koilocytes may be smaller but often show more irregularity and degenerative change (D).

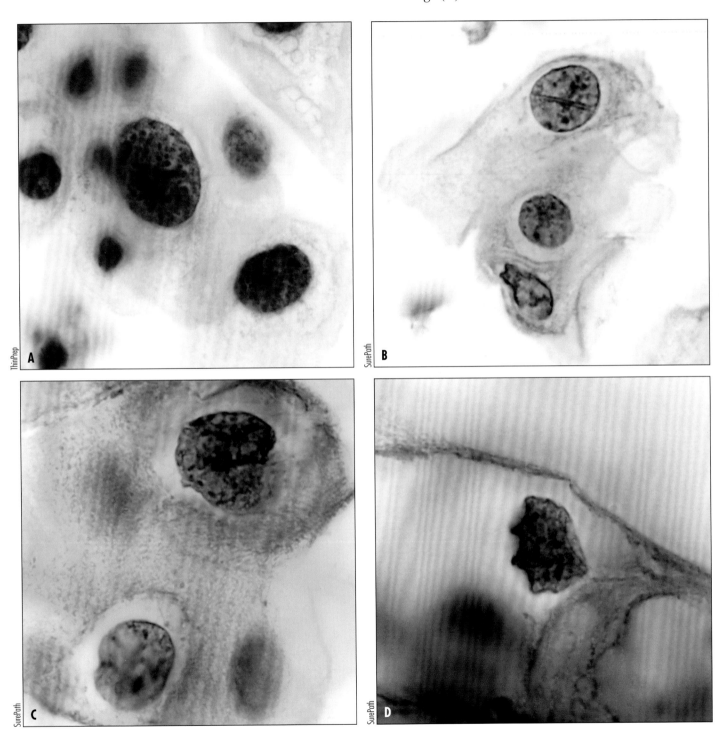

Figure 5-12. HSIL: Nuclear morphology.

The hallmarks of HSIL are cells with large nuclei (two to four times the size of an intermediate nucleus), immature squamous cytoplasm, and increased N:C ratios. The nuclei are usually smaller than those of LSIL, with increased nuclear abnormalities. In fact, nuclei derived from carcinoma in situ, especially in liquid-based preparations, are often only slightly larger than an intermediate nucleus (H). At the lower ends of the HSIL spectrum, the N:C ratio is lower and the nuclei are larger, with hyperchromatic, evenly distributed chromatin and significant nuclear membrane irregularity, often resulting in sharply defined notches (A, B, and E). Nucleoli are absent or inconspicuous, but chromocenters may be seen (E and F). At the upper end of the HSIL spectrum, nuclei may be round with minimal nuclear membrane wrinkling. In these cells (I), the clue to the origin is the markedly increased nuclear size and very scant rim of cytoplasm.

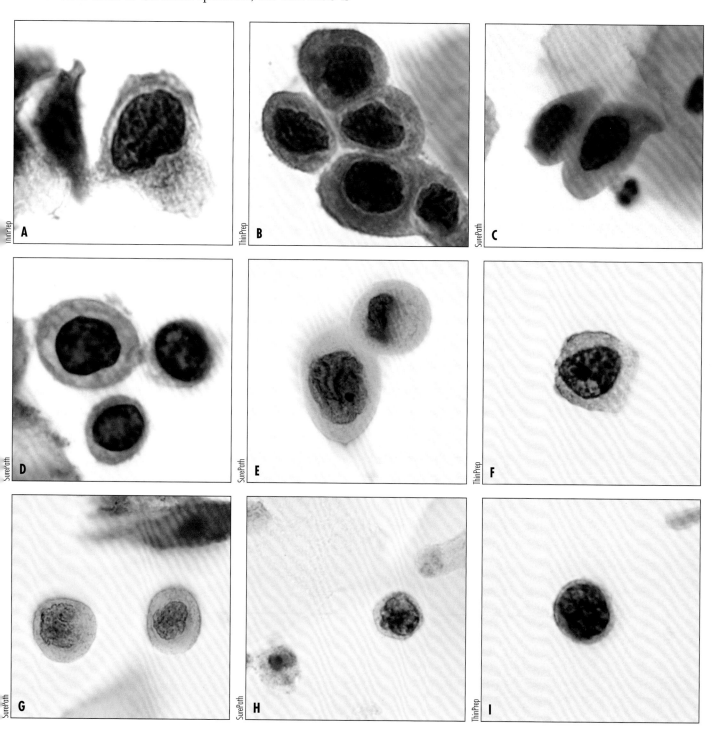

Figure 5-13. HSIL: Cellular morphology, single cell pattern.

The cells of HSIL occur as single dispersed cells or in sheets or clusters. The cells present represent the single dispersed-cell pattern. Especially in liquid-based specimens, these single cells are randomly distributed, often hiding "in plain sight" in the white (blank) areas between normal cells (B, E, and F). The cellular features of HSIL, such as increased nuclear size, increased N:C ratios, irregular nuclear mem- branes, and hyperchromasia, help to make the correct interpretation. Nuclear hyperchromasia may not be evident in all cells (E and J), but the membrane wrinkling and notching combined with the N:C ratios satisfy the cellular criteria for HSIL. Look for these single dispersed cells in cases with LSIL-type cells, as these represent a higher-grade lesion. When LSIL is present, it easily distracts from the smaller, less conspicuous cells of an HSIL component.

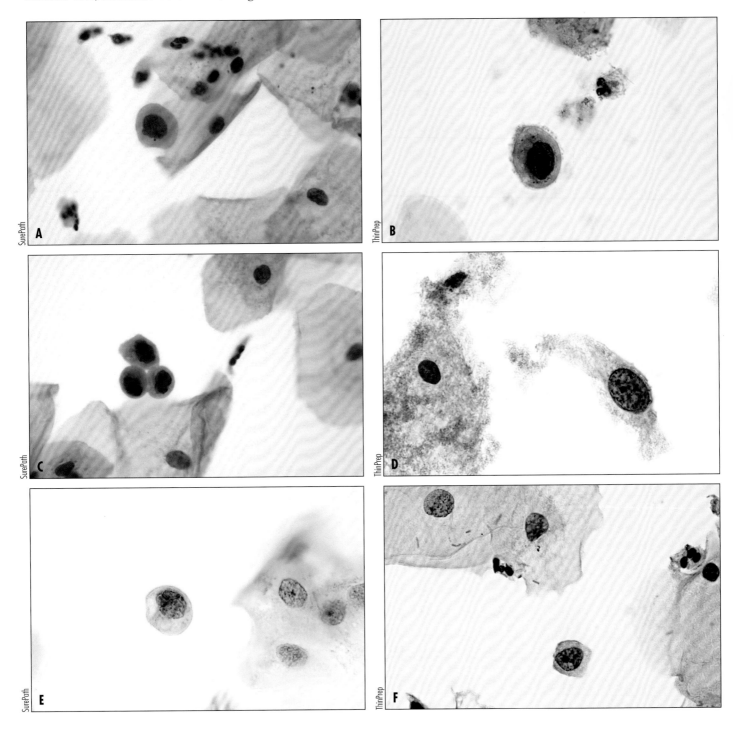

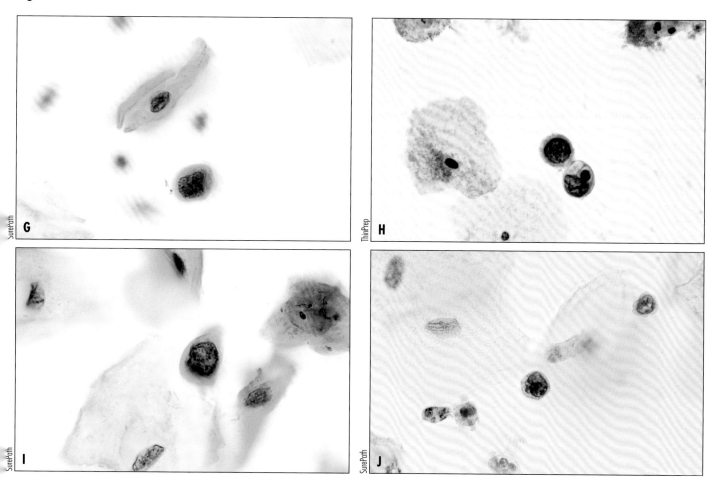

Figure 5-13 continued.

G

H

I

J

Figure 5-14. HSIL: Cellular morphology, sheets.

The cells of HSIL may present in sheets or clusters as well as single dispersed cells. The cells illustrated here show the sheet-type arrangement commonly seen in HSIL. The cells demonstrate all of the previously described nuclear features of SIL. Within the sheets, the cells show significant nuclear size variation (anisonucleosis) and a random, jumbled distribution or loss of polarity with overlapping of the nuclei. Increased N:C ratios are evident and can be appreciated best at the periphery of the sheets (A, B, E, and L).

Mitotic figures or apoptotic bodies (arrows in F and G) are commonly seen. At the upper end of the HSIL spectrum, the cellular groups may resemble glandular cells (I and K). The anisonucleosis and membrane wrinkling is visible with close inspection and should prompt an interpretation that will lead to a colposcopic evaluation of the patient. The cells at the periphery of these sheets may help to distinguish squamous from glandular origin. Squamous sheets will often contain cells with a polygonal shape and a more horizontal peripheral arrangement (E and L).

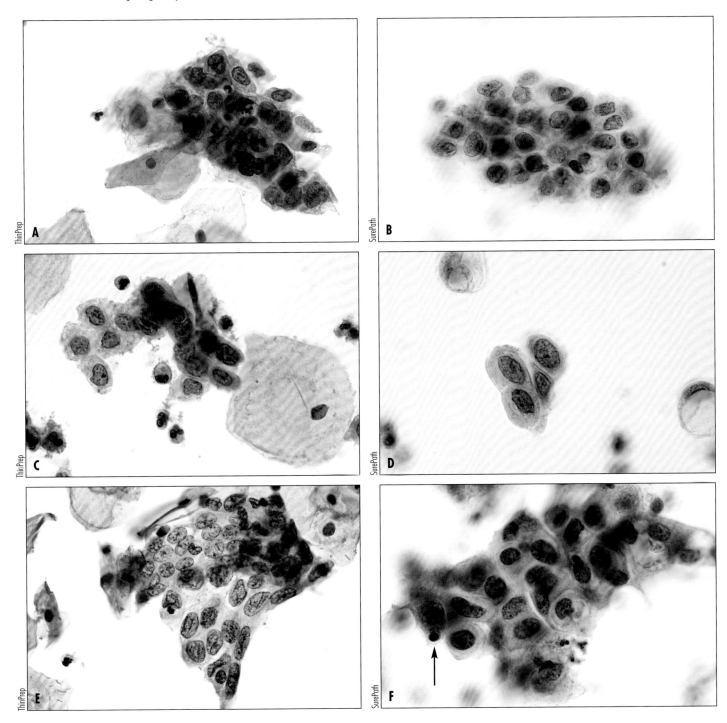

Figure 5-14 continued.

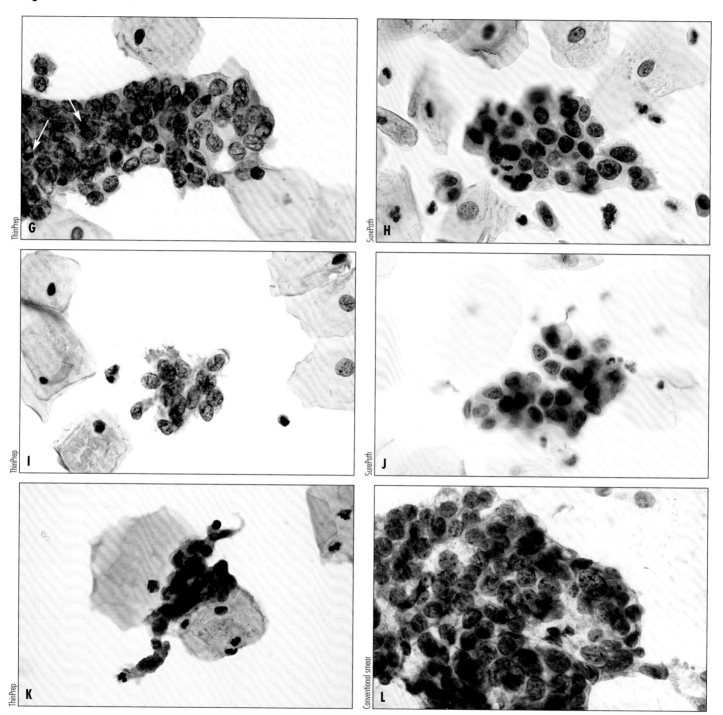

Figure 5-15. HSIL: Cellular morphology, hyperchromatic crowded groups.

When the sheets and clusters of HSIL become more three-dimensional, the thickness of the groups and resultant hyperchromasia can make evaluation difficult. These cellular groups may be derived from HSIL extending into endocervical glands that are pulled out intact, or represent full-thickness surface epithelium removed intact by the collecting device. The hyperchromatic crowded groups seen in HSIL are composed of cells with all of the diagnostic features of HSIL, as described previously. The cells have scant cytoplasm and hyperchromatic nuclei with coarse chromatin. There is nuclear size variation (anisonucleosis), and, when visible, the nuclear membranes are wrinkled, with occasional notches. Apoptotic bodies and mitoses (arrow in A and D) are often seen in these groups. Examining the cells at the periphery of the groups for a horizontal arrangement may help distinguish them from an abnormal glandular cluster.

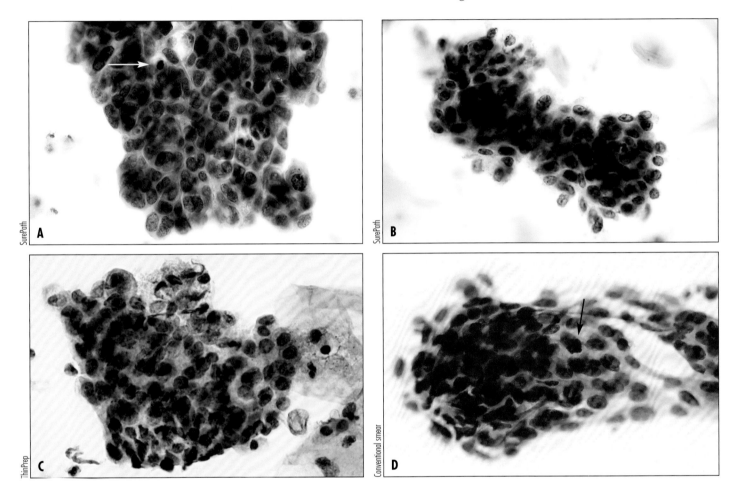

A — SurePath
B — SurePath
C — ThinPrep
D — Conventional smear

Figure 5-16. HSIL: Cellular morphology, keratinizing dysplasia.

Keratinizing dysplasia is an uncommon variant of HSIL that demonstrates many of the features of keratinizing squamous cell carcinoma. Characteristically, these samples will contain a mixture of abnormal cells with a significant degree of abnormal keratinization. These cells have a high N:C ratio, with degenerated pyknotic nuclei (A, C, and D). As noted in D, the cells may demonstrate either dense eosinophilic or cyanophilic cytoplasm. Bizarre cellular shapes with elongated cytoplasmic tails are common (A and D). The cells are often mixed with more typical HSIL cells (B). In comparison to the atypical parakeratosis sometimes seen in LSIL with HPV cytopathic effect, the cells in keratinizing dysplasia have larger abnormal nuclei and a significantly increased N:C ratio (B). The only difference between keratinizing dysplasia (HSIL) and keratinizing squamous carcinoma is the lack of a tumor diathesis and lack of nucleoli within the abnormal cells in HSIL. The cells present in C suggest the possibility of invasive carcinoma, as there appears to be a thin "clinging" diathesis. Specimens with these findings should be interpreted with the Bethesda category of HSIL with features suspicious for invasion.

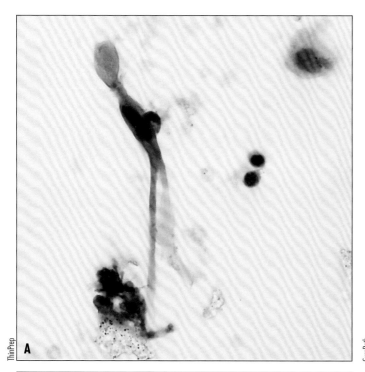

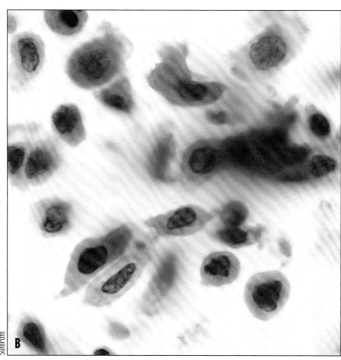

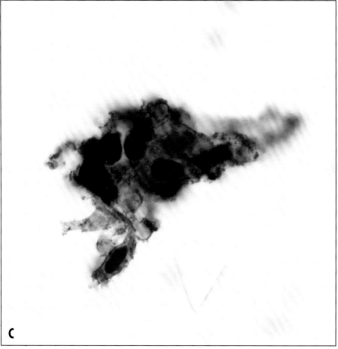

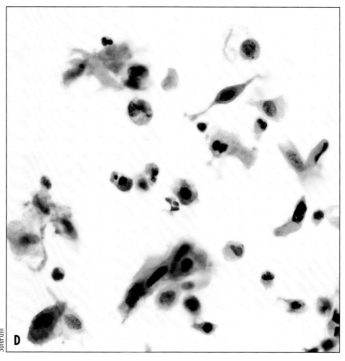

Figure 5-17. HSIL: Small HSIL cells in liquid-based preparations.

As noted in Figures 5-13 and 5-14, HSIL cells seen in liquid-based preparations—ThinPrep, SurePath, and the more recent MonoPrep—are often smaller than their counterparts noted on conventional smears. As present in A and B, these cells may resemble endometrial glandular cells, but the lack of nucleoli and significant membrane wrinkling or notching (arrow in B) help define them as squamous in origin. These cells, when present singly, may resemble histiocytes (D). Again the significant nuclear membrane wrinkling with notches, hyperchromasia, and very high N:C ratios are helpful in making a proper interpretation.

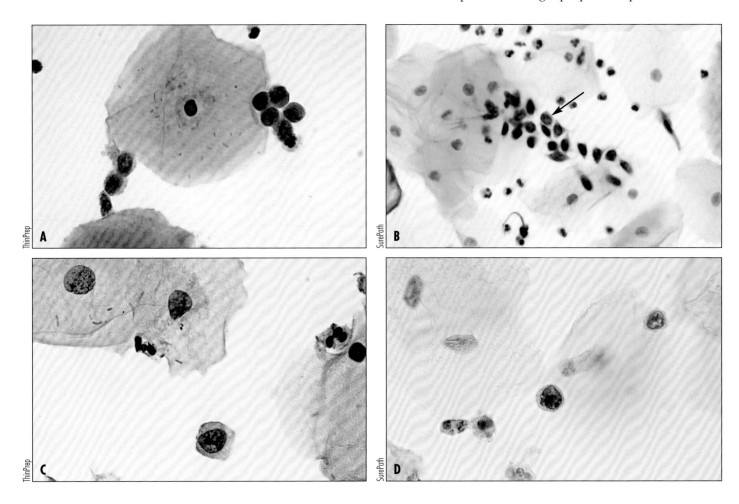

Figure 5-18. HSIL: Pale (hypochromatic) or normochromatic cells in liquid-based preparations.

Another feature noted in liquid-based preparations—although much less pronounced in cells stained for the ThinPrep Imaging System—is relative hypochromasia in the nuclei of dysplastic cells. As noted in Figure 5-17, these cells can be difficult to distinguish from histiocytes or small benign metaplastic squamous cells. The cells do retain the other criteria of HSIL, such as increased nuclear size and N:C ratio, and significant nuclear membrane wrinkling (A, B, and D). At times the membrane wrinkling can be subtle (C), and a close examination of the slide for other HSIL cells may increase confidence in the HSIL interpretation.

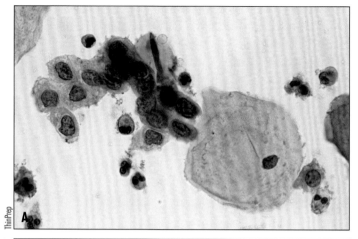

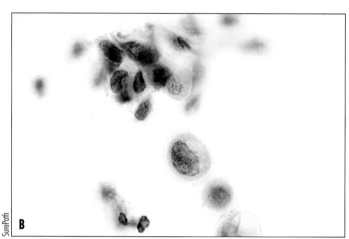

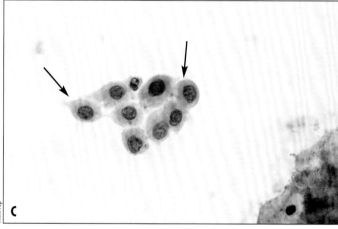

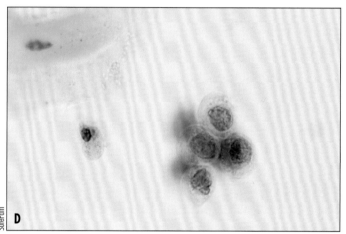

Figure 5-19. Invasive carcinoma: Nuclear features.

The hallmarks of invasive carcinoma include nucleoli and irregular chromatin clearing. Nucleoli can be variably sized, from small and angulated (C and D) to large and round (E and G). The irregular chromatin distribution is especially noted in C and H but is present to lesser degrees in most of the other nuclei as well. Marked degenerative features with nuclear fragmentation are also common (B). The irregular membranes of dysplasia are retained and even accentuated in carcinoma.

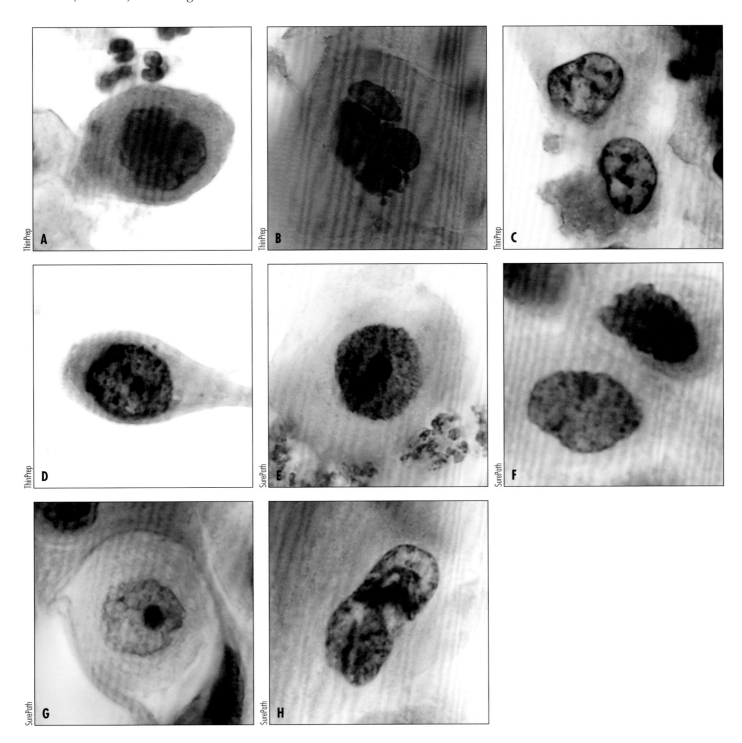

Figure 5-20. Nonkeratinizing squamous cell carcinoma.

The hallmarks of invasive carcinoma are nuclei with open, irregularly distributed chromatin and prominent nucleoli. Unlike repair, the cells are present in thicker, jumbled, loose groups with single abnormal cells (D and E). Other features include dense cyanophilic cytoplasm, high N:C ratios, and nuclei with irregular nuclear membranes. These cells may be seen in loose or syncytial groups or as single cells. An additional feature that may be useful in making the diagnosis is a background diathesis focally present in E and also illustrated in Figure 5-22.

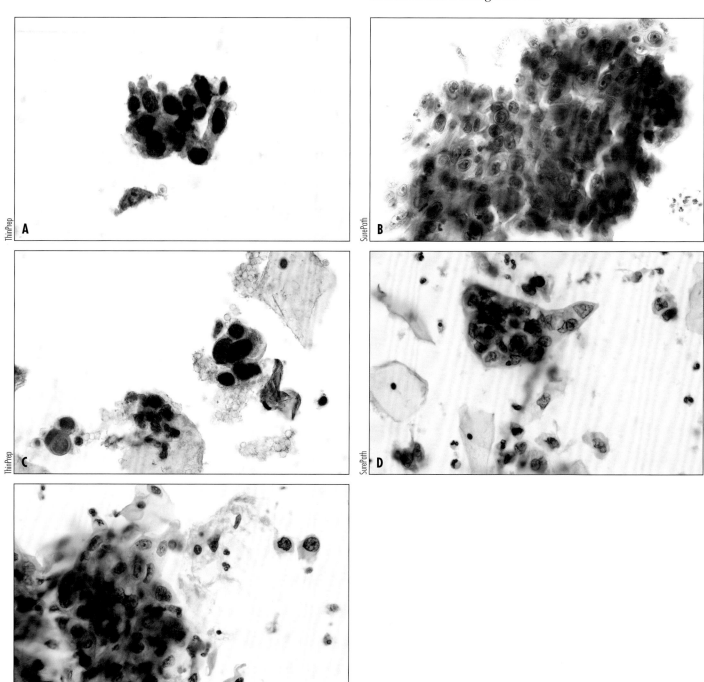

Figure 5-21. Keratinizing squamous cell carcinoma.

The only difference between keratinizing dysplasia (HSIL) and keratinizing invasive squamous cell carcinoma is the additional presence of a tumor diathesis and nucleoli. As is illustrated here, nucleoli are often absent. The malignant cells have hyperchromasia and pyknotic nuclei, but do not have nucleoli. The denseness of nuclei also hides the irregular chromatin seen in the nonkeratinizing carcinomas. The cell size is variable and may demonstrate bizarre shapes (C). The cytoplasm is dense and may be deeply eosinophilic (A and B) or cyanophilic (C, D, and F).

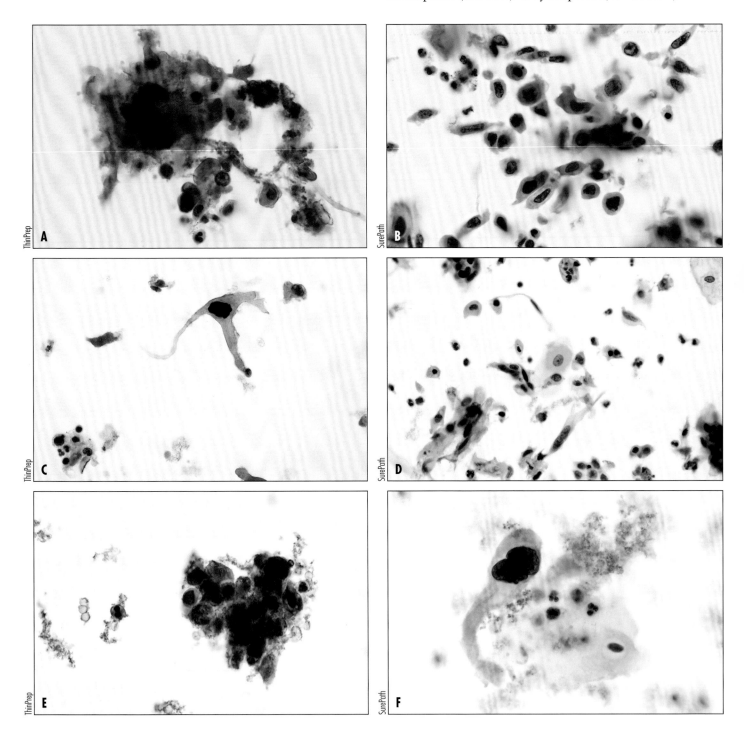

Figure 5-22. Tumor diathesis.

A tumor diathesis is composed of blood with lysed red blood cells, inflammation, and proteinaceous debris, often with embedded degenerated malignant cells (C and D). In conventional Pap smears, the material is present throughout the background of the sample. In liquid-based preparations, the diathesis is still present but is patchy and most often displayed as discreet aggregates of debris (B and F).

The diathesis material may also surround clusters of malignant cells in a halo, a pattern which has been referred to as clinging diathesis (E). In ThinPrep samples, the diathesis material may occlude the filter, resulting in samples where the malignant cells and diathesis are relegated to the periphery of the sample circle. A prewashing of the sample with acetic acid in these instances often results in a more cellular, well-dispersed sample.

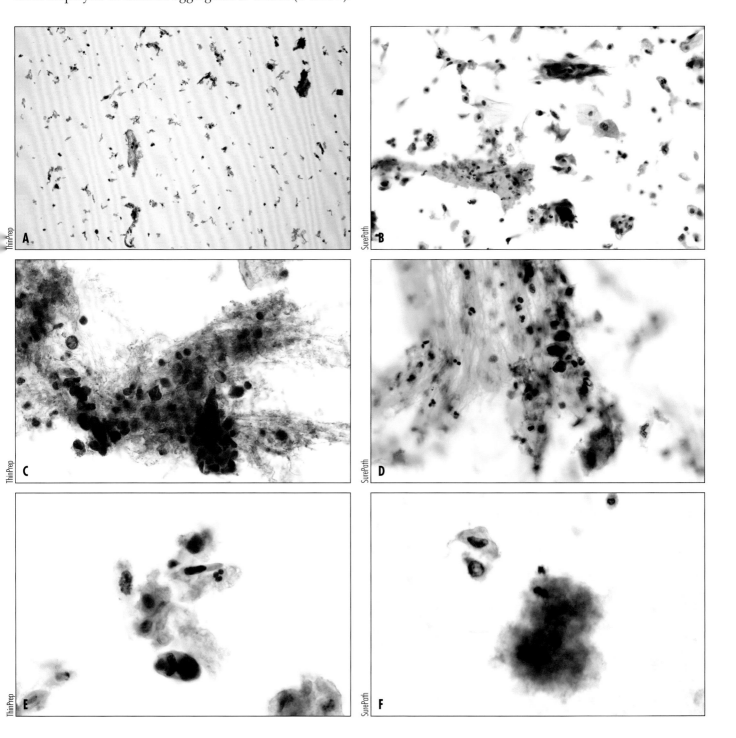

References

1. Kurman RJ, Solomon D. *The Bethesda System for Reporting Cervical/Vaginal Cytologic Diagnoses. Definitions, Criteria, and Explanatory Notes for Terminology and Specimen Adequacy.* New York: Springer-Verlag; 1994.

2 Kurman RJ, Malkasian GD Jr, Sedlis A, Solomon D. From Papanicolaou to Bethesda: the rationale for a new cervical cytologic classification. *Obstet Gynecol.* 1991;77:779-782.

3. Pitman MB, Cibas ES, Powers CN, Renshaw AA, Frable WJ. Reducing or eliminating use of the category of atypical squamous cells of undetermined significance decreases the diagnostic accuracy of the Papanicolaou smear. *Cancer.* 2002;25;96(3):128-134.

4. Kinney WK, Manos MM, Hurley LB, Ransley JE. Where's the high-grade cervical neoplasia?: the importance of minimally abnormal Papanicolaou diagnoses. *Obstet Gynecol.* 1998; 91(6):973-976.

5. ASCUS-LSIL Traige Study (ALTS) Group. Results of a randomized trial on the management of cytology interpretations of atypical squamous cells of undetermined significance. *Am J Obstet Gynecol.* 2003;188(6):1383-1392.

6. Solomon D, Nayar R. *The Bethesda System for Reporting Cervical Cytology. Definitions, Criteria, and Explanatory Notes.* 2nd ed. New York: Springer; 2004

7. Wright TC Jr, Cox JT, Massad L, Dunton CJ, Wilkinson EJ, Solomon D. 2006 Consensus Guidelines for the management of women with abnormal cervical cancer screening tests. *Am J Obstet Gynecol.* 2007;197(4):346-355.

8. Frable WJ. Litigation cells: definition and observations on a cell type in cervical vaginal smears not addressed by the Bethesda System. *Diagn Cytopathol.* 1994;11:213-215.

9. Hatem F, Wilbur DC. High grade squamous cervical lesions following negative Papanicolaou smears: false-negative cervical cytology or rapid progression. *Diagn Cytopathol.* 1995; 12(2):135-141.

10. Mitchell MF, Tortolero-Luna G, Wright T, et al. Cervical human papillomavirus infection and intraepithelial neoplasia: a review. *J Natl Cancer Inst Monogr.* 1996;21:17-25.

11. Wilbur DC, Dubeshter B, Angel C, Atkison KM. Use of thin-layer preparations for gynecologic smears with emphasis on the cytomorphology of high-grade intraepithelial lesions and carcinomas. *Diagn Cytopathol.* 1996;14:201-211; 1996.

12. Renshaw AA, Mody DR, Wang E, Haja J, Colgan TJ; Cytopathology Resource Committee, College of American Pathologists. Hyperchromatic crowded groups in cervical cytology - differing appearances and interpretations in conventional and ThinPrep preparations: a study from the College of American Pathologists Interlaboratory Comparison Program in Cervicovaginal Cytology. *Arch Pathol Lab Med.* 2006;130(3):332-336.

13. Clark SB, Dawson AE. Invasive squamous-cell carcinoma in ThinPrep specimens: diagnostic clues in the cellular pattern. *Diagn Cytopathol.* 2002;26(1):1-4.

Glandular Epithelial Abnormalities

Amy C. Clayton, MD

Introduction

Reliable detection and classification of glandular abnormalities on cervical Pap specimens have lagged behind the more common and longer-studied squamous lesions. However, in the last decade, the increased incidence of endocervical adenocarcinomas, new sampling methods that allow for greater representation from the endocervical canal, as well as increased awareness of and interest in glandular abnormalities, have led to an increasing number of cases of glandular cell abnormalities in Pap tests. Before the 1980s, glandular abnormalities were infrequent in Pap smears because of the spatula and swab method of sampling. In the 1980s, endocervical brush sampling was introduced. The brush bristles would not only scrape the surface epithelium of the transformation zone, but would often sample more anatomically remote regions, such as the upper endocervical canal, deep glandular crypts, and even the lower uterine segment. This efficacious sampling technique dramatically increased the frequency of malignant or premalignant glandular cells observed and produced a sometimes-confusing array of nonneoplastic cellular changes that had not previously been recognized in cervical specimens. These changes led to a classification system (Bethesda) that encompasses all glandular alterations that cannot be assessed as benign or reactive, and that fall short of a definitive glandular neoplasm, as "atypical glandular cells" (AGC). Unfortunately, because of the large number of cytological mimics, the AGC category also includes a large number of normal and benign reactive conditions, as well as particular variant presentations of squamous abnormalities. In many cases, there is no documented abnormality identifiable on histologic follow-up examinations generated by AGC Pap interpretations. Histologic follow-up of an AGC Pap interpretation may include reactive/reparative change, tubal metaplasia, lower uterine segment endometrium, endocervical or endometrial polyps, and high-grade squamous intraepithelial lesion (HSIL)—especially when the latter involves endocervical glands.

Adenocarcinoma In Situ

The prototypic endocervical glandular neoplastic lesion is adenocarcinoma in situ (AIS). The cytologic features of AIS have both characteristic low-magnification architectural and high-magnification cytoplasmic and nuclear features. The majority of AIS cases have a number of abnormal groups readily apparent with a low-magnification scan-ning objective. These groups are noticeable because of their crowded hyperchromatic appearance (hyperchromatic crowded groups or HCGs). They may present as small sheets, short strips (palisades) (Figure 6-1, A), or large microbiopsy fragments, all with tightly crowded and pseudostratified nuclei. Distinctive features include gland openings or a branched glandular pattern (Figure 6-1, B) in large fragments, or smaller fragments arranged in acini (gland-like structures with a three-dimensional appearance) (Figure 6-1, C) or rosettes (flattened two-dimensional grouping with palisaded nuclei at the periphery and cytoplasm towards the center of the group) (Figure 6-1, D). True feathering (nuclei at the periphery protruding beyond the confines of the cell, due to extreme nuclear crowding and cohesion to the basement membrane) is fairly specific for AIS (Figure 6-1, E) and is a particularly useful scanning magnification feature. False feathering (cytoplasmic tufts creating a feathered outline) is nonspecific and is found in a variety of benign and premalignant entities. The nuclei of AIS in cytologic specimens are similar to the appearance in histologic material: cigar-shaped and hyperchromatic with moderately coarse chromatin granules (Figure 6-1, F). The variation in size and shape within a given case is usually slight. Nucleoli are generally inconspicuous. The nuclear diameter can range in size from 8 to 10 μm (endometrioid type) to 20 to 30 μm. The nuclei are palisaded, with the long axis pointing in the same direction. The nuclei are polarized to one end of the cytoplasm, but pseudostratification from the polarized end is characteristic (Figure 6-1, G). Despite the highly organized architectural and nuclear structures, extreme nuclear crowding is present (Figure 6-1, H). Three-dimensionality of the groups is often apparent as the field focus is changed toward or away from the microscopic viewer. Mitotic figures and apoptotic bodies are helpful diagnostic features and are very common in AIS; however, they are not essential for the diagnosis and can be present in benign processes as well.

Endocervical Adenocarcinoma

The cytologic features of invasive endocervical adenocarcinoma most often reveal a departure from the orderly cellular arrangements of AIS, with the common additional feature of a background diathesis (Figure 6-2, A), although all of these changes may be subtle. The cells present singly, as loosely cohesive sheets (Figure 6-2, B), or as three-dimensional clusters (Figure 6-2, C). A key feature distinguishing adenocarcinoma from AIS or reactive endocervical cells is the irregular placement of the nucleus within the cell and in relationship to adjacent nuclei (Figure 6-2, D). The nuclei are large and variably sized, with irregular chromatin distribution and parachromatin clearing (Figure 6-2, E). Macronucleoli are typically present. The cytoplasm is more abundant than that seen in endometrial carcinoma and is cyanophilic or eosinophilic. If any of these features are noted in smears with the other cytologic criteria for AIS, invasive adenocarcinoma should be suggested. A columnar shape is often retained in tumors that are well to moderately differentiated (Figure 6-2, F). As endocervical adenocarcinoma becomes less differentiated, the cells lose their endocervical cellular features and become difficult to distinguish from other poorly differentiated adenocarcinomas or even from nonkeratinizing squamous cell carcinoma (Figure 6-2, G).

Endometrial Adenocarcinoma

Pap tests have a low sensitivity for the detection of endometrial adenocarcinoma. Although cells from these tumors may exfoliate and subsequently be identified in cervical specimens, cell numbers are generally low (Figure 6-3, A). At times a finely granular, watery, tumor diathesis may be present. The cells seen in well-differentiated endometrial adenocarcinoma are usually present in small three-dimensional groups of 5 to 10 cells (Figure 6-3, B). The nuclei are slightly enlarged, with mild anisonucleosis and slight hyperchromasia (Figure 6-3, C). Small to medium sized nucleoli are visible in better preserved groups, but degenerative changes are frequent in exfoliated endometrial cells, and the nucleoli may be obscured. The cytoplasm is scant and may be vacuolated, with ill-defined cell borders. Higher-grade endometrial adenocarcinomas will have similar features but with increasingly larger nuclear size and more prominent nucleoli (Figure 6-3, D and E). Endometrial adenocarcinoma that extends to the endocervix may be directly sampled. Because endometrial and endocervical carcinomas both present in their native (nonexfoliated) state with pseudostratified columnar architecture, the cells directly sampled from each of these lesions will demonstrate cytologic features that are very similar. Endometrial cancers will generally show a smaller overall cell and nuclear size compared to endocervical tumors of similar grade. However, the endometrial origin may only be discovered following surgical biopsy or resection.

Atypical Glandular Cells: Endocervical

Atypical glandular cells have abnormal features that may mimic true abnormalities or lack sufficient diagnostic criteria for a definitive diagnosis of carcinoma. The most common cytologic mimics of AIS and endocervical adenocarcinoma include nonspecific reactive glandular changes (including the cells associated with cervicitis and endocervical polyps), tubal metaplasia, SIL involving glands, and cells from the lower uterine segment.

Features of cervicitis include moderately crowded sheets of either metaplastic or glandular epithelium.

Although the architectural arrangements are most often flat (two-dimensional, sheet-like), cases that mimic AIS may contain palisaded nuclei with pseudostratification and "pseudofeathers" (Figure 6-4, A). The background is often inflammatory. The nuclei are enlarged, with vesicular to stippled chromatin, single or multiple nucleoli, and intracytoplasmic neutrophils. The presence of nucleoli can lend a markedly atypical appearance to the cells (Figure 6-4, B). However, smooth thick nuclear borders and lack of nuclear disarray (irregular placement of nuclei within the cell group) help to support a benign reactive etiology. Some cases will show overlapping features with neoplastic glandular cells, as described previously, and a designation of "atypical glandular cells" is appropriate in these circumstances.

Endocervical polyps produce cellular groups with squamoid cytoplasm and reparative features (Figure 6-4, C). The cells appear to be streaming within the group but maintain polarity. The groups may exhibit a perceptible depth of focus. Some polyps can produce cytologic features more worrisome for AIS, including tightly crowded groups with pseudorosettes, feathering, and irregularly distributed chromatin. The nuclei are enlarged but have vesicular chromatin with prominent nucleoli (Figure 6-4, D). These changes can become very pronounced in cases of cervical polyps with ulcerated surfaces, a common feature leading to bleeding. When the nuclei become hyperchromatic with smudged chromatin or demonstrate nuclear disorder within the cell group, glandular neoplasia might be considered. Endocervical polyps may also show degenerative changes of vacuolization with intracytoplasmic inflammatory cells. These changes may mimic the "oxyphil" cells encountered in endometrial adenocarcinoma (Figure 6-4, E). Comparison to the histologic morphology (if available) may help to reassure the observer about the benign nature of these types of cellular changes.

Tubal metaplasia (TM) is also frequently mistaken for AIS in cytologic specimens. Studies by Novotny (1992) and Ducatman (1993) have characterized some of the features of TM in cervical cytology specimens. TM is characterized by small to medium sized groups of glandular type cells with enlarged hyperchromatic nuclei, as compared to benign endocervical cells (Figure 6-5, A). The chromatin is finely granular, with usually small, inconspicuous nucleoli. The most useful features that distinguish TM from AIS are the pallor and fine granularity of nuclear chromatin, and cytologists should avoid making outright interpretations of AIS when the classic coarse hyperchromasia associated with AIS is absent. The nuclei of TM are oval to round and of different sizes. This heterogeneity in combination with a disordered crowded arrangement imparts a "clumsy" appearance to these cell groups (Figure 6-5, B). The cytoplasm is moderately abundant and denser than what is usually seen in benign endocervical or AIS cells. Novotny (1992) has described a sharp, flat, somewhat thickened apical border as being characteristic of TM cells. If cilia and terminal bars are readily apparent, the diagnosis is straightforward; however, these features may be absent or only present focally (Figure 6-5, C).

In TM, wide variations in architecture and nuclear features can lead one to consider an interpretation of glandular neoplasia, in particular, AIS. The nuclei can become more orderly in their arrangements, forming rosettes or gland openings. Palisading and pseudostratification with nuclear overlap can be seen. When the nuclei are degenerated, hyperchromasia and coarsening of the chromatin can be enhanced. When all of these features are present, AIS is often considered, and sometimes this differential diagnosis cannot be resolved on cytology alone (Figure 6-5, D).

Selvaggi (1994, 2002) and Drijkoningen (1996) have published helpful cytologic features for distinguishing high-grade squamous dysplasias involving endocervical glands from AIS in Pap specimens. While many HSIL patterns would not be confused with AIS, occasionally endocervical gland involvement by cervical intraepithelial neoplasia (CIN) II/III presents with polarization of the cells at the gland periphery with nuclear pseudostratification, a feature not classically described for squamous lesions (Figure 6-6, A). The nuclei can assume more elongated shapes and palisade within the cell group, lending an appearance of some of the architectural features present in AIS (Figure 6-6, B).

Another potential pitfall in this differential diagnosis is the identification of the presence of glandular cells at the edges of abnormal groups and concluding that the entire group is of endocervical glandular origin (Figure 6-6, C). It should be recognized that dysplastic squamous groups can be sampled while still attached to adjacent benign glandular epithelium. In addition, one can become distracted by numerous reactive glandular groups (some with pronounced atypia), with just a few clearly abnormal squamous cells (SIL), often closely associated with the reactive glandular groups. The chromatin in these abnormal cells will be very coarsely granular, and the nuclei are oval to round, as would be expected for HSIL. While these cells would most likely have been assessed as squamous in nature if viewed in isolation, the close association with glandular groups and the predominance of "atypical" glandular cells on the smear are pitfalls in assessing the abnormality as one of glandular origin. The association of reactive glandular or metaplastic cells with SIL has also been described by Bose (1994). Careful attention should be given in order to distinguish the reactive glandular cells from sometimes-scant dysplastic squamous cells.

Occasionally, SIL can assume vague or poorly formed acinar or rosette-like structures (Figure 6-6, D). This presentation is most often noted in the setting of glandular involvement by SIL, where it appears as if the glandular location may impart some influence on the arrangement of cells within the glandular crypt. When these cells are removed from the glandular crypt, they may still demonstrate vague glandular arrangements.

Finally, the chromatin of dysplastic squamous cells can depart from the characteristic granular dark chromatin pattern (Figure 6-6, E). When dysplastic squamous cells

involve endocervical glands, the chromatin can appear pale and uniformly dispersed. Nucleoli, sometimes large and prominent, can also be seen. This nuclear appearance more closely approximates that of glandular epithelium. If the subtle nuclear membrane irregularities or abnormal crowded architecture is not appreciated, the group can be mistaken for reactive glandular cells.

Lower uterine segment (LUS) sampling may also produce HCGs, which can be mistaken for AIS on Pap specimens. De Peralta-Venturino (1995) has described in detail the cytologic features of LUS sampling and has discussed the potential misinterpretations. LUS is characterized by numerous large, irregular, branched HCGs on low-magnification microscopy (Figure 6-7, A). The groups tend to have fishhook shapes and an elongate pulled-out appearance. A biphasic pattern of glands and stroma is usually present (Figure 6-7, B). The pattern is entirely different from spontaneously exfoliated endometrium. Exfoliated endometrial cells form rounded three-dimensional groups with degeneration and pyknosis of the nuclei, which occur as part of the degenerative process. The stroma of directly sampled LUS is composed of uniform, oval to spindled nuclei with minimal atypia (Figure 6-7, C). The scant cytoplasm creates a very crowded hyperchromatic appearance. The cells are very disorderly, with the long axes of the nuclei pointing in all directions. Capillaries can often be seen traversing the stromal cells. The glandular cells have extremely crowded nuclei but are ordered, with branched gland formations and palisading (Figure 6-7, D). Mitotic figures can be found in both the glandular and stromal cells during the proliferative phase of the menstrual cycle. Intact organoid features may be noted, especially tube-like structures indicative of sampled intact endometrial glands. Key features distinguishing directly sampled LUS from AIS include recognition of the characteristic branched and curved shapes of LUS seen at low magnification, with both glandular and stromal components being present. Despite the presence of mitotic figures, the nuclei have a bland chromatin distribution and smooth nuclear membranes.

Atypical Glandular Cells: Endometrial

Benign endometrial cells are most often seen in cervical smears as exfoliated clusters of small glandular cells. Benign exfoliated endometrial cells occur as small three-dimensional clusters. The nuclei are round and about the size of an intermediate squamous cell nucleus. They have inconspicuous nucleoli and scant basophilic, occasionally vacuolated cytoplasm. Endometrial stromal cells, especially superficial stromal cells, may occasionally be seen in cervical specimens. Deep stromal cells are round to spindle shaped, with oval dark nuclei and scant cytoplasm. Deep stromal cells are seldom present in cervical specimens and may be difficult to differentiate from a high-grade squamous lesion, given their high nuclear to cytoplasmic ratio and hyperchromatic irregular nuclei. Superficial stromal cells having decidual change are most often isolated and, with their foamy abundant cytoplasm, closely resemble histiocytes. These cells are often present surrounding the compact endometrial cells seen as part of the "exodus" phenomenon. Exfoliated histiocytes and stromal cells have not been correlated with a clinically significant endometrial lesion (Tambouret 2001).

Benign exfoliated endometrial cells are commonly present in cyclic women, most often in the first half of the cycle. The presence of exfoliated endometrial cells in women under the age of 40 is only rarely associated with significant endometrial pathology. However, benign-appearing endometrial cells may also be seen in older women. In postmenopausal women, exfoliated endometrial cells are most often due to hormone replacement therapy, chronic endometritis, endometrial polyps, or other benign processes. However, benign shed endometrial cells may occasionally be found in conjunction with endometrial hyperplasia or well-differentiated adenocarcinoma. Because of this possible relationship, the 2001 Bethesda System recommends that benign endometrial cells present in cervical cytology specimens from women over the age of 40 should be reported. Since the implementation of this recommendation into practice, studies have shown that the reporting of benign endometrial cells in all women older than 40 years, without regard to menstrual status, will increase the endometrial biopsy rate, without substantial additional identification of endometrial neoplastic lesions. Authors have therefore suggested that the recommendation might be modified to include assessments in the context of a known menstrual history to eliminate unnecessary endometrial biopsies in menstruating women in this age group (Bean 2006).

The changes in atypical endometrial cells are subtle and consist primarily of slightly increased nuclear size and more prominent nucleoli. Atypical endometrial cells may be associated with dysfunctional uterine bleeding (DUB), use of an intrauterine device (IUD), endometrial polyps, endometrial hyperplasia, or even endometrial adenocarcinoma. The changes associated with DUB can range from small three-dimensional clusters of cells with scant cytoplasm to cells that have increased cytoplasm, slight nuclear enlargement with small nucleoli, and occasional cytoplasmic vacuoles (degenerative in nature) (Figure 6-8, A). Shed endometrial cells in the setting of an IUD can appear very atypical, with overall cellular enlargement, numerous cytoplasmic vacuoles, nuclear chromatin clearing, and prominent nucleoli (Figure 6-8, B). Clinical history of IUD use (often with the presence of *Actinomyces* organisms) is often

the most helpful clue in assessing these groups as being from a benign process, as they can very closely resemble endometrial neoplasia. In cervical specimens, endometrial polyps can give rise to cells with a range of cytologic appearances, some of them resembling endometrial or endocervical neoplasms (Figure 6-8, C). The cells on the surface of polyps will often become degenerated or demonstrate reparative features. When the cell groups are shed spontaneously, they will round up as they pass through the mucus of the endocervical canal. This architecture, in combination with increasing degeneration after being shed, can lead to groups with a very dark, hyperchromatic, crowded appearance, sometimes indistinguishable from glandular neoplasia. The differences between endometrial hyperplasia, DUB, and well-differentiated endometrial adenocarcinoma are very subtle and often cannot be distinguished reliably. Hyperplasia of more complex and atypical types may demonstrate nuclear enlargement with visible nucleoli typical of endometrial adenocarcinoma, but the degenerative changes that occur from all spontaneously shed endometrial cells (regardless of type) can essentially mask the differences between benign, hyperplastic, and well-differentiated neoplasms (Figure 6-8, D).

Other Neoplasms, Including Metastasis

Other tumors found in Pap specimens can be derived either from direct extension (most commonly rectal) or metastasis involving the cervical or endocervical tissues, or from peritoneal-derived neoplasms (ovary or fallopian tube) that gain access to the fallopian tube lumen and float down through the endometrial cavity and endocervical canal (Figure 6-9, A through F). Neoplastic cells originating in the peritoneal cavity will commonly be associated with a very clean specimen background, as diathesis from any destructive stromal invasion is not in the vicinity of the Pap specimen. Metastatic tumors involving cervical or endocervical soft tissues should demonstrate proteinaceous debris, blood, and inflammatory cells typical of tumor diathesis. In addition, colon cancers may show evidence of fecal or vegetable material in the background due to rectovaginal fistula formation. Metastatic tumors will exhibit cytologic features characteristically seen in these tumors when sampled from other, more common, presenting sites. When cytologic features of atypical cells presenting in Pap specimens do not match those described previously for endocervical and endometrial origins, a metastatic tumor should always be considered in the differential diagnosis.

Figure 6-1, A. Adenocarcinoma in situ: Palisaded strips.

These cell groups are arranged in linear strips with palisaded nuclei demonstrating polarization to the basal end of cytoplasm. The nuclei axes are parallel to each other, characterizing the orderly architectural arrangements of AIS. The glandular cells of AIS most often do not demonstrate cytoplasmic mucin. The cytoplasm is slightly granular and varies from scant to moderate.

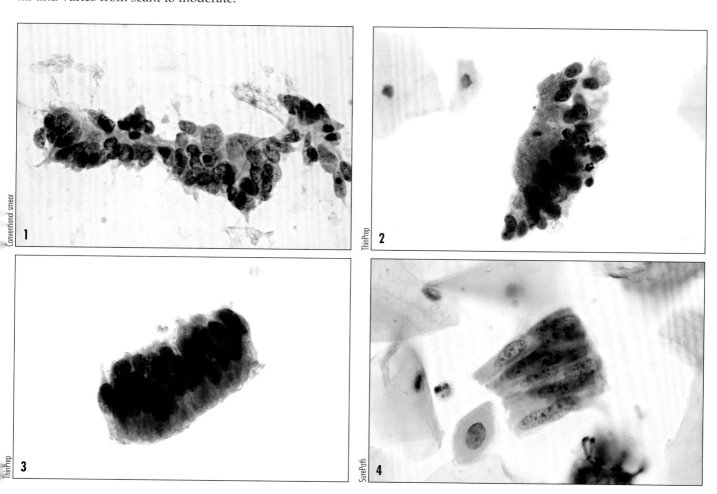

Figure 6-1, B. Adenocarcinoma in situ: Complex branched fragments.

AIS may demonstrate cellular groups with branched glands. Because of the fragmentation that occurs during processing, conventional preparations tend to have larger fragments than liquid-based preparations.

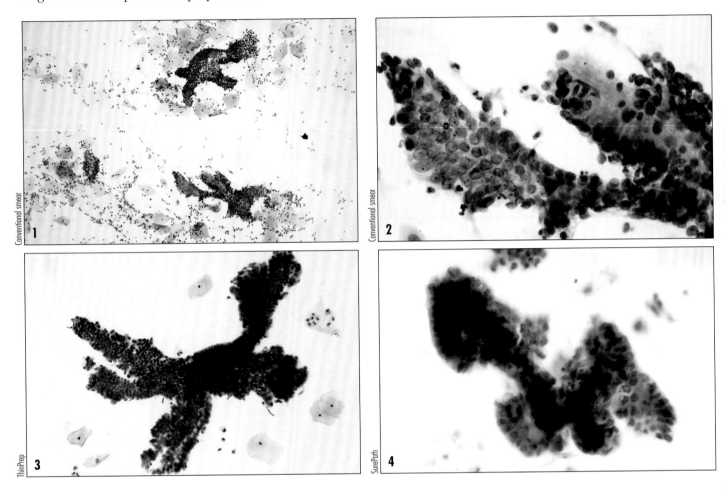

Figure 6-1, C. Adenocarcinoma in situ: Acinar architecture.

Acinar arrangement of cells within aggregates is demonstrated here. There is polarization of nuclei (a key architectural feature of AIS), both at the periphery of the groups and within the groups, leading to multiple gland-like structures.

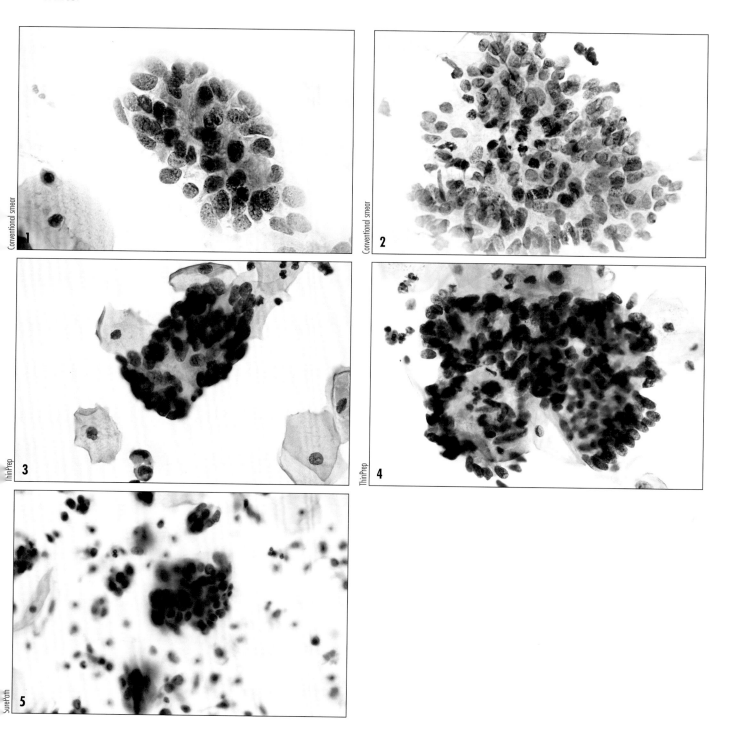

Figure 6-1, D. Adenocarcinoma in situ: Rosette architecture.

Rosette structures, created by nuclei emanating from a central point and radiating outward in a three-dimensional sphere, are characteristic of AIS. More depth of focus is appreciated in liquid-based preparations. Rosettes in conventional preparations may appear more like acinar structures because of the flattening effect of direct smears.

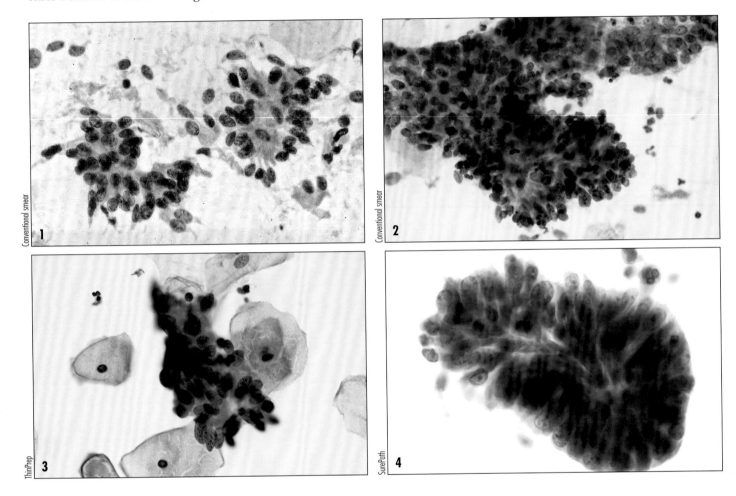

Figure 6-1, E. Adenocarcinoma in situ: Feathering.

True feathering architecture is very specific for AIS. Feathering is created by the release of nuclei from the confines of the cell group once it is removed from the glandular crypt attachment point. The nuclei of AIS are extremely crowded, with overlap when bounded by the basement membrane. Once the boundary is removed, the nuclei can protrude into the free space surrounding the cell group. A feathering appearance is created by the tips of the nuclei extending beyond the cytoplasm of the cell group. Feathering is most obvious in conventional preparations. Liquid-based preparations tend to blunt the feathering effect.

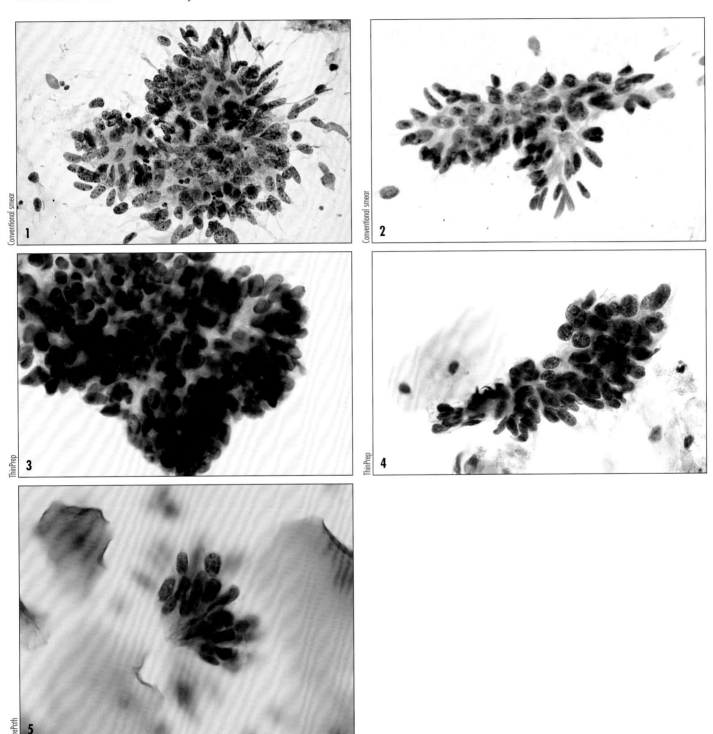

Figure 6-1, F. Adenocarcinoma in situ: Nuclear features.

The nuclei of AIS are most often elongated, with slightly granular chromatin (1, 2, and 3). Nucleoli are not commonly present. The size can vary from small (10 to 12 μm) to large (greater than 20 μm) but tends to be uniform within a given case. Variations do exist, however. A more open chromatin pattern, with small nucleoli and slightly rounded nuclei, is seen in 4, 5, and 6. The endometrioid variant of AIS is characterized by small, rounded to slightly oval nuclei and scant cytoplasm (7, 8, and 9).

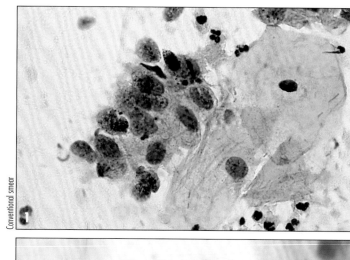

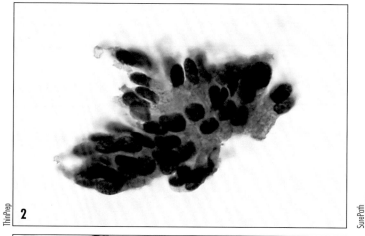

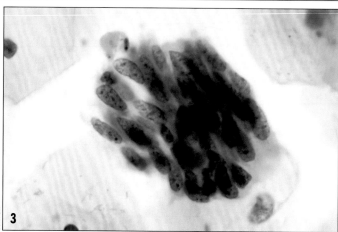

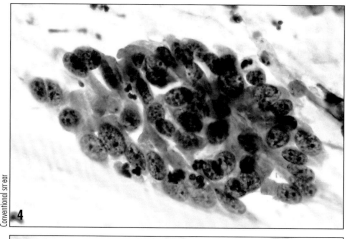

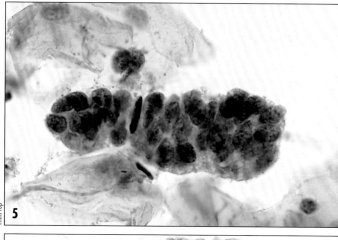

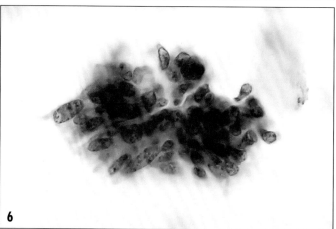

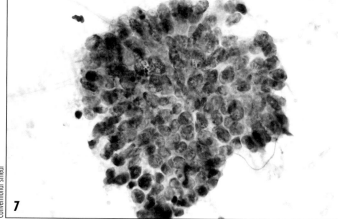

Figure 6-1, F continued.

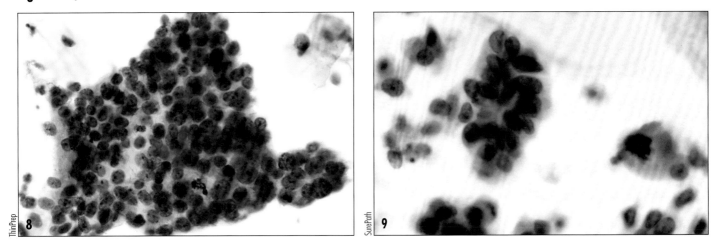

8 ThinPrep

9 SurePath

Figure 6-1, G. Adenocarcinoma in situ: Nuclear pseudostratification.

The nuclei of AIS can appear pseudostratified, reflecting the extreme crowding of nuclei within cell groups.

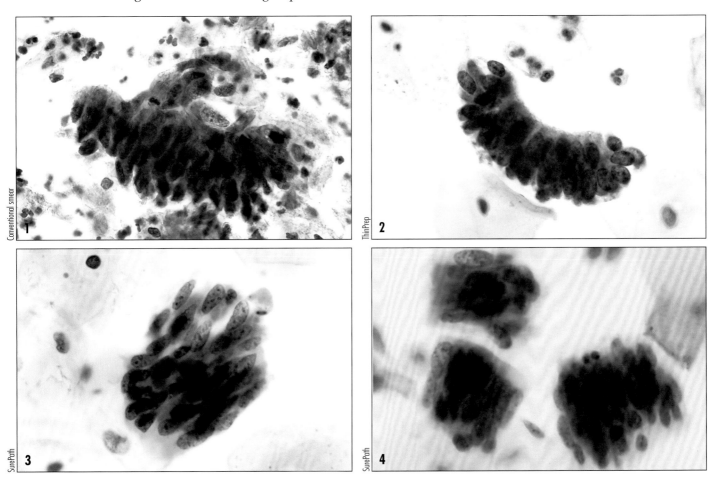

1 Conventional smear

2 ThinPrep

3 SurePath

4 SurePath

Figure 6-1, H. Adenocarcinoma in situ: Three-dimensional architecture.

The three-dimensional nature of AIS groups can make evaluation difficult if care is not taken to focus through the depth of the groups. One can appreciate the highly ordered nature of AIS cellular groups as acinar and rosette structures become apparent as one focuses through the different depths of field.

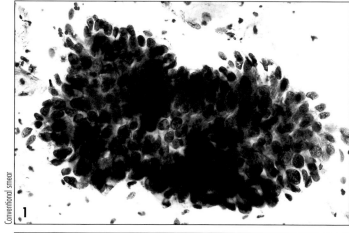

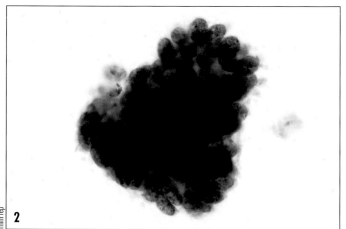

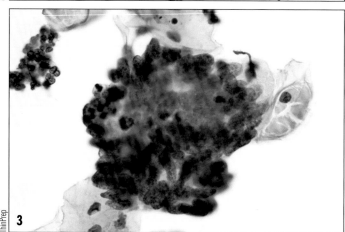

Figure 6-2, A. Endocervical adenocarcinoma: Diathesis.

The background of endocervical adenocarcinoma varies depending on the degree of associated tissue destruction and inflammation by the invasive neoplasm. Tumor diathesis can be bloody, proteinaceous, or mixed. On conventional preparations, the diathesis is uniformly distributed as a granular to bloody precipitate (1). Diathesis on liquid-based preparations can be obscuring (2 and 3) but most often is more subtle (4 and 5). In liquid samples, the diathesis can also cling to the cells without being obvious in the background (5). The quality of liquid-based tumor diathesis can be fluffy to granular or more wispy in nature.

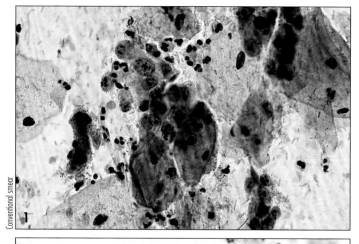

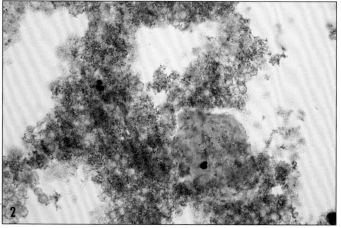

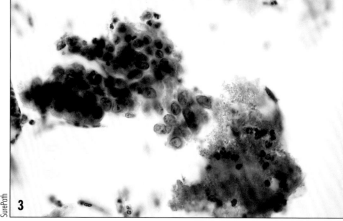

Figure 6-2, A continued.

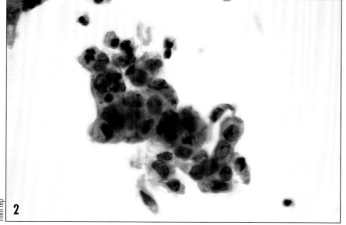

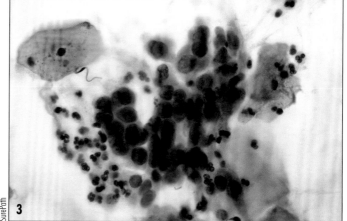

Figure 6-2, B. Endocervical adenocarcinoma: Loose architectural arrangement.

Loss of the specific architectural features seen in adenocarcinoma in situ often heralds the presence of invasion. Adenocarcinoma is more commonly characterized by loose and discohesive cell groupings.

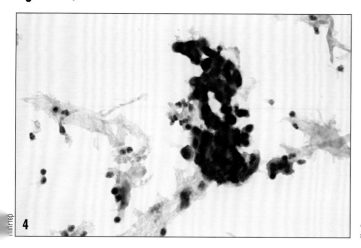

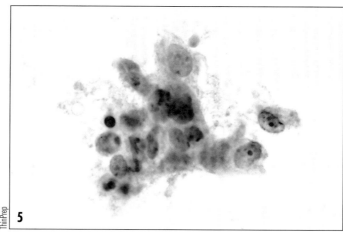

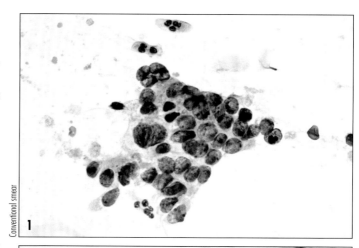

Figure 6-2, C. Endocervical adenocarcinoma: Three-dimensional architecture.

Three-dimensional arrangements characterize both adenocarcinoma in situ and endocervical adenocarcinoma, but invasive neoplasms demonstrate a more disorderly appearance within the crowded groups (palisading and parallel nuclear axes are less common in adenocarcinoma).

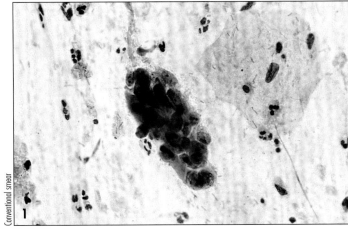

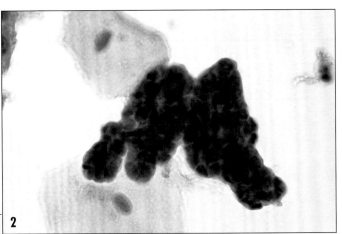

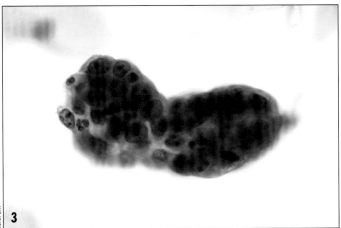

Figure 6-2, D. Endocervical adenocarcinoma: Nuclear disarray.

Nuclear disarray (loss of nuclear polarization and no orientation of nuclear axes) creates a disorderly appearance within cell groups of endocervical adenocarcinoma. This disarray is another indication of possible invasion.

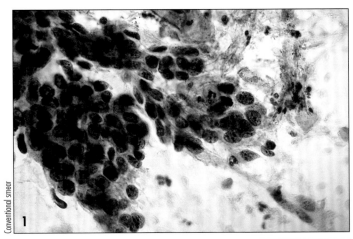

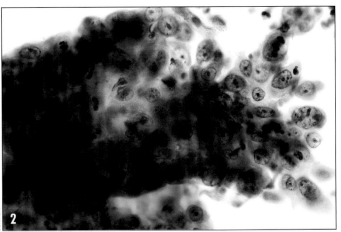

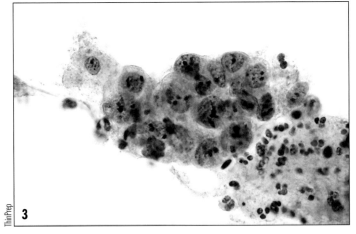

Figure 6-2, E. Endocervical adenocarcinoma: Nuclear pleomorphism.

Nuclear pleomorphism (variation in size and shape) is more prominent in adenocarcinoma and will be present to variable degrees within endocervical adenocarcinoma.

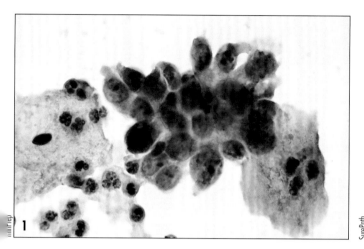
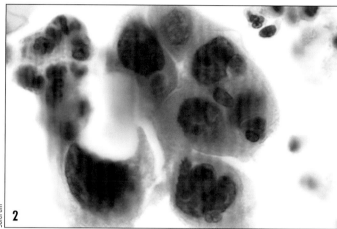

Figure 6-2, F. Endocervical adenocarcinoma: Well-differentiated

Well-differentiated endocervical adenocarcinoma can be very similar (architecture and nuclear features) to adenocarcinoma in situ (1 and 2), and the distinction between the two may not be possible. Some well-differentiated adenocarcinomas may demonstrate subtle nuclear changes (rounded nuclei, presence of nucleoli, slight nuclear disarray) or subtle diathesis, which are suggestive of invasion (3 and 4).

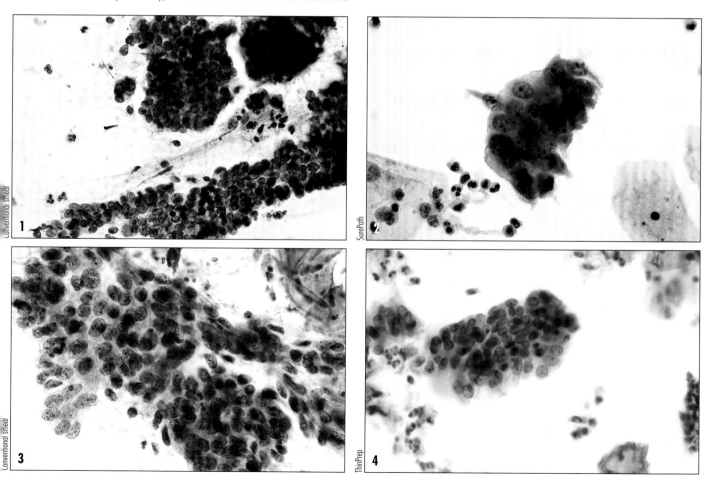

Figure 6-2, G. Endocervical adenocarcinoma: Moderate and poorly differentiated.

Moderate and poorly differentiated adenocarcinomas demonstrate increasing nuclear disarray, pleomorphism, and loss of glandular architectural features. Some tumors may be difficult to recognize as glandular in origin. Features favoring endocervical over endometrial origin include irregular cell cluster outline and variable thickness of the cell group (indicative of direct sampling from endocervical wall rather than passive flotation of cell groups down through the endocervical canal) and moderate to abundant cytoplasm. Features favoring glandular over squamous derivation include nuclear polarization or vague acinar architecture (5). Some endocervical adenocarcinomas are exceedingly difficult to distinguish from squamous carcinoma, and indeed, some may be classified as adenosquamous (4).

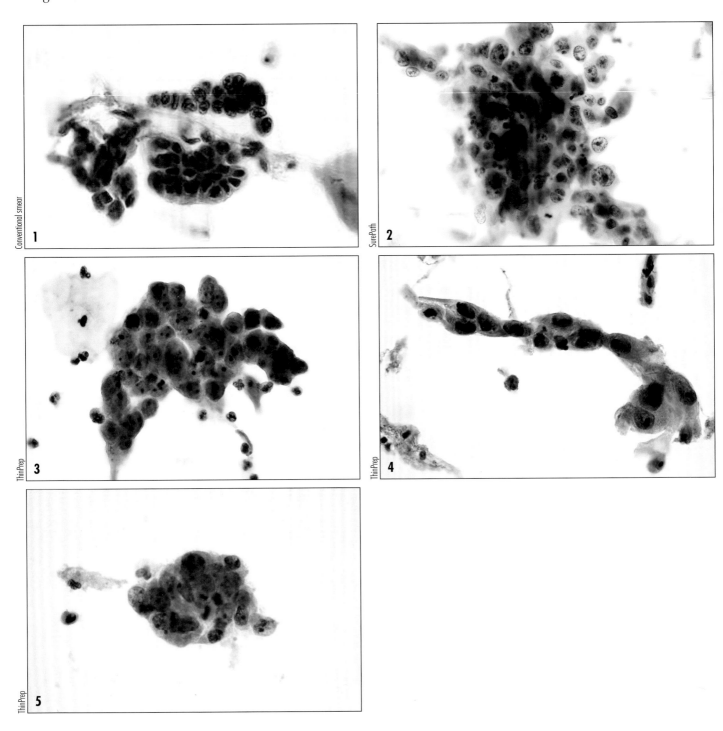

Figure 6-3, A. Endometrial adenocarcinoma: Background and low-magnification appearance.

The low-magnification appearance of endometrial adenocarcinoma can be subtle. Shedding neoplastic endometrial cells are generally small three-dimensional clusters or single cells and can be easily overlooked on low-magnification examination (1, 2, and 3). A clue may be the presence of diathesis: watery to bloody on conventional preparations (4); stringy and clinging on liquid-based preparations (5 and 6). On conventional preparations, the neoplastic cells tend to stream together in collections of mucous material and are closely associated with histiocytes, presumably of endometrial origin (4). This association of cellular elements is lost in liquid-based preparations due to homogenization of the cells.

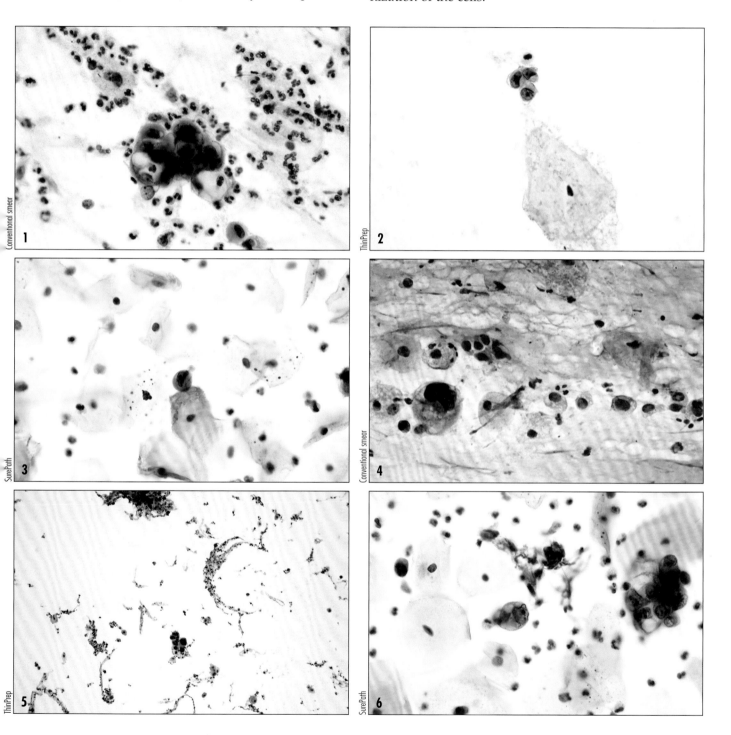

Figure 6-3, A continued.

Occasionally, the tumor cells demonstrate marked degeneration or are obscured by mucus or inflammatory debris, such that recognition becomes very difficult (7, 8, and 9).

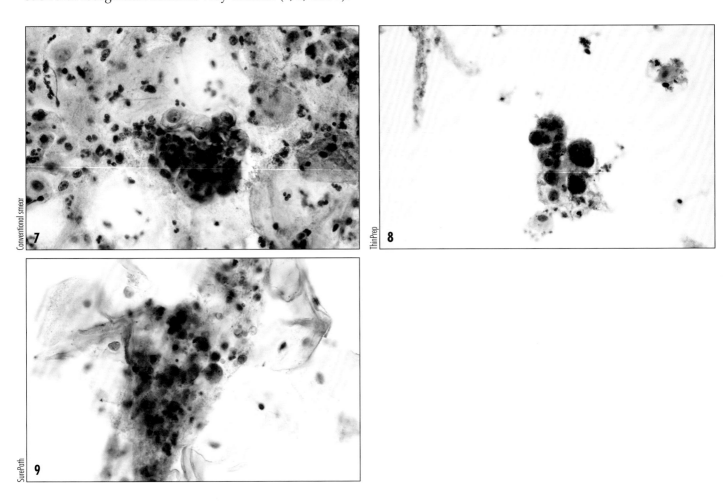

Conventional smear 7

ThinPrep 8

SurePath 9

Figure 6-3, B. Endometrial adenocarcinoma: Small three-dimensional groups.

The most characteristic architectural feature of endometrial adenocarcinoma is a three-dimensional cluster of neoplastic cells. As the cells are spontaneously shed from the endometrial cavity, the cells round up in the fluid within the endometrial cavity and endocervical canal (1 and 2). This architecture helps to distinguish endometrial lesions from directly sampled tumors (tumors involving the endocervix or cervical tissues), which will have an irregular outline and variable thickness within the cell group. It is not uncommon to have cytoplasmic vacuoles (degenerative in nature) (3) or intracytoplasmic neutrophils (4).

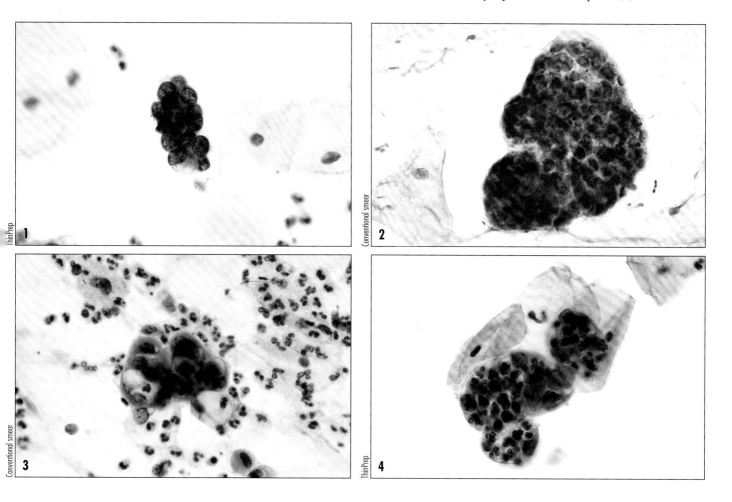

Figure 6-3, C. Endometrial adenocarcinoma: Well-differentiated.

Well-differentiated endometrial adenocarcinomas are most often characterized by small nuclei (8 to 10 μm) with scant cytoplasm. The nuclei may demonstrate degeneration with nuclear condensation, such that nuclear details are difficult to appreciate (1, 2, and 3). The presence of nucleoli is a worrisome feature in shed endometrial cells and may indicate neoplasia (4). Some well-differentiated tumors may exhibit a moderate amount of cytoplasm and increased nuclear size (5, 6, and 7).

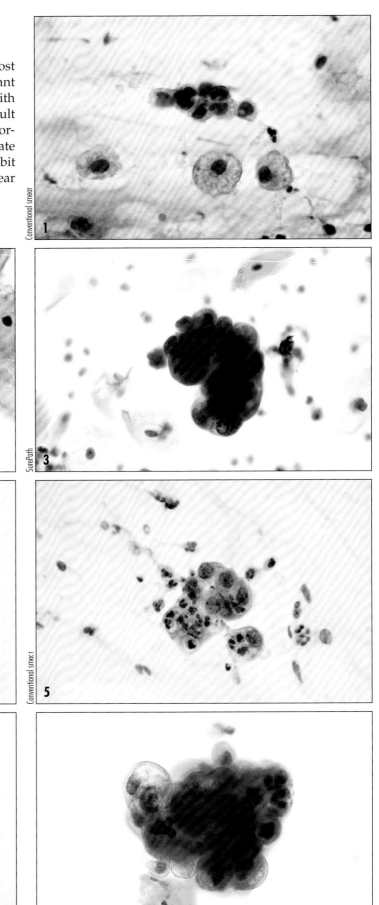

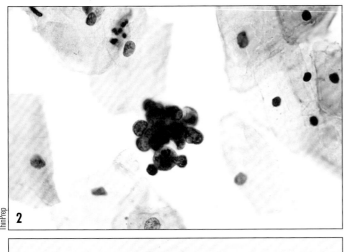

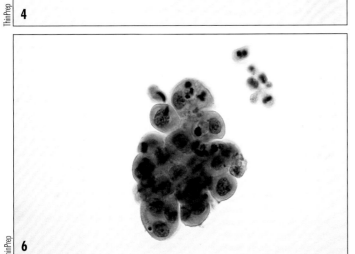

Figure 6-3, D. Endometrial adenocarcinoma: Moderately differentiated.

Moderately differentiated adenocarcinoma will demonstrate increasing nuclear size and more abundant cytoplasm. Nucleoli and irregular nuclear contours become more evident with increasing grade.

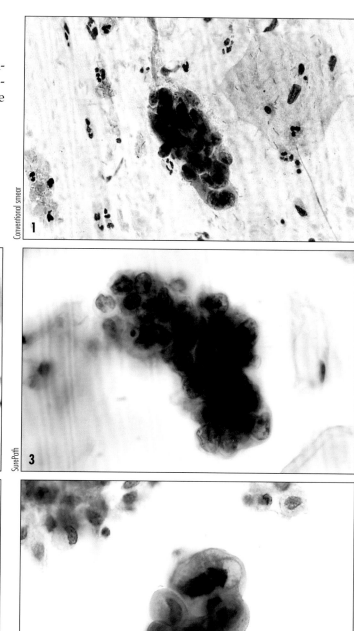

Conventional smear 1

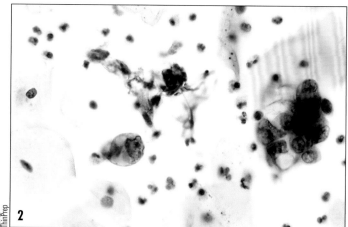

ThinPrep 2

3 SurePath

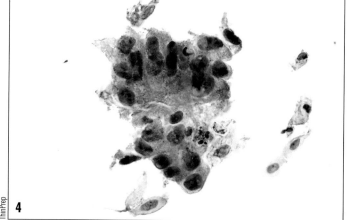

ThinPrep 4

5 SurePath

Figure 6-3, E. Endometrial adenocarcinoma: Poorly differentiated.

Poorly differentiated endometrial adenocarcinomas include both endometrioid, clear cell, serous (1, 2, and 3, respectively), and undifferentiated types, and will demon- strate marked nuclear pleomorphism and a tendency to lose the typical tightly clustered architecture. It may be difficult to appreciate the glandular nature of the neoplasm (4, 5, and 6).

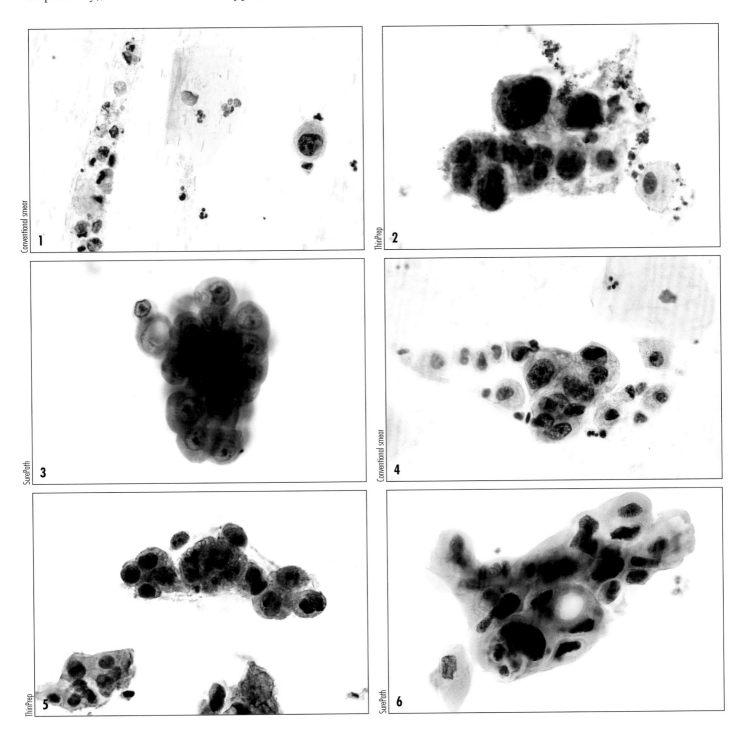

Figure 6-4, A. Atypical endocervical cells: Architectural features of cervicitis.

Reactive endocervical cells can demonstrate nuclear crowding and architectural features similar to adenocarcinoma in situ. "Pseudofeathering" (1 and 2) is likely the result of mechanical disruption during sampling rather than true feathering (the result of extreme nuclear crowding). However, marked crowding can occur as a result of reactive and inflammatory conditions, creating architectural patterns that may not be readily distinguishable from adenocarcinoma in situ: marked crowding (3), palisading nuclei (4 and 6), and acinar formations (5 through 8).

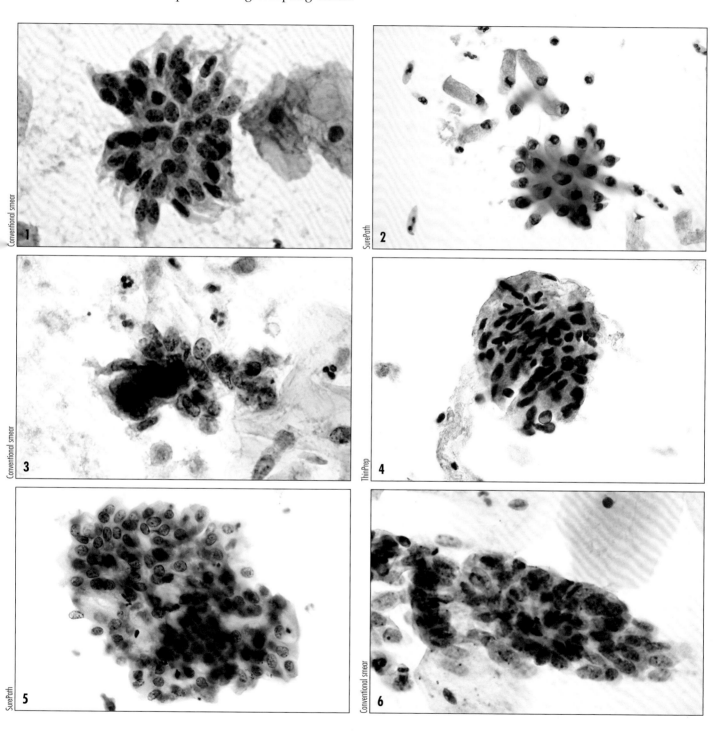

Figure 6-4, A continued.

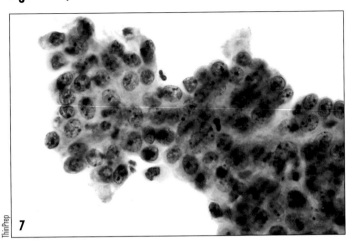

7 · ThinPrep

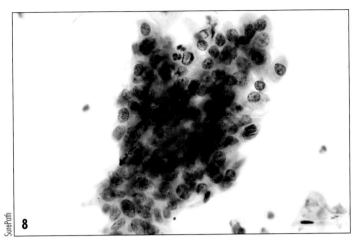

8 · SurePath

Figure 6-4, B. Atypical endocervical cells: Nuclear features of cervicitis.

The nuclei of cervicitis will most often demonstrate a vesicular chromatin pattern with prominent nucleoli (1 through 4). The degree of nuclear enlargement (2) or membrane irregularity (3 and 4) may bring adenocarcinoma into consideration. Some reactive endocervical cell groups may demonstrate nuclear hyperchromasia without visible nucleoli and architectural patterns that simulate adenocarcinoma in situ (5 and 6). Hyperchromatic crowded groups of reactive endocervical cells with even nuclear distribution (7) and moderate nuclear disarray may mimic both glandular and squamous lesions (8).

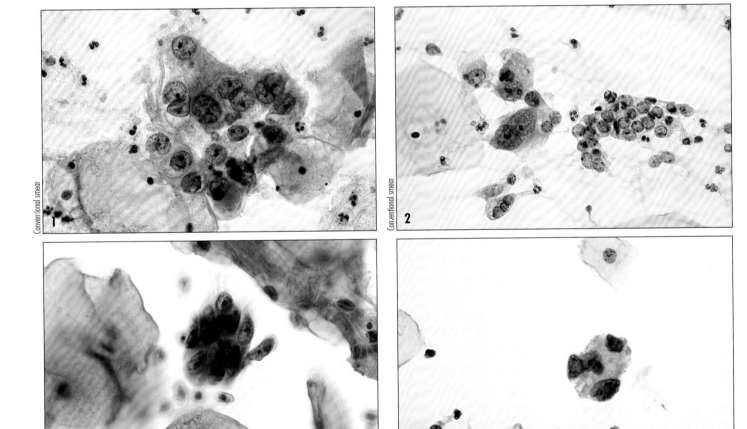

1 · Conventional smear

2 · Conventional smear

3 · SurePath

4 · ThinPrep

Figure 6-4, B continued.

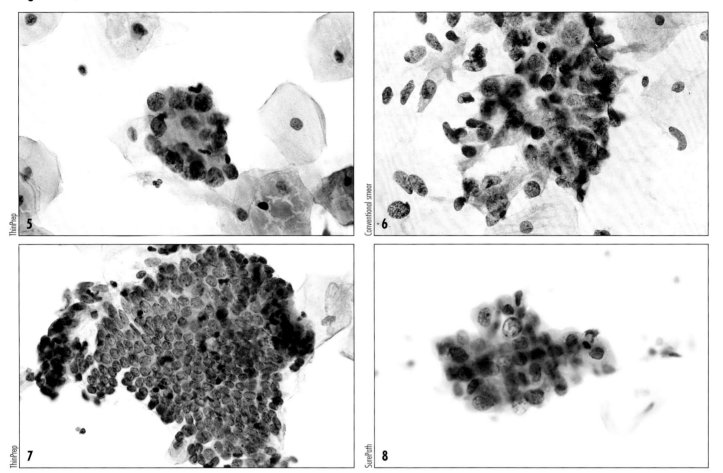

Figure 6-4, C. Atypical endocervical cells: Architectural features of endocervical polyp.

Endocervical polyps are most commonly associated with reparative-type groups of cells on cervical samples with variable degrees of squamoid or glandular features. The streaming appearance in flat sheet-like groups is easy to recognize as benign and reactive (1 and 2). However, departure from a flat architecture to three-dimensional groupings is not uncommon in patients with endocervical polyps (3 and 4).

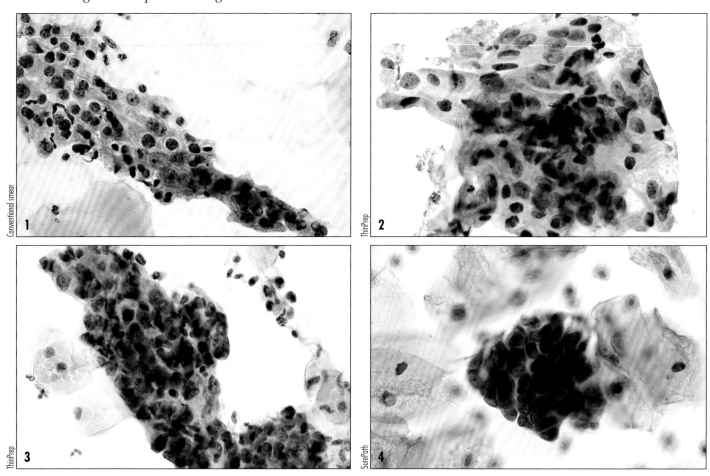

Figure 6-4, D. Atypical endocervical cells: Nuclear features of endocervical polyp.

The nuclear features of endocervical polyps include multinucleation (1), nuclear enlargement with vesicular chromatin and prominent nucleoli (2, 3, and 4), and marked degenerative change with hyperchromatic smudgy chromatin and cytoplasmic vacuolization (5 and 6). Cells with neutrophils within cytoplasmic vacuoles may be present in association with endocervical polyps. These cells mimic the "oxyphil" cells present in association with endometrial adenocarcinoma (7). Comparison to concurrent biopsies may provide correlation for abnormal-appearing cells from these specimens (8, endocervical polyp).

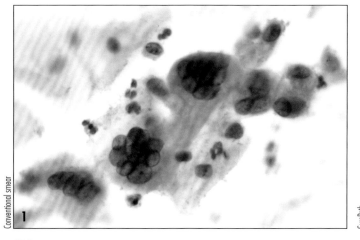

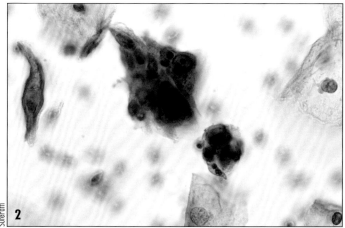

Figure 6-4, D continued.

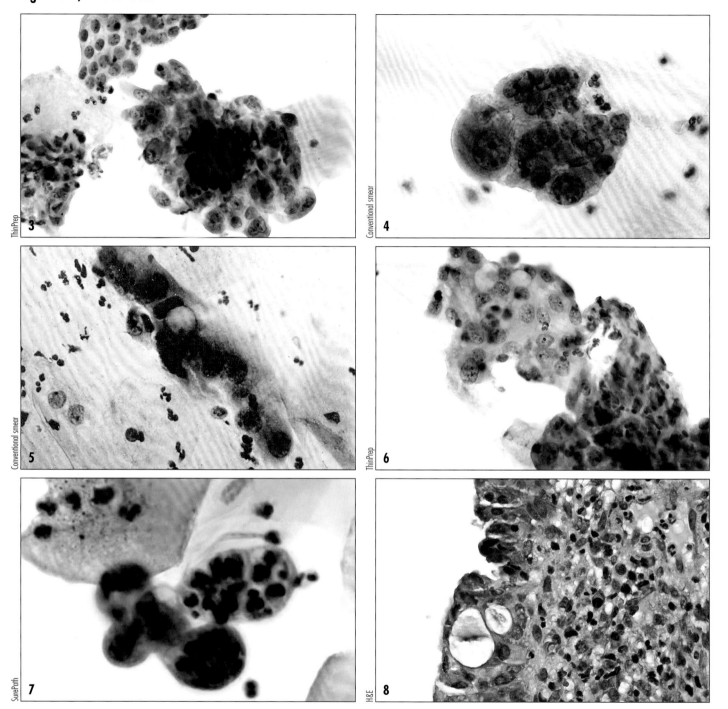

Figure 6-5, A. Tubal metaplasia: Nuclear features.

The presence of cilia confirms tubal metaplasia. Unfortunately this feature is often lost due to mechanical disruption. The nuclei of tubal metaplasia are characterized by rounded to slightly oval shapes, and chromatin that is decidedly darker than endocervical cell chromatin (1). The quality of the chromatin is most often finely granular (2 through 5). Small nucleoli may or may not be visible. Associated inflammatory or reactive conditions may cause the nuclei of tubal metaplastic cells to show increasing nuclear hyperchromasia (6, 7, and 8). Tubal metaplastic cells are heterogeneous in nature (ciliated, nonciliated, and intercalated) (9). The ciliated and nonciliated cells have

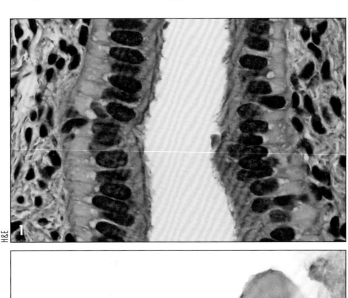

H&E — 1

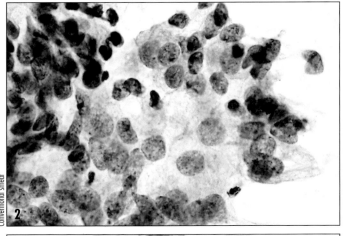

Conventional smear — 2

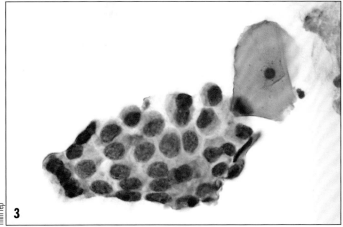

ThinPrep — 3

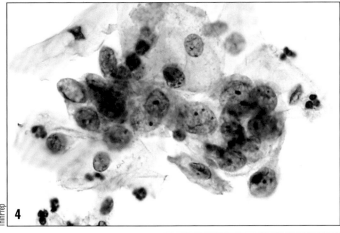

ThinPrep — 4

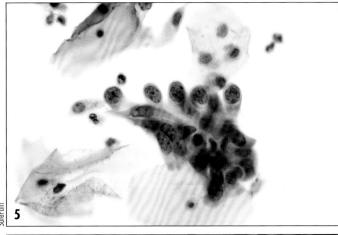

SurePath — 5

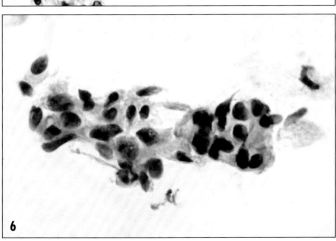

Conventional smear — 6

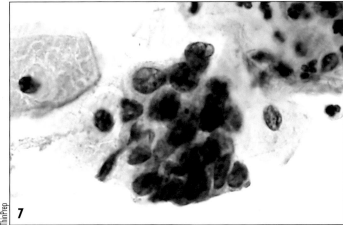

ThinPrep — 7

Figure 6-5, A continued.

more rounded nuclei, while the intercalated cells have elongate nuclei and less cytoplasm. This leads to a heterogeneous appearance within the cell groups (2, 4, 6, and 7).

Note the absence of cytoplasmic mucin in the cells of tubal metaplasia.

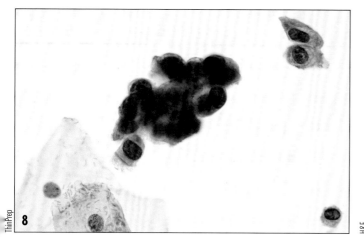

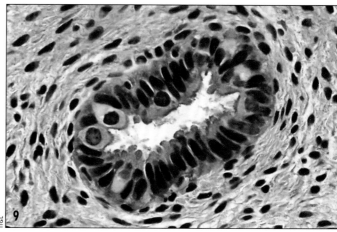

Figure 6-5, B. Tubal metaplasia: Sharp apical borders and clumsy architectural arrangement of nuclei.

Even when cilia are absent, the presence of a well-defined apical border may be the clue to the benign nature of the cell groups. The terminal bar lends more rigidity to the api-

cal surface than is seen in endocervical cells, providing this distinguishing feature (see arrows). Another characteristic feature of tubal metaplasia is the haphazard clumsy arrangement of nuclei within the cell group. The nuclear axes will point in different directions, and the nuclei may overlap, but not because of excessive crowding (1, 2, and 3).

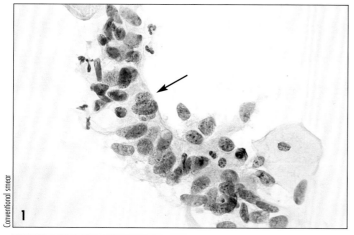

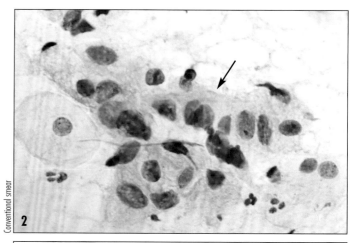

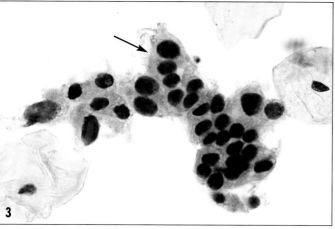

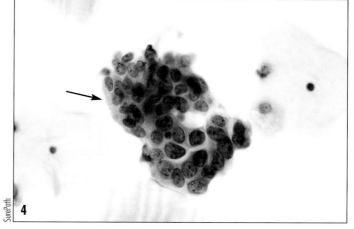

Figure 6-5, C. Tubal metaplasia: Absence of visible cilia in hyperchromatic crowded groups.

Unfortunately, tubal metaplasia can give rise to hyperchromatic crowded groups that do not demonstrate visible cilia, sharp apical borders, or the characteristic heterogeneous nuclear appearance. These groups bring differential diagnoses that include both adenocarcinoma in situ and squamous carcinoma in situ. When the cells maintain a flat architecture with minimal nuclear overlap, it is easier to assess as reactive and degenerative in nature (1, 2, and 3). However, increasing nuclear crowding, slight air-drying artifact (4), or increased depth of focus within the cell group (5 and 6) can make these indistinguishable from glandular or squamous neoplastic lesions.

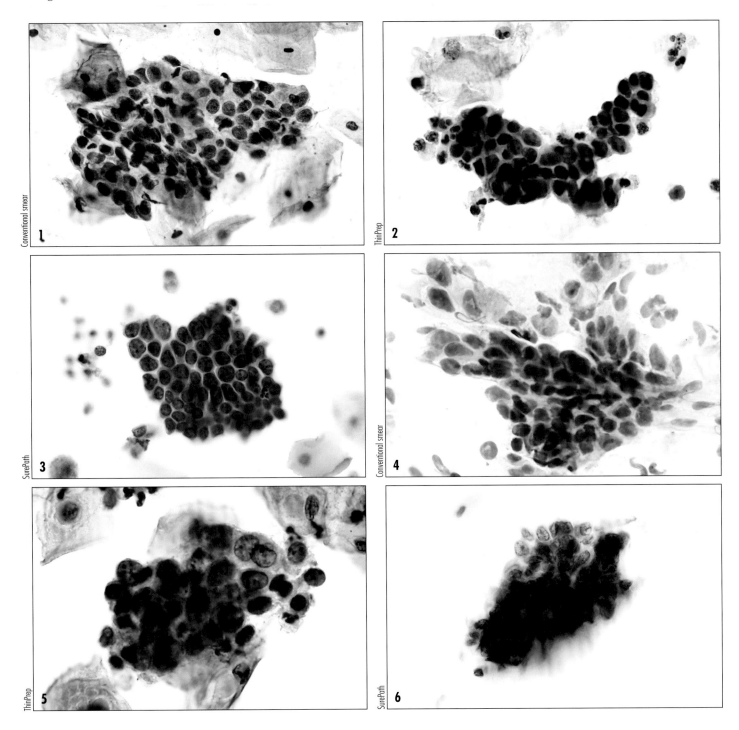

Figure 6-5, D. Tubal metaplasia: Atypical glandular cells indistinguishable from AIS.

Rarely tubal metaplasia can exhibit most, if not all, of the features of adenocarcinoma in situ, including acinar arrangements, feathering, nuclear elongation with hyperchromasia, palisading, and marked nuclear crowding. Recognizing that tubal metaplasia in tissue sections can be similar in morphology to adenocarcinoma in situ helps one to understand the spectrum of change seen in cytology specimens (9). Liquid-based preparations produce tighter and thicker groups because of the tendency of the cells to contract and become more three-dimensional (4, 5, 6, and 8).

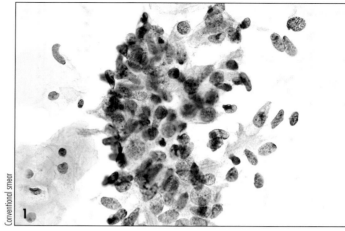

Conventional smear

1

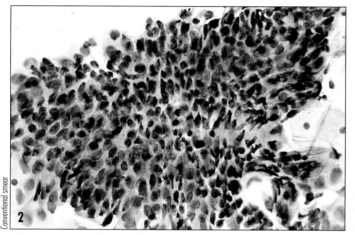

Conventional smear

2

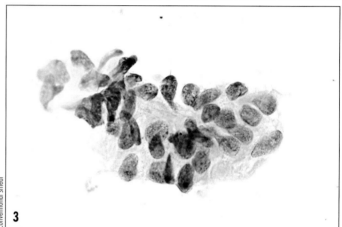

Conventional smear

3

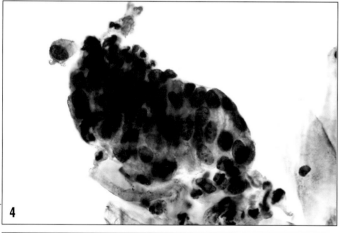

ThinPrep

4

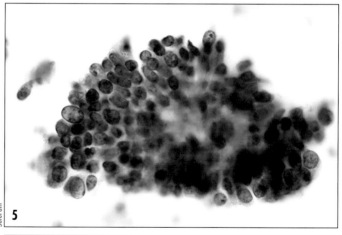

SurePath

5

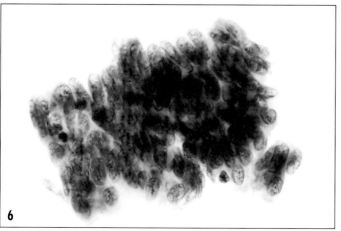

SurePath

6

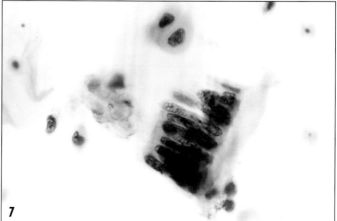

SurePath

7

Figure 6-5, D continued.

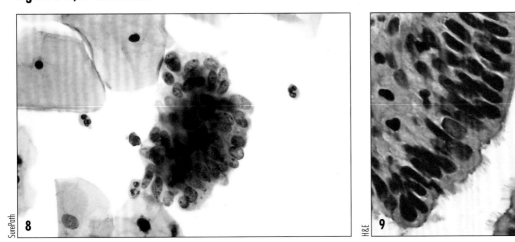

Figure 6-6, A. HSIL involving glands:
Nuclear palisading at the periphery of the cell group.

When high-grade squamous lesions involve glands, they
will often take on glandular features, such as palisading of
the nuclei at the edge of the group (1 and 2) or nuclear
polarization, creating a pseudoacinar-type architecture (3
and 4).

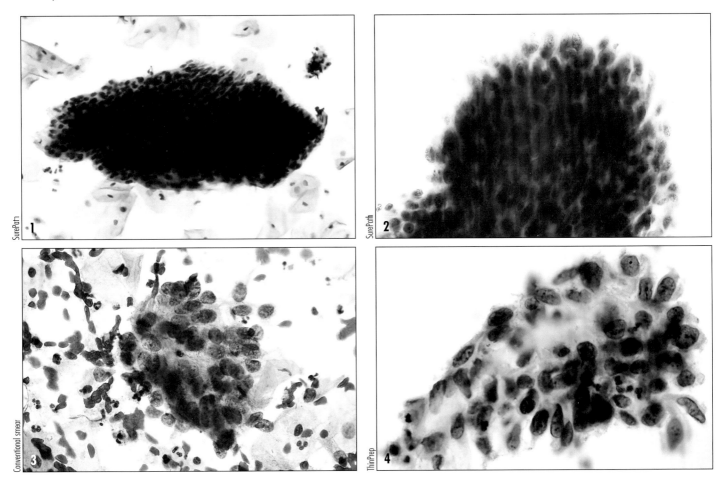

Figure 6-6, B. HSIL involving glands:
Nuclear palisading within the cell group.

Squamous high-grade dysplasias may be characterized by elongate nuclei with nuclear axes parallel to one another (1), leading to a "palisaded" appearance in cytology specimens, which may be misinterpreted as glandular in nature.

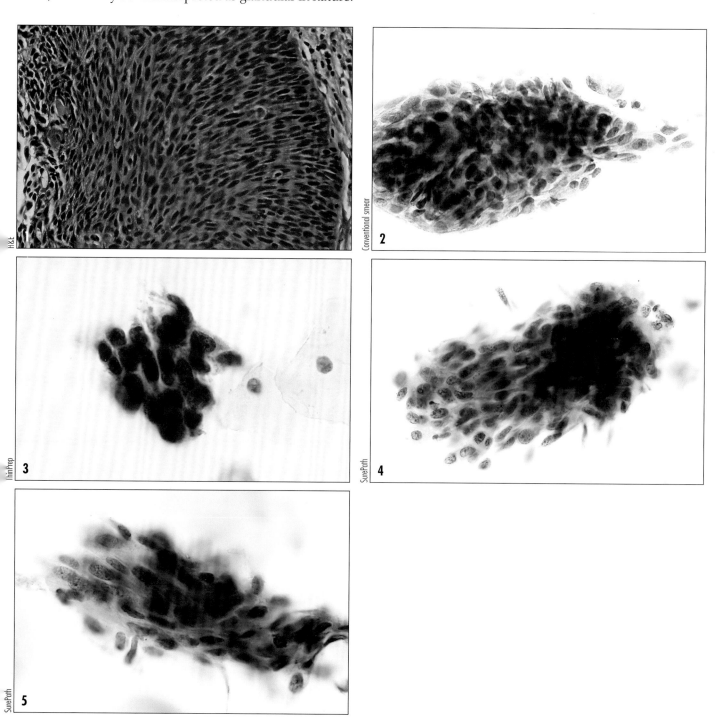

Figure 6-6, C. HSIL involving glands: Glands and SIL within the same cell group.

When HSIL involving glands is cytologically sampled, the cell groups may contain both glandular and squamous elements because of the adjacency within the gland crypt (1). On the cervical cytology specimen, the glandular portion may be more readily visualized within a crowded group, leading one to conclude that the entire group is glandular (2, 3, and 4). As well, sometimes the cells of HSIL will take on glandular features when present within a gland crypt. These features include more abundant cytoplasm with nuclei pushing to the basilar side of the cell and amphophilic to vacuolated cytoplasm (5 through 8). These groups are sometimes mistaken for reactive glandular cells.

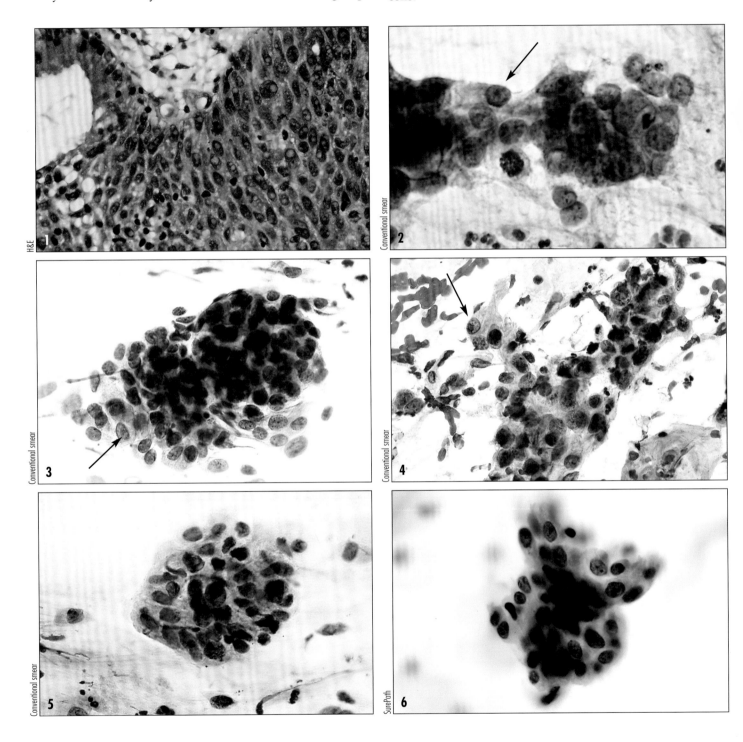

Figure 6-6, C continued.

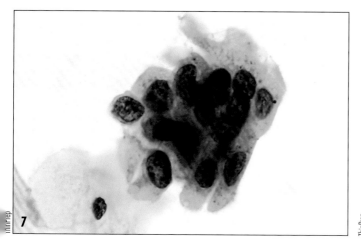

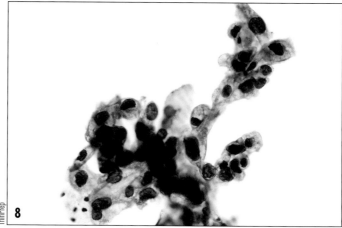

Figure 6-6, D. HSIL involving glands:
Acinar architectural arrangements.

Acinar arrangements within the squamous epithelium can sometimes be seen in tissue sections when high-grade dysplasia involves gland crypts (1). This explains the acinar formations that can be seen in HSIL lesions on cytology specimens. This can be appreciated in both conventional Pap smears and liquid-based preparations.

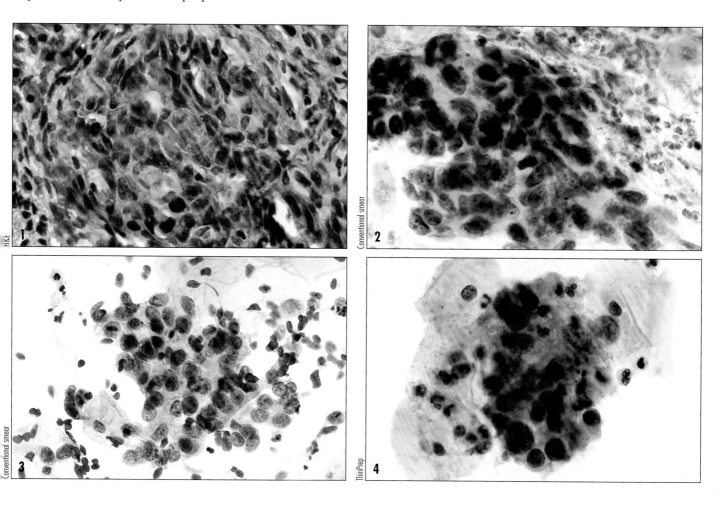

Figure 6-6, D continued.

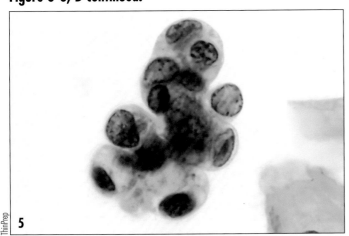

ThinPrep 5

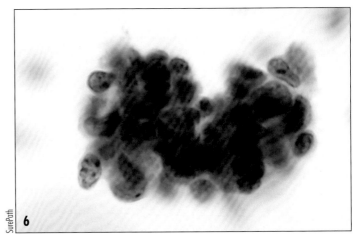

SurePath 6

Figure 6-6, E. HSIL involving glands: Pale chromatin with small nucleoli.

One of the more disconcerting features of squamous lesions involving glands is the occasional loss of nuclear chromatin coarseness and hyperchromasia that typically characterizes SIL (1). This can lead to crowded groups on cervical cytology specimens that may not be remarkably hyperchromatic. The rounded nuclei and occasional acinar arrangements lead one to conclude that the groups are glandular, sometimes erroneously thought to be reactive in nature.

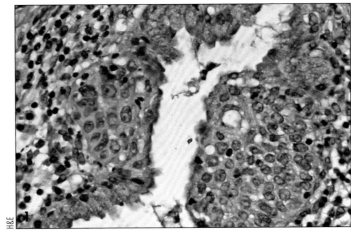

H&E

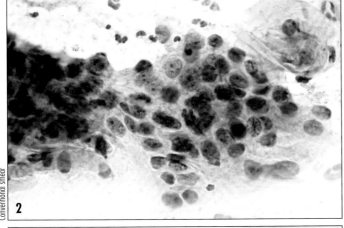

Conventional smear 2

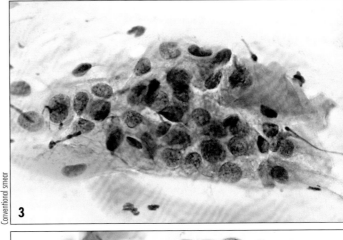

Conventional smear 3

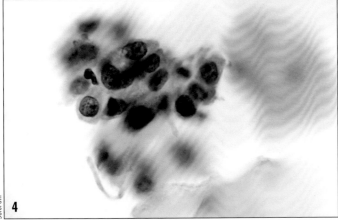

SurePath 4

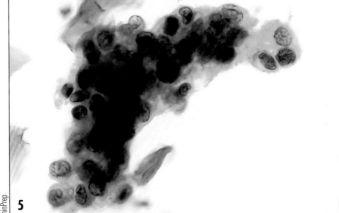

ThinPrep 5

Figure 6-7, A. Lower uterine segment sampling: Low-magnification architectural features.

The low-magnification architecture of the lower uterine segment differs between conventional preparations and liquid-based samples. Conventional preparations allow for larger fragments to remain preserved. The cell groups are irregular in shape and demonstrate a stretched or "pulled taffy" configuration (1, 2, and 3). The thickness of the group is greatest in the center, while the periphery appears thin and frayed. LUS fragments in liquid-based preparations are smaller and demonstrate less of the "stretched" configuration, although the frayed edges are still apparent (4 and 5). Very small, wispy fragments are not uncommon in liquid-based preparations (6).

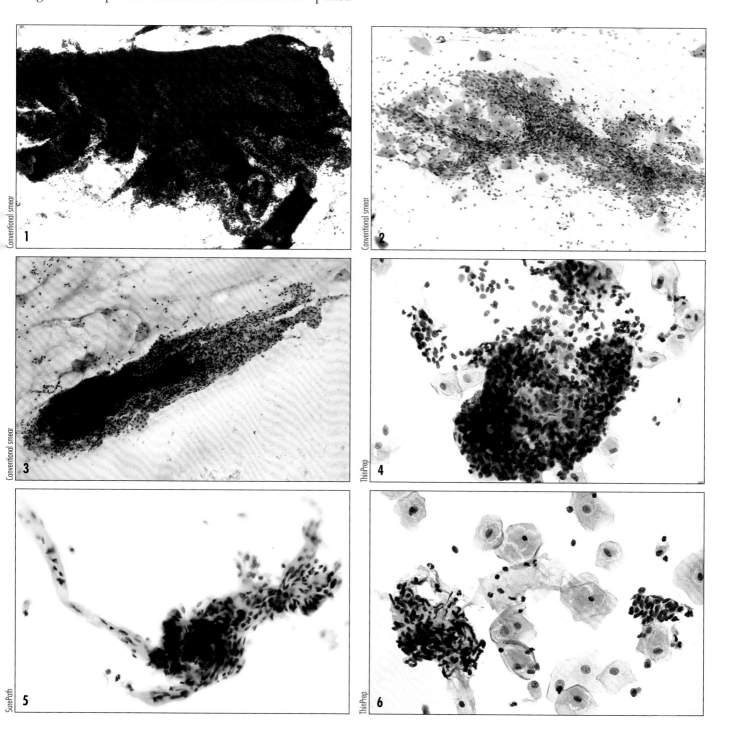

Figure 6-7, B. Lower uterine segment sampling: Biphasic pattern.

Very elaborate, complex branched groups with both tubular glandular components and the more disorderly appearing stromal components are found on conventional preparations (1, 2, and 3). The glandular component may be mistaken for adenocarcinoma in situ, given the branched configuration and very tightly crowded epithelial cells. The biphasic nature of the cell sample is a clue to the benign nature of the group. This biphasic configuration is much less common in liquid-based preparations, as the groups are relatively disaggregated during processing. When present in a liquid-based sample, LUS usually presents as smaller groups with minimal branching (4 and 5).

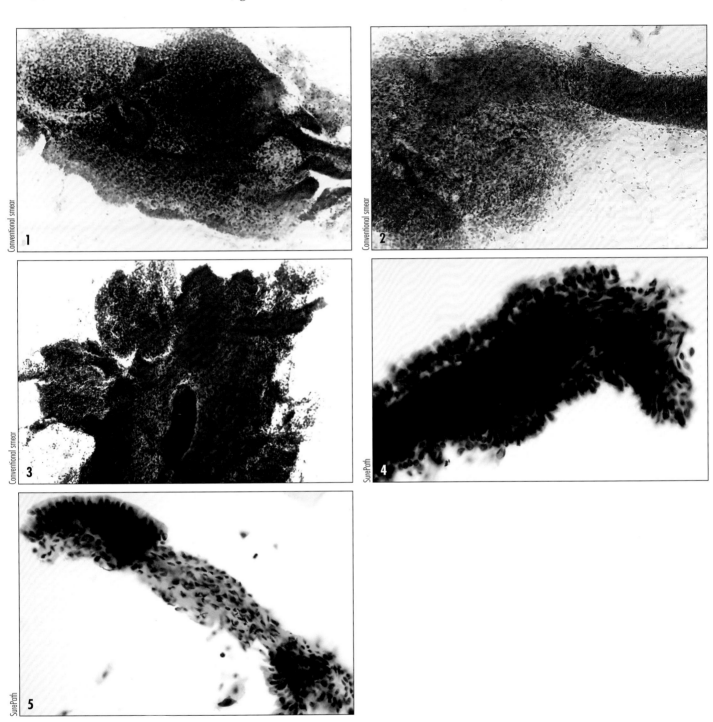

Figure 6-7, C. Lower uterine segment sampling: Stromal component.

The stromal component on high-magnification examination is seen as bland, slightly elongate to oval cells arranged in a disorderly pattern. The cells are most often associated with small amounts of stromal matrix (1, 4, and 6), although this can vary. When the matrix is scant (3 and 5) the groups are more likely to be interpreted as a glandular abnormality, especially when the small groups lend a feathered appearance to the groups (2 and 5). Careful inspection may reveal the presence of penetrating capillaries (3), confirming the stromal nature of the cell group.

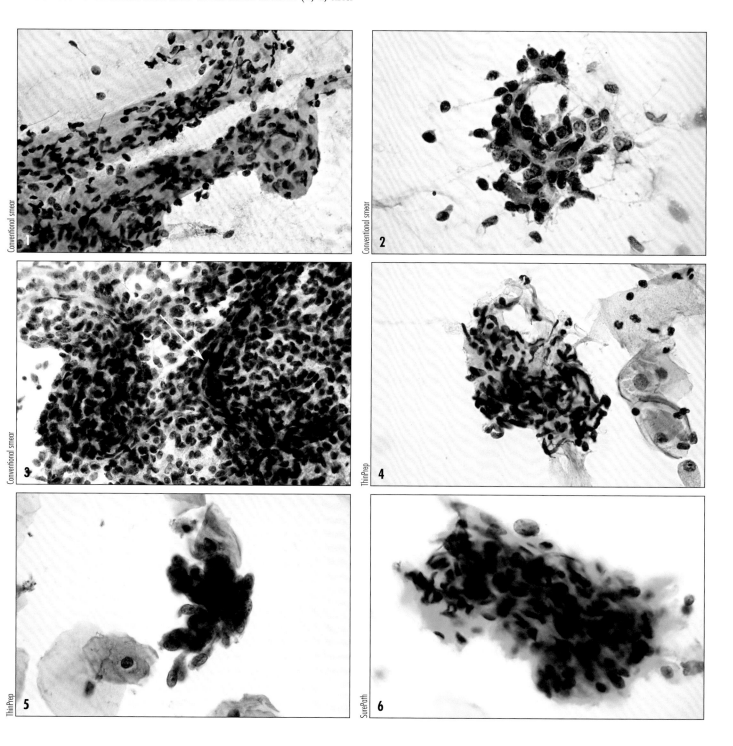

Figure 6-7, D. Lower uterine segment sampling: Epithelial component.

The most troubling presentation of LUS is when the glandular component presents without attachment to the stromal cells. The glandular cells are slightly oval and will be very crowded, with nuclear overlap (1 and 2). Some of the architectural arrangements of adenocarcinoma in situ, including peripheral palisading within the group and acinar formations, can be seen (3 and 4). Unfortunately mitotic figures can also be seen in LUS, making the distinction even more challenging. If the specimen is well preserved, the bland chromatin and small nuclear size of LUS may help to serve as the only distinguishing features separating AIS or HSIL involving glands from LUS.

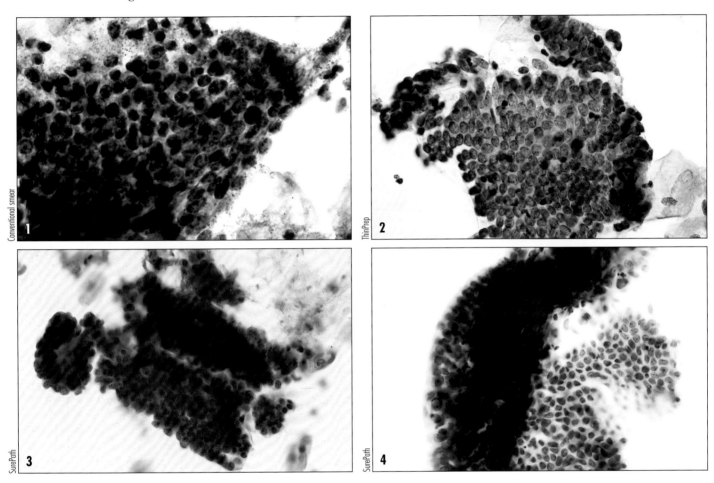

Figure 6-8, A. Atypical endometrial cells: Dysfunctional uterine bleeding.

Shedding endometrial cells will most often present as small three-dimensional clusters of endometrial cells with scant cytoplasm (1, 2, and 3). However, the endometrial cells may exhibit cellular alterations that match the changes present in the endometrium associated with abnormal bleeding, including stromal pseudodecidual

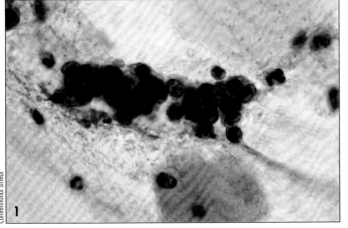

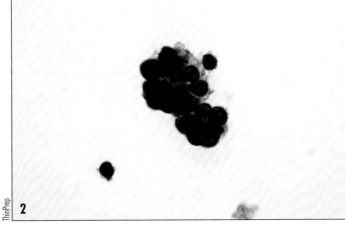

Figure 6-8, A continued.

change (4 and 5) or surface reactive atypia (6), with more abundant cytoplasm and visible nucleoli. Larger groups resembling the exodus pattern of menstrual endometrium are occasionally present (7 and 8). The morphologic changes may be very similar to well-differentiated endometrial adenocarcinoma.

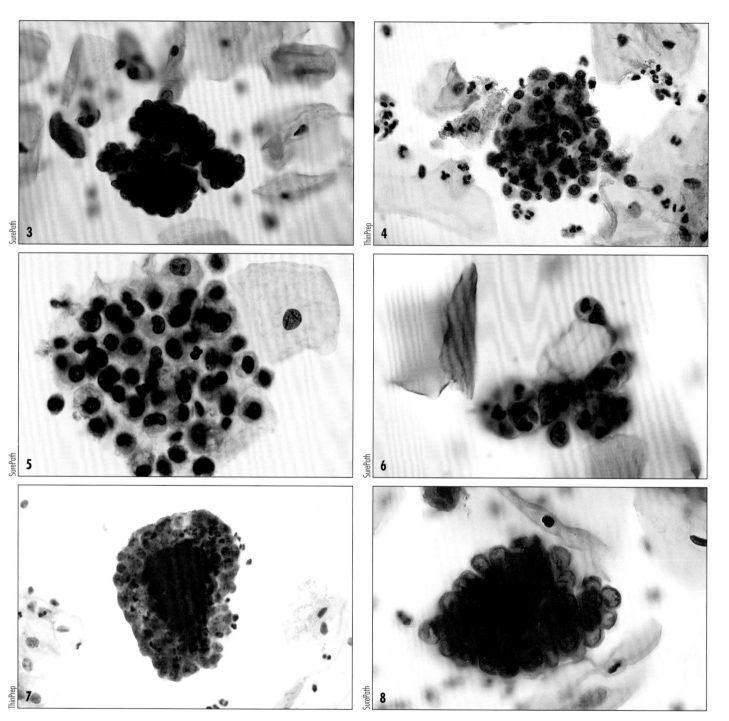

Figure 6-8, B. Atypical endometrial cells: Intrauterine device effect.

Shedding endometrial cells produced in the setting of an intrauterine device are remarkable for the degree of cytologic atypia that they exhibit. Cellular enlargement, with cytoplasmic vacuoles (degenerative in nature), and nuclear enlargement, with prominent nucleoli, characterize these cellular groups (1 and 2). The reactive change to the implanted device may include nuclear hyperchromasia with membrane irregularity (3) and increased nuclear to cytoplasmic ratio (4 and 5). These features are identical to well- to moderately differentiated endometrial adenocarcinomas. Clinical correlation is important in assessing the clinical significance of atypical glandular groups arising in a woman with an IUD in place.

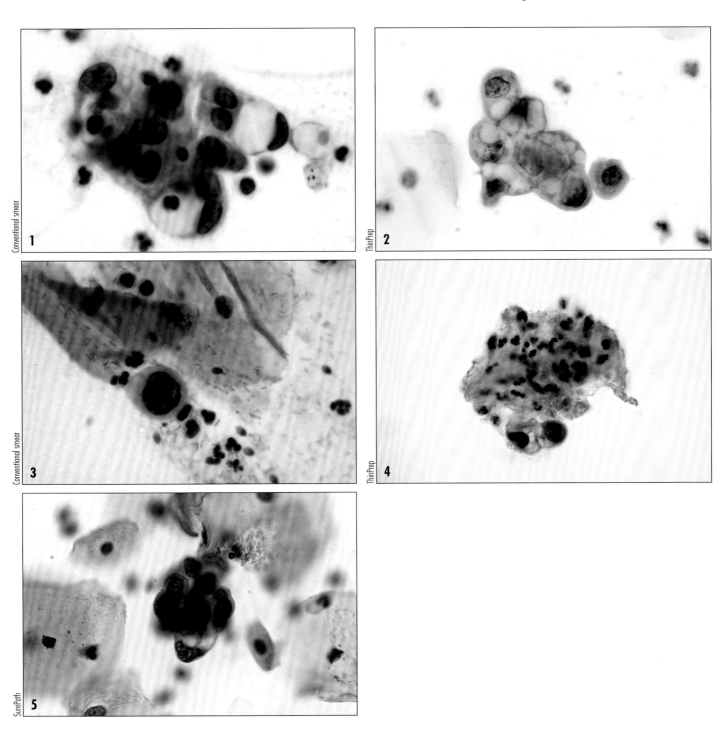

Figure 6-8, C. Atypical endometrial cells: Endometrial polyp.

Cells shedding from endometrial polyps produce a similar spectrum of morphologies, as does dysfunctional uterine bleeding. The cell groups range from small clusters with scant cytoplasm (1), to irregularly shaped, three-dimensional groups with branching (2 and 3), to clusters that demonstrate cellular and nuclear enlargement with cytologic atypia (4).

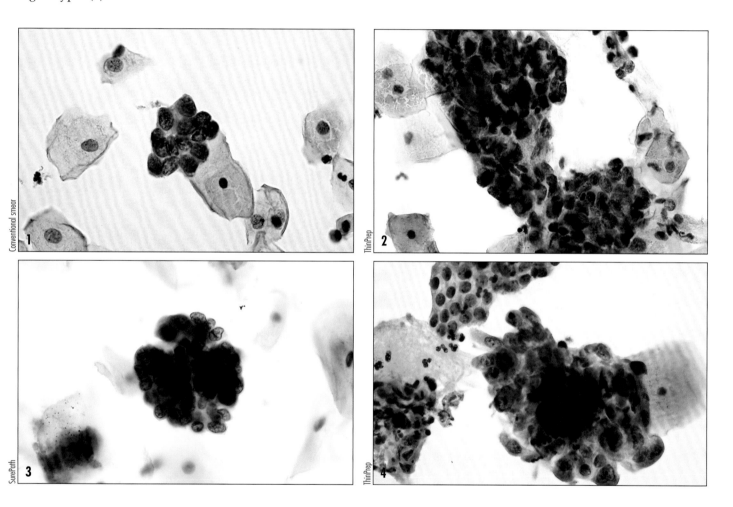

Figure 6-8, D. Atypical endometrial cells: Endometrial hyperplasia.

The presentation of endometrial hyperplasia in cervical cytologic specimens will depend on the type and degree of hyperplasia within the endometrial cavity. The cells range from small clusters with scant cytoplasm (1 and 2), to larger clusters with scant cytoplasm (3), to clusters with irregular architecture and increasing cytologic atypia (4 and 5). Degenerating blood can mimic a diathesis (3). These clusters can also be indistinguishable from well-differentiated endometrial adenocarcinoma.

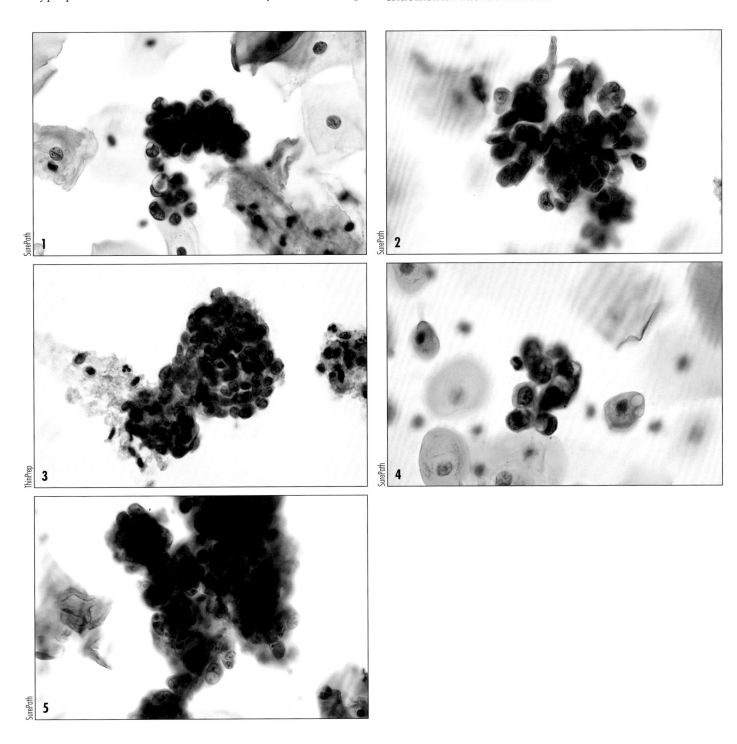

Figure 6-9, A. Metastatic adenocarcinoma: Colon/rectal.

Adenocarcinomas from colon or rectal origin (either direct extension through the rectovaginal septum or metastatic to the cervical/vaginal tissue) will most often produce a necrotic background in the cytologic specimen (1). The cell clusters most often demonstrate typical features of colorec- tal carcinoma: hyperchromatic columnar groups with elongate palisaded nuclei (2 and 3). Poorly differentiated tumors may lose the discrete columnar appearance but will maintain hyperchromasia within the disorganized groups (1 and 4). Colon cancers with rectovaginal fistulas may show vegetable material in the background (5).

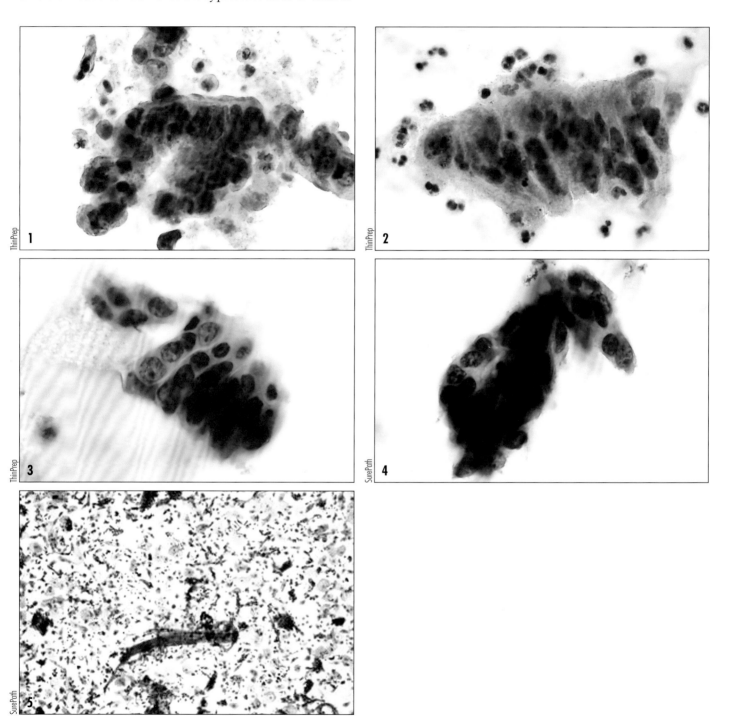

Figure 6-9, B. Metastatic adenocarcinoma: Ovarian.

Ovarian adenocarcinoma will most often gain access to cervical Pap specimens by floating through the fallopian tubes and endometrial cavity. The background is therefore most often clean. The cell clusters are sphere-like and often contains "soap-bubble–like" cytoplasmic vacuoles (2).

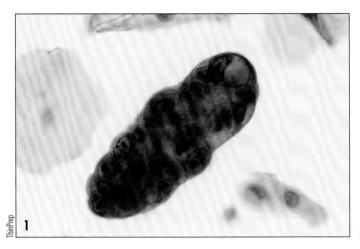

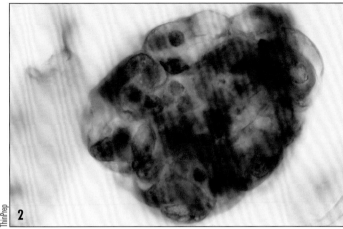

Figure 6-9, C. Metastatic adenocarcinoma: Breast.

Metastatic breast adenocarcinoma may present in a cervical cytologic specimen as a result of endometrial metastasis (indirect access to the Pap specimen by shedding) or through direct involvement of cervical or vaginal tissues.

The background will vary depending on the degree of tissue destruction associated with the tumor but is most often clean. Metastatic breast carcinoma will typically produce small three-dimensional clusters of relatively monotonous cells. Metastatic lobular breast carcinoma may present as single cells or small chains.

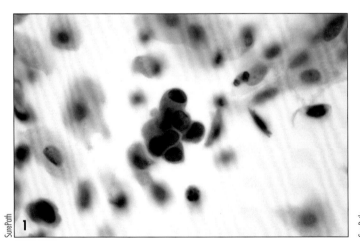

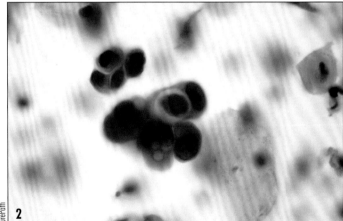

Figure 6-9, D. Metastatic adenocarcinoma: Fallopian tube.

Fallopian tube adenocarcinoma is identical in appearance to ovarian adenocarcinoma. The background is clean, with three-dimensional tumor clusters, sometimes exhibiting "soap-bubble–like" cytoplasmic vacuoles.

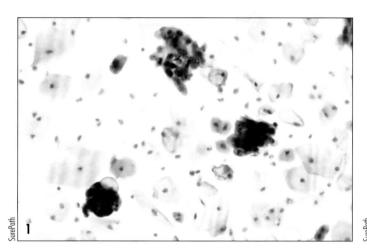

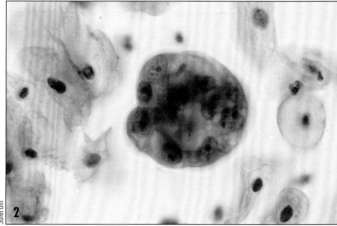

Figure 6-9, E. Malignant mixed Mullerian tumor.

Malignant mixed Mullerian tumor (most often of endometrial origin) is a high-grade neoplasm composed of both malignant stromal and epithelial components. A biphasic pattern may be recognizable on the Pap specimen (if shed from the endometrial cavity or by direct sampling of the polypoid mass, which may extend into the endocervical canal); however, most often the cells appear poorly differentiated and not clearly recognizable as either epithelial or stromal.

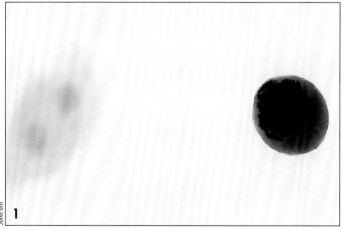

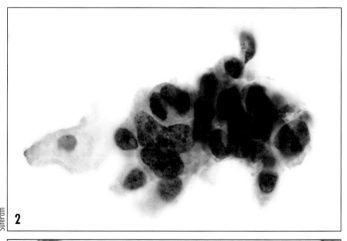

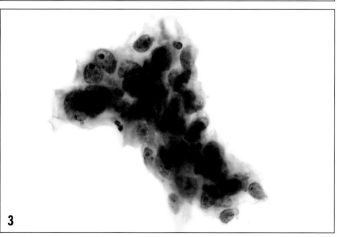

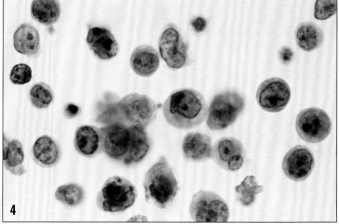

Figure 6-9, F. Metastatic adenocarcinoma: Pancreatic.

Rarely, other metastatic carcinomas may present in cervical specimens. Metastatic pancreatic adenocarcinoma is illus-

trated here, demonstrating loose sheets and cords of malignant glandular cells in a clean background. The nuclei exhibit typical glandular features, including nuclear polarization and vesicular chromatin with a single prominent nucleolus.

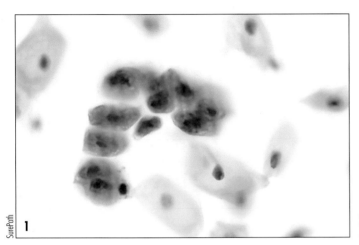
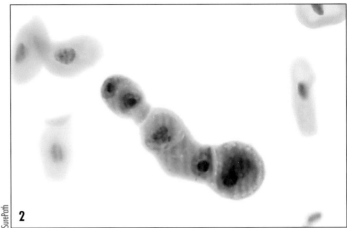

Bibliography

Ashfaq R, Gibbons D, Vela C, Saboorian MH, Iliya F. ThinPrep Pap Test: accuracy for glandular disease. *Acta Cytol.* 1999; 43:81-85.

Bean SM, Connoly K, Roberson J, Eltoum I, Chhieng DC. Incidence and clinical significance of morphologically benign-appearing endometrial cells in patients age 40 years or older: the impact of the 2001 Bethesda System. *Cancer (Cancer Cytopathol).* 2006;108:39-41.

Betsill WL, Clark AH. Early endocervical glandular neoplasia, I: histomorphology and cytomorphology. *Acta Cytol.* 1986; 30:115-126.

Bose S, Kannan V, Kline T. Abnormal endocervical cells. Really abnormal? Really endocervical? *Am J Clin Pathol.* 1994; 101:708-713.

Cangiarella JF, Chhieng DC. Atypical glandular cells: an update. *Diagn Cytopathol.* 2003;29:271-279.

Chang A, Sandweiss L, Bose S. Cytologically benign endometrial cells in the Papanicolaou smears of postmenopausal women. *Gynecol Oncol.* 2001;80:37-43.

DePeralta-Venturino MN, Purslow MJ, Kini SR. Endometrial cells of the "lower uterine segment" (LUS) in cervical smears obtained by endocervical brushings: a source of potential diagnostic pitfall. *Diagn Cytopathol.* 1995;12:263-271.

Di Tomasso JP, Ramzy I, Mody DR. Glandular lesions of the cervix: validity of cytologic criteria used to differentiate reactive changes, glandular intraepithelial lesions and adenocarcinoma. *Acta Cytol.* 1996;40:1127-1135.

Drijkoningen M, Meertens B, Lauweryns J. High grade squamous intraepithelial lesions (CIN 3) with extension into the endocervical clefts: difficulty of cytologic differentiation from adenocarcinoma in situ. *Acta Cytol.* 1996;40:889-894.

Ducatman BS, Wang HH, Jonasson JG, et al. Tubal metaplasia: a cytologic study with comparison to other neoplastic and non-neoplastic conditions of the endocervix. *Diagn Cytopathol.* 1993;9:98-105.

Goff BA, Atanasoff P, Brown E, et al. Endocervical glandular atypia in Papanicolaou smears. *Obstet Gynecol.* 1992;79:101-104.

Gray JA, Nguyen GK. Cytologic detection of endometrial pathology by Pap smears. *Diagn Cytopathol.* 1999;20:181-182.

Hecht JL, Sheets EE, Lee KR. Atypical glandular cells of undetermined significance in conventional cervical/vaginal smears

and thin-layer preparations. *Cancer (Cancer Cytopathol).* 2002;96:1-4.

Kurman RJ, Solomon D. *The Bethesda System for Reporting Cervical/Vaginal Cytologic Diagnoses. Definitions, Criteria and Explanatory Notes for Terminology and Specimen Adequacy.* New York: Springer-Verlag; 1994.

Lee KR, Manna EA, St. John T. Atypical endocervical glandular cells: accuracy of cytologic diagnosis. *Diagn Cytopathol.* 1985;13:202-208.

Lee KR, Minter LJ, Granta SR. Papanicolaou smear sensitivity for adenocarcinoma in situ of the cervix: a study of 34 cases. *Am J Clin Pathol.* 1997;107:30-35.

National Cancer Institute Workshop Report: the 1988 Bethesda system for reporting cervical/vaginal cytologic diagnoses. *JAMA.* 1989;262:931.

Nguyen TN, Bourdeau JL, Ferenczy A, Franco EL. Clinical significance of histiocytes in the detection of endometrial adenocarcinoma and hyperplasia. *Diagn Cytopathol.* 1998;19:89-93.

Novotny DB, Maygarden SJ, Johnson DE, Frable WJ. Tubal metaplasia: a frequent pitfall in cytologic diagnosis of endocervical glandular dysplasia. *Acta Cytol.* 1992;36:1-10.

Rimm DL, Gmitro S, Frable WR. Atypical reparative change on cervical/vaginal smears may be associated with dysplasia. *Diagn Cytopathol.* 1996;14:374-379.

Roberts JM, Thurloe JK, Bowditch RC, Humcevic J, Laverty CR. Comparison of ThinPrep and Pap smear in relation to prediction of adenocarcinoma in situ. *Acta Cytol.* 1999;43:74-80.

Selvaggi SA. Cytologic features of squamous cell carcinoma in situ involving endocervical glands in endocervical cytobrush specimens. *Acta Cytol.* 1994;38:687-692.

Selvaggi SA. Cytologic features of high-grade squamous intraepithelial lesions involving endocervical glands on ThinPrep cytology. *Diagn Cytopathol.* 2002;26:181-185.

Solomon D, Davey D, Kurman R, et al. The 2001 Bethesda System: terminology for reporting results of cervical cytology. *JAMA.* 2002;287:2114-2119.

Solomon D, Nayar R. *The Bethesda System for Reporting Cervical Cytology. Definitions, Criteria, and Explanatory Notes.* 2nd ed. New York: Springer; 2004.

Tambouret RH, Bell DA, Centeno BA. Significance of histiocytes in cervical smears from peri/postmenopausal women. *Diagn Cytopathol.* 2001;24:271-275.

Look-Alikes and Morphologic Spectrums of Change

Michael R. Henry, MD
Amy C. Clayton, MD
Camilla J. Cobb, MD

Introduction

It is remarkable that such a small area of the body, the cervix, provides such a broad range of cytologic findings. The previous chapters have delineated the various epithelial abnormalities, organisms, benign changes, and artifacts that can be found on cytologic specimens from the cervical/vaginal area. This chapter will look at some of these same findings in a different way.

First, almost all of the previously described entities share similar cytologic features with other entities or artifacts. These look-alikes must always be considered when evaluating Pap slides, and the next pages will focus on some of the more common and significant entities and their mimickers.

Second, all of the epithelial abnormalities found on Pap slides fall within spectrums of cytologic change that range from benign to frankly malignant. Our diagnostic classification schemes, both historical and current (the Bethesda System), set up well-defined categories, but, in reality, many cellular presentations fall into gray zones between these specific diagnoses. It has always been recognized that

epithelial abnormalities, especially squamous lesions, begin with minimal abnormal cytologic change and progress over time to more significant findings and eventually to invasive carcinoma. As our knowledge of the role of human papillomavirus (HPV) in cervical disease has evolved, we can now recognize why some morphologic changes look as they do. This has allowed for the development of nomenclature (the Bethesda System) that enables clinical follow-up in a standardized appropriate fashion (American Society for Colposcopy and Cervical Pathology [ASCCP] guidelines). These morphologic spectrums occur both between diagnostic categories (such as NILM [negative for intraepithelial lesion or malignancy] – ASC-US [atypical squamous cells of undetermined significance] – LSIL [low-grade squamous intraepithelial lesion] – HSIL [high-grade squamous intraepithelial lesion]) as well as within a specific diagnosis (eg, the spectrum of nuclear changes in AIS [adenocarcinoma in situ]). Recognition of the existence of these spectrums is necessary for an understanding of the practice of gynecologic cytology and will aid the cytologist in formulating appropriate diagnostic interpretations.

Look-Alikes: Organisms

Figure 7-1. Trichomonas vaginalis.

Characteristic morphology allows for easy recognition of *Trichomonas vaginalis* (TV) in the vast majority of cases. The most distinctive feature is the organism's elliptical nucleus, which must be identified for definitive diagnosis. Red cytoplasmic granules are also fairly characteristic but are not always present. The flagella, seen routinely in wet-mount preparations, may be seen in liquid-based slides but are almost never observed in conventional Pap smears (A). Look-alikes of TV include cytoplasmic fragments, debris, bare nuclei, and degenerated inflammatory or epithelial cells.

Cytoplasmic fragments (B) and degenerated cells (C) are sometimes misidentified as TV. This confusion is most like-ly to occur in Pap slides showing cytolysis, or marked inflammation. Likewise, inspissated mucus, lubricant material, or other debris can also be confused with TV (D). Cytoplasmic fragments, mucus, and lubricant material will typically have variable shapes and sizes and irregular borders, compared to the uniform size and smooth outlines of TV. *Trichomonas* organisms can vary in size, but in an individual case, the organisms tend to be uniform. Noting the absence of the distinctive TV elliptical nuclei in suspicious structures or material avoids misdiagnosis. Bare nuclei can also be mistaken for TV and are also typically seen in the background of cytolysis (E). Bare nuclei tend to be rounded or slightly ovoid, instead of the usual appearance of pear-shaped TV, and lack the surrounding cytoplasm with granules. Bare nuclei usually have a small nucleolus, which again should not be confused with the elliptical nucleus of TV.

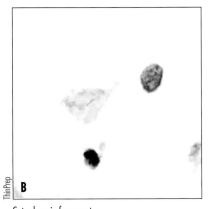

ThinPrep **B**

Cytoplasmic fragments

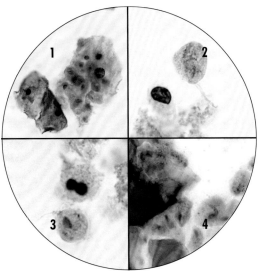

A. *Trichomonas vaginalis*
1,2. ThinPrep
3. SurePath
4. Conventional smear

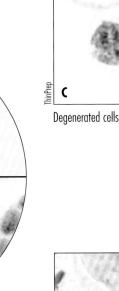

ThinPrep **C**

Degenerated cells

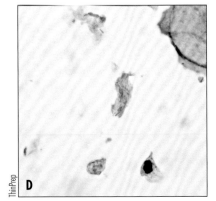

ThinPrep **D**

Mucous and debris

ThinPrep **E**

Naked nuclei

Figure 7-2. Herpes.

Herpes viral changes, characterized by multinucleation, nuclear molding, and chromatin margination (the "3 M's") (A), along with "ground-glass" nuclei and nuclear enlargement, can resemble reactive nuclear changes or the nuclear features of SIL. Multinucleation in squamous and endocervical cells may be seen as a nonspecific reactive change that can mimic herpes, especially when the affected cells degenerate (B). However, compared to herpes, these reactive nuclei are smaller, tend to overlap rather than mold, and do not show chromatin margination. Also, reactive nuclei retain a chromatin pattern and usually have small nucleoli, instead of having ground-glass–like change or large inclusions. Degenerating multinucleated cells can be a morphologic difficulty, because the chromatin may appear washed out and can simulate the homogenous appearance of herpes-infected nuclei.

The cells of LSIL are often multinucleated, and if the large dark nuclei are undergoing degeneration, they can be confused with the homogenous ground-glass appearance of herpes cytopathic changes (C). Again, classic cytopathic change must be present in order to diagnose herpes. Occasionally, herpetic changes are seen in singly nucleated cells, and when these cells are of parabasal or squamous metaplastic origin, there can be confusion with CMV (cytomegalic virus) infection or HSIL. CMV usually infects glandular cells or immature squamous cells, and infected cells are much larger than their normal counterparts (D). Singly, nucleated cells with herpetic changes are usually not significantly enlarged, and multinucleated forms are generally present elsewhere on the slide.

Herpes can be associated with marked reactive/reparative epithelial changes that can mimic carcinoma (Figure 7-10). Reactive cells are distinguished by their fine, evenly distributed chromatin, smooth nuclear borders, uniform appearance, and arrangement in orderly sheets (E).

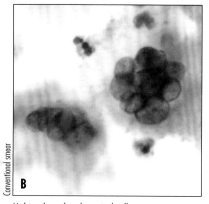

B

Multinucleated endocervical cells

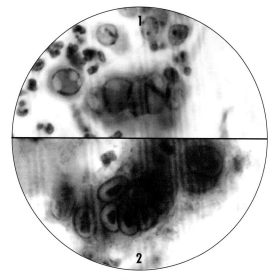

A. Herpes
1. ThinPrep
2. Conventional smear

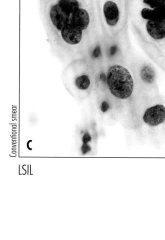

C

LSIL

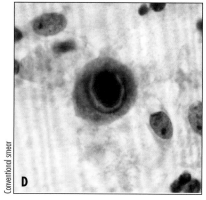

D

Cytomegalovirus

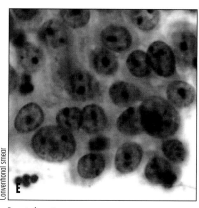

E

Repair/reactive

Figure 7-3. Candida albicans.

The organisms of *Candida albicans* consist of budding yeasts and pseudohyphae (A), and can be confused with other organisms, as well as other native and foreign structures found in Pap slides. Mucus strands are sometimes confused with the pseudohyphae of *Candida* (B). Mucus strands are commonly seen in liquid-based preparations and are usually pleomorphic, whereas *Candida* has a more uniform appearance of parallel walls that are typically rounded at the distal end, tapered at the branching end, and are associated with budding yeast forms. Fibers and threads vary in thickness (generally thicker than *Candida*), can be very long, may curl and knot, and are solid. *Candida* hyphae are usually not as long, do not curl as tightly or knot, and appear hollow. Trichomes are hairy growths of diverse structure that grow on the surfaces of some plants and can present in Pap slides as a contaminant (C). The divergent morphology of the trichome, often showing multiple arms and the absence of yeast forms, are helpful discriminators in the differential diagnosis. Other fungal hyphae, such as *Geotrichum* (D) or *Aspergillus*, may rarely be seen in Pap slides, most often as a contaminant. These hyphae show true septation and are not associated with budding yeast. *Leptothrix* is a thin long bacteria often associated with *Trichomonas* infection. *Leptothrix* is thinner than *Candida* hyphae and also shows no budding yeast forms (E).

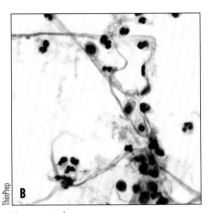

ThinPrep
B

Mucous strands

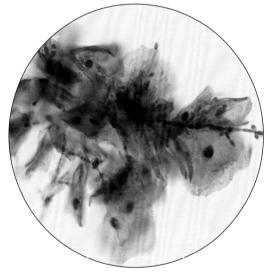

A. Candida
SurePath

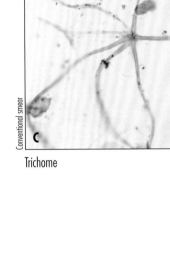

Conventional smear
C

Trichome

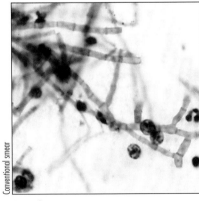

Conventional smear

Geotrichum

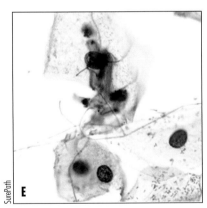

SurePath
E

Leptothrix

Reactive Changes

Figure 7-4. Follicular cervicitis.

Follicular cervicitis (FC) typically involves only a portion of the Pap slide and is composed of a polymorphic population of lymphocytes and a few tingible body macrophages (ie, macrophages with phagocytized debris) (A). FC is readily recognized in well-preserved preparations, but confusion with other small cell lesions is a problem when there is poor preservation and/or degeneration. In cases of lymphoma or leukemia, which rarely present in Pap slides and almost always as a metastatic rather than primary malignancy, tumor cells usually dominate the specimen and show a more monomorphic population of large lymphoid cells with irregularly distributed granular chromatin and prominent nucleoli (B). Apoptotic cells are also often seen in cases of lymphoma/leukemia and are typically absent in FC. Likewise, small cell carcinoma would also dominate the Pap slide and show small tumor cells singly and in cell clusters, with molding and chain formation (C). Because of their cohesiveness and epithelial attachments, rather than the loose cluster formation seen in follicular cervicitis, hyperchromatic crowded groups of squamous cells (eg, HSIL [D] or endometrial cells [E]) are less often confused with FC.

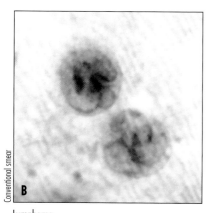

Conventional smear

B

Lymphoma

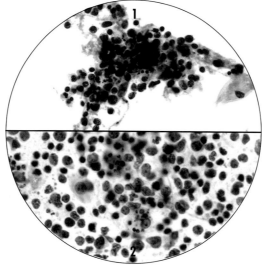

1

2

A. Follicular cervicitis
1. ThinPrep
2. Conventional smear

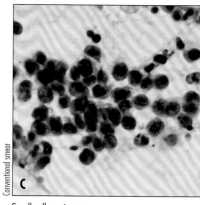

Conventional smear

C

Small cell carcinoma

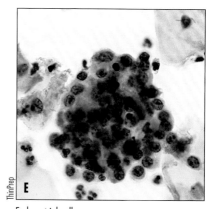

ThinPrep

E

Endometrial cells

ThinPrep

D

HSIL

Figure 7-5. Reparative changes.

Reparative change is characterized by orderly sheets of uniform streaming cells (like a "school of fish"), showing nuclear enlargement, absent to mild hyperchromasia, prominent nucleoli, and rare mitotic figures (A). Many of these cellular features are also present in malignant cells, such as adenocarcinoma (B) and nonkeratinizing squamous cell carcinoma (C), but the malignant cells also show significant cellular and nuclear pleomorphism, single and loosely clustered abnormal cells, and loss of polarity within groups of cells. Malignant nuclei are also darker and have irregularly distributed chromatin and irregular nuclear borders. On the other hand, reparative cells have evenly distributed chromatin and smooth nuclear borders. Reparative changes are usually observed in a minority of cells on a slide, except in rare cases, such as radiation-induced change, in which many or most of the cells may be affected (A3). In most cases of malignancy, the abnormal cells dominate the smear and are sometimes the only cells present. Reparative/reactive change may be seen in conjunction with SIL, and rarely dysplastic cells with these additional reactive changes may be seen (D). As mentioned in Figure 7-2, cells infected with Herpes virus may contain large eosinophilic intranuclear inclusions, which may rarely be mistaken for the large nucleoli of repair (E).

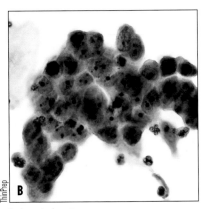

ThinPrep

B

Endocervical carcinoma

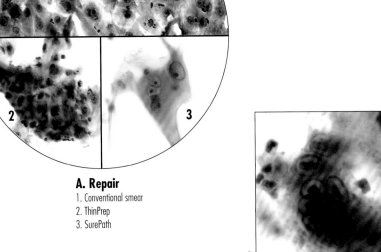

Conventional smear

C

Nonkeratinizing squamous cell carcinoma

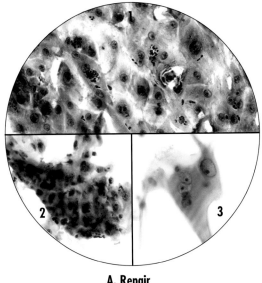

A. Repair
1. Conventional smear
2. ThinPrep
3. SurePath

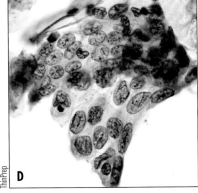

ThinPrep

D

HSIL

Conventional smear

E

Herpes with intranuclear inclusions

Squamous Lesions

Figure 7-6. ASC-US.

Many benign changes in a cervical/vaginal sample may resemble those cellular changes which fall into the ASC-US category (A). Benign nuclear enlargement may be seen in perimenopausal women as well as in women with folate or vitamin B_{12} deficiency (B). These squamous cells have very low nuclear to cytoplasmic (N:C) ratios and no evidence of HPV cytopathic effect. Benign perinuclear halos are often seen in inflammatory conditions and especially in *Trichomonas* infections (C). These halos are smaller than those in koilocytes and do not have peripheral cytoplasmic thickening or significant associated nuclear abnormalities. Glycogenated squamous cells may resemble koilocytes, but the halos often contain yellow or refractile material and again do not show nuclear abnormalities (D). Other benign entities may resemble the dyskeratotic changes associated with HPV infection. Benign parakeratosis consists of miniature squamous cells with round pyknotic nuclei and no evidence of koilocytic change (E1). Parakeratotic-like degenerated cells may rarely be seen in women taking oral contraceptives (E2). Keratotic changes may also be present in *Candida* infections (F). These cells may have some nuclear irregularity and size and shape variation, but do not demonstrate koilocytic halos.

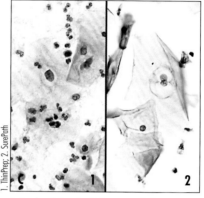

Perinuclear halos: 1. *Trichomonas*; 2. Reactive

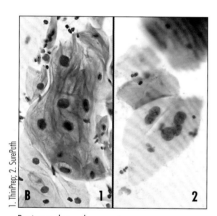

Benign nuclear enlargement:
1. Perimenopausal change; 2. Folate deficiency

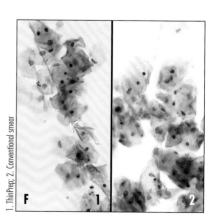

Glycogen

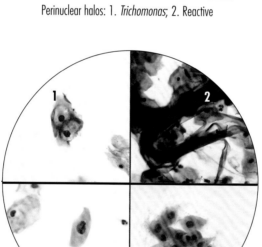
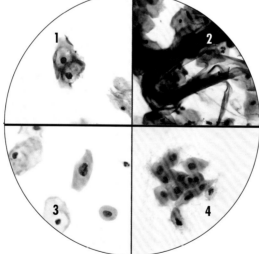

A. ASC-US
1. Changes suggestive of koilocytotic change
2. Atypical parakeratosis
3. Changes suggestive of mild dysplasia
4. Dyskeratotic change suggestive of HPV

1,2. SurePath
3,4. ThinPrep

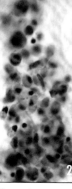

Parakeratosis: 1. Benign parakeratosis;
2. Degenerative "pill" effect

Reactive keratotic change with *Candida*

Figure 7-7. LSIL: Mild squamous dysplasia.

The characteristic features of LSIL include diagnostic nuclear features of dysplasia (increased size, hyperchromasia, membrane irregularity) or diagnostic evidence of HPV infection (koilocytosis). These changes are seen in mature large squamous cells with low N:C ratios (A). Look-alikes for LSIL include benign epithelial cells with large nuclei,

such as in perimenopausal change (B) or folate deficiency (C), benign decidualized stromal cells (D), or abnormal epithelial cells such as ASC-US (E) or borderline HSIL (F). Changes in large cells that can mimic the halos seen with HPV cytopathic effect include glycogen (G) or reactive halos (H) (see also Figure 7-17). These changes are described in detail in chapters 4 and 5.

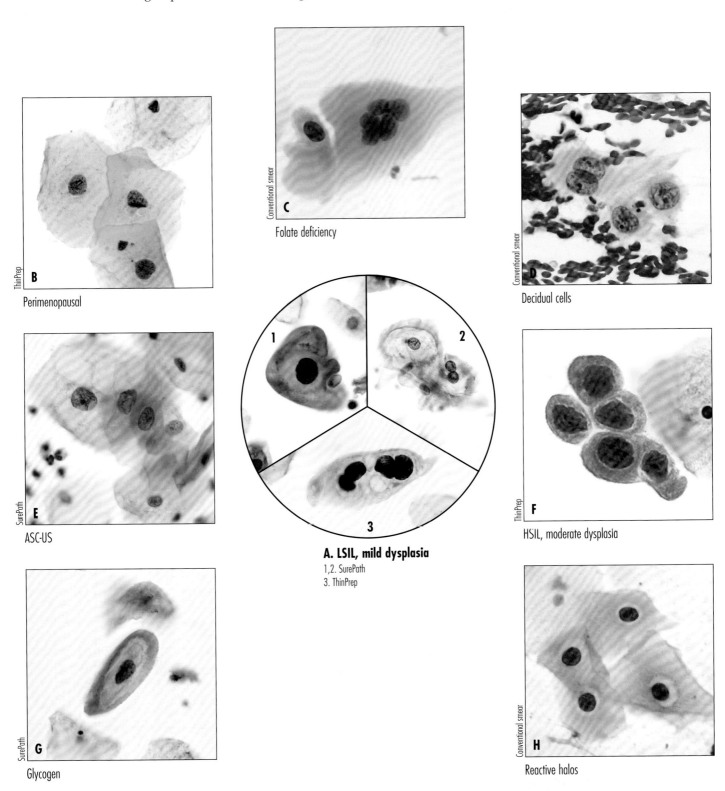

B — ThinPrep
Perimenopausal

C — Conventional smear
Folate deficiency

D — Conventional smear
Decidual cells

E — SurePath
ASC-US

A. LSIL, mild dysplasia
1,2. SurePath
3. ThinPrep

F — ThinPrep
HSIL, moderate dysplasia

G — SurePath
Glycogen

H — Conventional smear
Reactive halos

Figure 7-8. HSIL: Single small cells.

The cells of HSIL may present as single cells, sheets, crowded groups, or most often as a combination of all three. One of the characteristics of dysplasia is the loss of cohesion in the cells and thus the tendency for isolated single cells. A hallmark of HSIL is the decreasing overall size of the cell as the grade of the lesion increases, with a concomitant increase in the N:C ratio. In conventional Pap smears, these single cells were often geographically located in loose groups or within strands of mucous. With the advent of liquid-based preparations, these single cells are much more evenly disbursed throughout the preparation and are often difficult to identify on screening (see Figure 5-18).

More germain to this section, there are many types of small isolated cells derived from other entities that may mimic HSIL. These include nonepithelial cells such as histiocytes or lymphocytes. Histiocytes (B) have small nuclei with even chromatin and often a coffee-bean shape with a prominent longitudinal groove. Small lymphocytes with their characteristic, very small nuclei should not be mistaken for HSIL. However, larger germinal center lymphocytes (C1) or lymphoma (C2 and 3) may be mistaken for squamous dysplasia. Germinal center cells are often accompanied by tingible body macrophages as seen in follicular cervicitis (see Figure 4-6). These cells do not have the membrane notching of HSIL and often have a more coarsely granular chromatin pattern.

Epithelial cells that may be confused with HSIL include reserve cells, parabasal cells, and immature squamous metaplastic cells (D). These cells are cytologically quite similar to each other and can be distinguished from HSIL by the lower N:C ratios, lack of significant membrane notching or irregularity, and normochromasia. Singly, the cells of ASC-H (atypical squamous cells, cannot exclude HSIL) may be indistinguishable from those of HSIL, as they have, by definition, features of HSIL but are qualitatively or quantitatively insufficient for a definitive diagnosis. Other single epithelial cells that can mimic HSIL include cells derived from IUD (intrauterine device) effect (E), single-cell pattern in AIS (F), and, rarely, metastatic tumors such as from breast (G). All of these are described in detail in chapters 4 and 6.

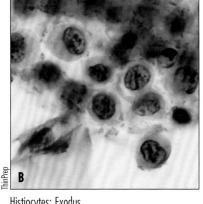

ThinPrep

B

Histiocytes: Exodus

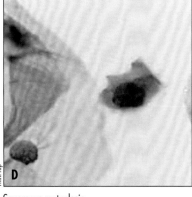

ThinPrep

D

Squamous metaplasia

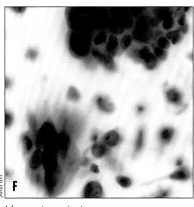

SurePath

F

Adenocarcinoma in situ

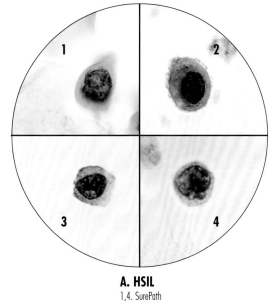

A. HSIL
1,4. SurePath
2,3. ThinPrep

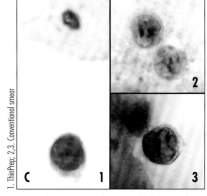

1. ThinPrep; 2,3. Conventional smear

C   **1**   **2**   **3**

1. Lymphocyte, germinal center cell; 2,3. Lymphoma

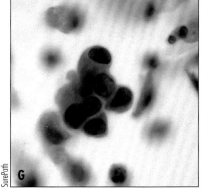

Conventional smear

E

Intrauterine device

SurePath

G

Metastatic breast carcinoma

153

Figure 7-9. HSIL: Hyperchromatic crowded groups.

As mentioned in chapter 5, HSIL may present as single cells, sheets, or thick three-dimensional clusters of immature cells sometimes known as hyperchromatic crowded groups (A). There are several entities that may resemble these hyperchromatic crowded groups. Clusters of atrophic parabasal-type cells are commonly seen in the background of atrophy. These cells have lower N:C ratios, little nuclear variation, and no mitoses (B). Glandular elements often present as crowded groups. Benign endocervical cells show basally located nuclei and mucin vacuoles as well as little nuclear size and shape variation (C). Groups of tubal metaplasia may be quite crowded, with increased N:C ratios, but often demonstrate apical cilia on close examination and again show little variation in nuclear size or shape (D). Benign exfoliated endometrial cells often have cytoplasmic vacuoles and regular small nuclei (E). Fragments of lower uterine segment (LUS) have nuclei similar to exfoliated endometrial cells and may be seen in tubular arrangements or associated with stromal cells (F). The cells of endocervical AIS are similar to HSIL, with nuclear membrane irregularity, anisonucleosis, and frequent mitoses (G). However, in AIS, these fragments often show a columnar arrangement at the periphery of the group.

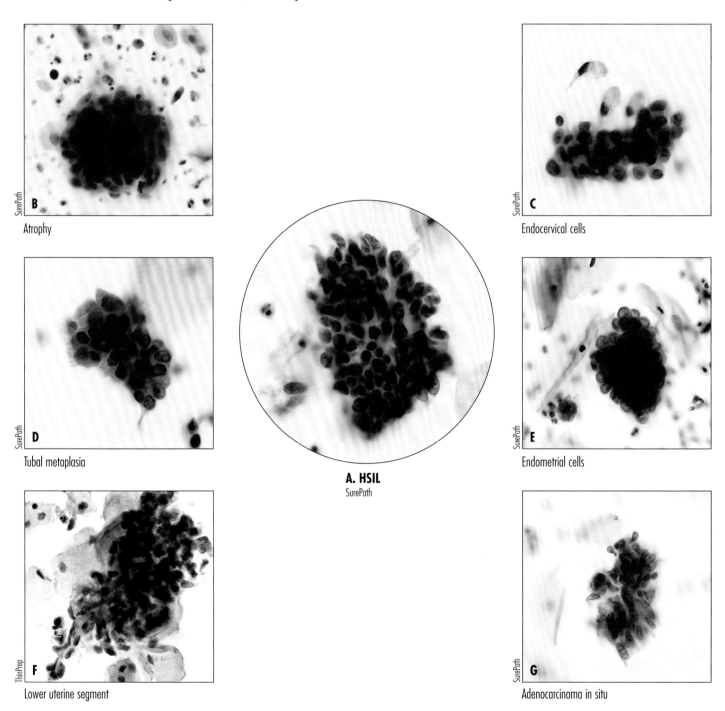

B SurePath
Atrophy

C SurePath
Endocervical cells

D SurePath
Tubal metaplasia

A. HSIL
SurePath

E SurePath
Endometrial cells

F ThinPrep
Lower uterine segment

G SurePath
Adenocarcinoma in situ

Figure 7-10. Nonkeratinizing squamous cell carcinoma.

Nonkeratinizing squamous cell carcinoma is characterized by discohesive cells of variable size with malignant nuclear features, including irregular chromatin clearing, prominent variable nucleoli, nuclear membrane irregularities, and abnormal mitoses (A). Some of these changes may be present to variable degrees in other malignant and benign lesions. Reparative epithelial changes demonstrate prominent nucleoli but maintain cohesion, with nuclear streaming in two-dimensional sheets (B). Atypical reparative change (C) has features between repair and carcinoma and should be flagged as atypical (see Figure 5-6). While herpetic or CMV viral change is not often mistaken for carcinoma (D1), when seen in the background of degeneration and ulcerative necrosis, these changes may be difficult to distinguish from malignancy (see Figures 4-14 and 4-15). Similarly, the reactive cells seen in pemphigus, with their prominent nucleoli, may be mistaken for carcinoma (D2). The cells derived from atrophy may occasionally contain nucleoli and be present in a background of marked inflammation and degeneration. The overall atrophic pattern with a blended spectrum of atrophic change is helpful in arriving at the correct interpretation (E). Finally, moderately or poorly differentiated adenocarcinoma from the cervix, endometrium, or metastasis can be essentially indistinguishable from squamous carcinoma (F). Close attention to the cellular patterns and patient history may be useful in arriving at the proper interpretation.

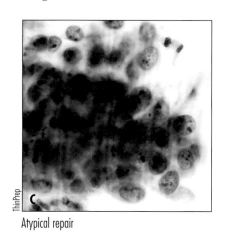

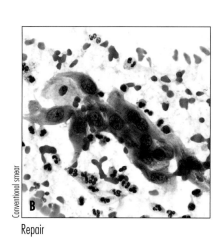

C
ThinPrep
Atypical repair

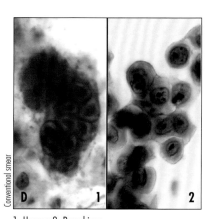

Conventional smear
D

1. Herpes; 2. Pemphigus

Conventional smear
B
Repair

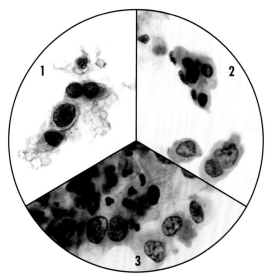

A. Squamous cell carcinoma
1,3. ThinPrep
2. SurePath

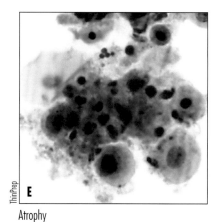

ThinPrep
E
Atrophy

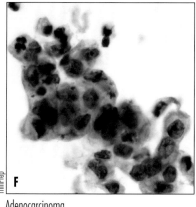

ThinPrep
F
Adenocarcinoma

Figure 7-11. Diathesis

As described in chapter 4, a tumor diathesis is composed of a mixture of degenerative material, including blood with lysed red blood cells, inflammation, and proteinaceous debris, often with embedded degenerated malignant cells (A). A number of materials may closely mimic a diathesis, and, in fact, material derived from ulceration in a benign condition may be indistinguishable from a true tumor diathesis. When this material is identified on a slide, a careful inspection should be under taken for malignant or atypical cells. Inflammatory debris is often seen in the back-

ground of infection, such as with *Trichomonas* (B), where the organisms may be buried in the debris, or as a generic finding composed of neutrophils and degenerating cytoplasmic fragments (C). Atrophic samples are often composed of fragile parabasal-type cells in the background of inflammatory debris, mucin, and blood, which can closely mimic a diathesis (D and E). Degenerated blood is commonly seen in samples taken during or just after menses (F). Clumps of bacteria may be seen in liquid-based samples, which may mimic cellular debris (G). Rarely, lubricant may be seen in the background, also mimicking a diathesis (H).

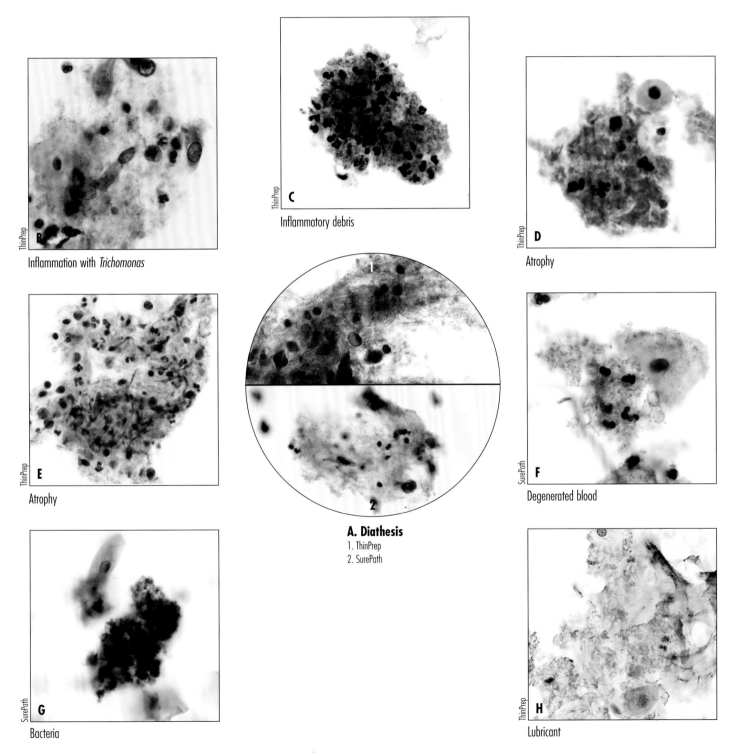

ThinPrep

Inflammation with *Trichomonas*

ThinPrep C

Inflammatory debris

ThinPrep D

Atrophy

ThinPrep E

Atrophy

A. Diathesis
1. ThinPrep
2. SurePath

SurePath F

Degenerated blood

SurePath G

Bacteria

ThinPrep H

Lubricant

Glandular Lesions: Adenocarcinoma In Situ

Figure 7-12. Classic AIS look-alikes.

Many different lesions can exhibit some of the characteristic features of adenocarcinoma in situ, including nuclear elongation, palisading, and rosette or acinar architecture (A). These look-alike lesions can include tubal metaplasia (B), directly sampled lower uterine segment (C), endocervical polyps (D), endocervical adenocarcinoma (E), endometrial adenocarcinoma (F), squamous carcinoma in situ (G). The specific cytologic characteristics of these entities are more fully described in chapters 5 and 6, but, briefly, the benign lesions listed above lack increased mitoses, apoptosis, and significant nuclear hyperchromasia. Additional features that help to differentiate benign lesions from AIS include cilia in tubal metaplasia and biphasic stromal and glandular component in LUS. Dysplastic squamous lesions tend to demonstrate more irregular nuclei with a horizontal instead of vertical cell orientation, and invasive adenocarcinoma may show more discohesion, prominent nucleoli, and a tumor diathesis.

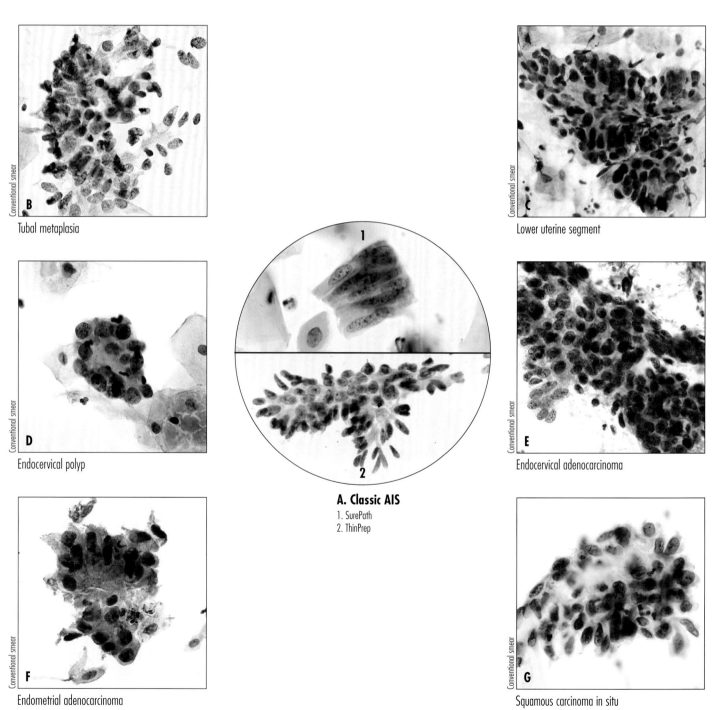

Conventional smear

B Tubal metaplasia

Conventional smear

C Lower uterine segment

Conventional smear

D Endocervical polyp

1

2

A. Classic AIS
1. SurePath
2. ThinPrep

Conventional smear

E Endocervical adenocarcinoma

Conventional smear

F Endometrial adenocarcinoma

Conventional smear

G Squamous carcinoma in situ

Figure 7-13. Variant AIS look-alikes.

The variations of adenocarcinoma in situ that will have the most impact on differential diagnoses include relatively bland-appearing AIS, in which the nuclei demonstrate less nuclear crowding and hyperchromasia (A1); the pleomorphic variant of AIS, in which the nuclei are more angulated and irregular in shape and demonstrate a more open chromatin pattern with visible chromocenters (A2); and the intestinal variant of AIS, which has cytologic features similar to colonic carcinoma, including the presence of prominent goblet cells (A3, arrow).

The minimally atypical form of AIS will most often be confused with benign reactive conditions including endocervical polyp, reactive endocervical cells (B), and tubal metaplasia (C). Squamous carcinoma in situ derived from glandular crypts can also appear uncharacteristically bland, exhibiting pale chromatin with small nucleoli (D). In most cases, other areas of the slide will have more charac-teristic AIS architecture and nuclear changes, which should allow for an appropriate final interpretation.

The pleomorphic form of AIS will most often be mistaken for another type of malignancy including endometrioid adenocarcinoma (E), endocervical adenocarcinoma (F), or squamous carcinoma in situ (G). Atypical-appearing benign conditions, such as a markedly inflamed endocervical polyp (H), may also have features very similar to AIS. Degenerative chromatin patterns in the presence of ulcerative diathesis can be noted in ulcerated benign endocervical polyps and mimics similar changes found in neoplastic glandular abnormalities.

The intestinal variant of AIS closely resembles colonic adenocarcinoma with prominent goblet cells. There are still increased mitoses and apoptotic bodies, but true goblet cells with prominent cytoplasmic vacuoles that displace the nucleus to one side of the cell are also seen. Metastatic or contiguously invasive colon cancer (I) would have similar features. Cellular clusters derived from a recto-vaginal fistula (J) contain goblet cells but have much less nuclear abnormality.

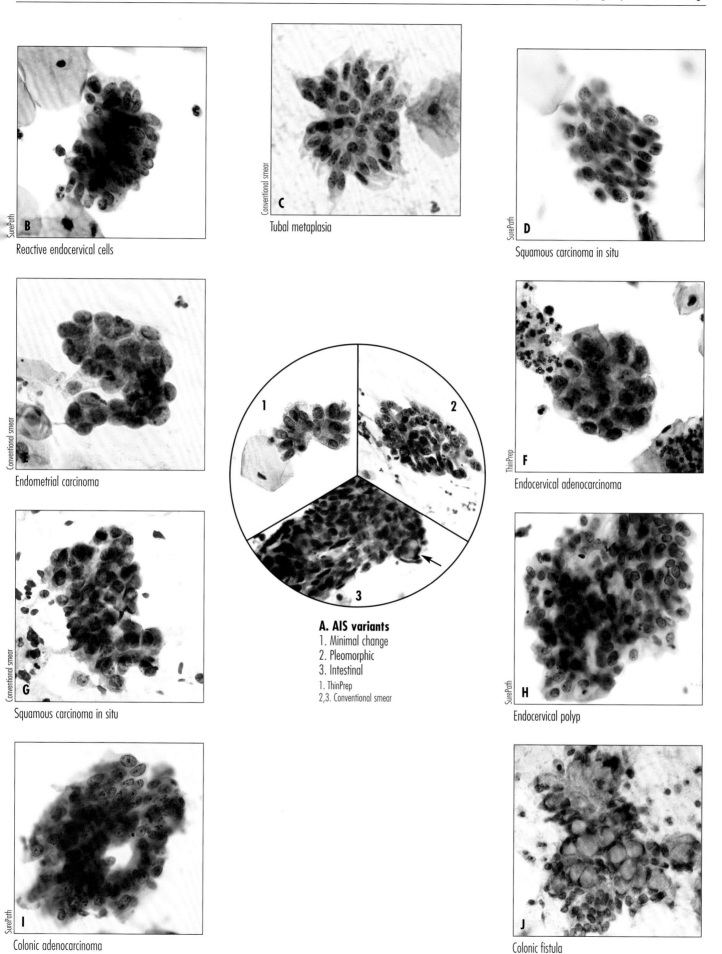

B
SurePath
Reactive endocervical cells

C
Conventional smear
Tubal metaplasia

D
SurePath
Squamous carcinoma in situ

E
Conventional smear
Endometrial carcinoma

F
ThinPrep
Endocervical adenocarcinoma

G
Conventional smear
Squamous carcinoma in situ

A. AIS variants
1. Minimal change
2. Pleomorphic
3. Intestinal
1. ThinPrep
2,3. Conventional smear

H
SurePath
Endocervical polyp

I
SurePath
Colonic adenocarcinoma

J
Colonic fistula

Figure 7-14. Well-differentiated endocervical adenocarcinoma look-alikes.

Well-differentiated endocervical adenocarcinoma demonstrates loosely cohesive aggregates of glandular cells with mild nuclear atypia and disarray within the cell group (A).

Similar features can be seen in tubal metaplasia (B), reactive endocervical cells (C), endocervical polyp (D), endometrial adenocarcinoma (E), and squamous carcinoma in situ (F). Refer to chapter 6 for a more complete description of these entities.

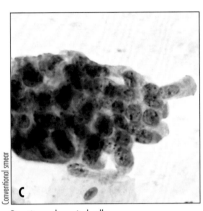

Reactive endocervical cells

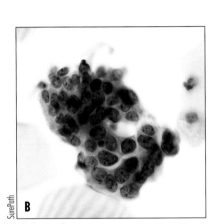

Tubal metaplasia

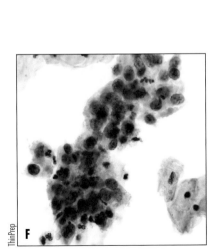

Endocervical polyp

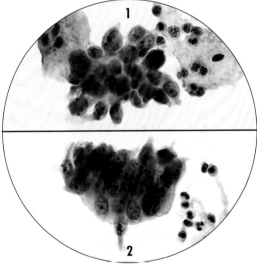

A. Endocervical adenocarcinoma
1,2. ThinPrep

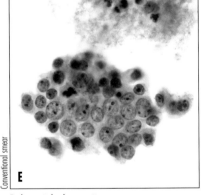

Endometrial adenocarcinoma

Squamous carcinoma in situ

Figure 7-15. Poorly-differentiated endocervical adenocarcinoma look-alikes.

Marked nuclear pleomorphism and disarray along with a three-dimensional architecture characterize poorly differentiated endocervical adenocarcinoma (A). These features can be seen to variable degrees in both benign and malignant conditions including IUD effect (B), endocervical repair (C), fallopian tube adenocarcinoma (D), high-grade endometrial adenocarcinoma (E), and squamous carcinoma (F). Refer to chapters 4, 5, and 6 for a more complete description of these entities.

Conventional smear

C

Endocervical repair

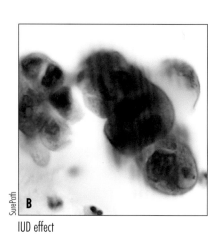

SurePath

B

IUD effect

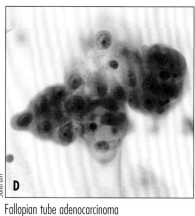

SurePath

D

Fallopian tube adenocarcinoma

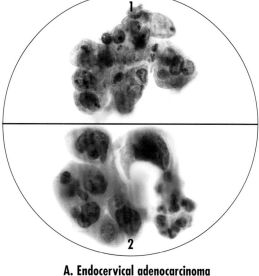

1

2

A. Endocervical adenocarcinoma
1. ThinPrep
2. SurePath

ThinPrep

E

Endometrial adenocarcinoma

ThinPrep

F

Squamous carcinoma

Figure 7-16. Well-differentiated endometrial adenocarcinoma look-alikes.

Well-differentiated endometrial adenocarcinoma can take on two different appearances: one with small nuclei and vacuolated cytoplasm (A1), and the second with small nuclei and scant cytoplasm (A2). Vacuolated cytoplasm with similar morphology can be seen in endocervical cells demonstrating Arias-Stella change (B), IUD effect (C), endometrial hyperplasia (D), and, rarely, squamous carcinoma in situ. Small cells with scant cytoplasm are features that can also be found in benign shedding endometrium (E), squamous carcinoma in situ (F), the stripped nuclei of parabasal cells in atrophic specimens (G), and the endometrioid variant of AIS (H). Refer to chapters 4, 5, and 6 for a more complete description of these entities.

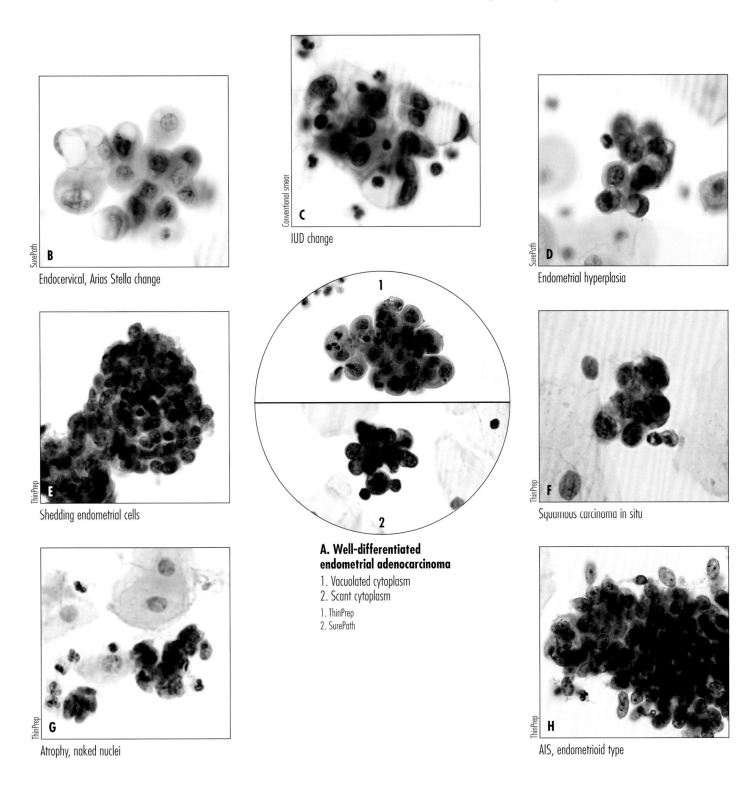

B — SurePath
Endocervical, Arias Stella change

C — Conventional smear
IUD change

D — SurePath
Endometrial hyperplasia

E — ThinPrep
Shedding endometrial cells

F — ThinPrep
Squamous carcinoma in situ

G — ThinPrep
Atrophy, naked nuclei

H — ThinPrep
AIS, endometrioid type

A. Well-differentiated endometrial adenocarcinoma

1. Vacuolated cytoplasm
2. Scant cytoplasm

1. ThinPrep
2. SurePath

Spectrums

It is interesting to look back over the history of gynecologic cytology and realize that from the beginning the pioneers in the field were able to define cytologic features that resulted in very detailed classification schemes. Early on it was recognized that there were spectrums of change, with dysplasia developing from different types of benign cells with increasing levels of abnormality ranging from benign to malignant. Even now, with our increased understanding of HPV and its role in the development of dysplasia and carcinoma, we recognize these spectrums of change and have integrated them into the most recent diagnostic nomenclature, the Bethesda System. However, there are overlaps in the cytologic characteristics between all of the diagnostic categories. At the simplest level, benign squamous nuclei have a range of nuclear size that overlaps with

ASC-US and even with LSIL and HSIL. All of the diagnostic features present in all of the cells on a slide must be integrated to come up with a final diagnosis.

The following series of figures will illustrate various morphologic spectrums of change in cervical/vaginal specimens. Some of these will demonstrate the spectrums seen in the development of squamous or glandular abnormalities, starting with benign cells and ending with dysplasia or carcinoma. Other types of spectrums will be shown, demonstrating the range of changes present within specific entities. It is important to recognize that the changes shown represent a morphologic spectrum and not necessarily a continuous biologic spectrum of progression from preneoplasia to intraepithelial neoplasia and finally to invasive carcinoma.

Morphologic Squamous Spectrums

Figure 7-17. Perinuclear halos: Benign to koilocytic.

Perinuclear halos are often present in squamous cells and, as detailed in chapter 5, may be associated with HPV infection. There is a morphologic spectrum seen in these halos, ranging from small perinuclear vacuoles in benign reactive cells to diagnostic koilocytic halos of LSIL. Reactive halos are small without peripheral condensation of the cytoplasm and are often seen in the background of acute inflammation or infection (A). Classically these halos are associated with *Trichomonas* (B), but they may also be seen with other infections, such as *Candida*. Larger halos may be present in intermediate squamous cells containing significant amounts of cytoplasmic glycogen (C). The halos of glycogenated cells tend to lack the optical clearing associated with true koilocytes and often contain yellow refractile material. Perinuclear halos, which are suggestive of but not diagnostic for LSIL, are included in the ASC-US category (D). At the dysplastic end of the halo spectrum, true koilocytes are defined by the large, optically clear, perinuclear halo with peripheral condensation of the cytoplasm (E).

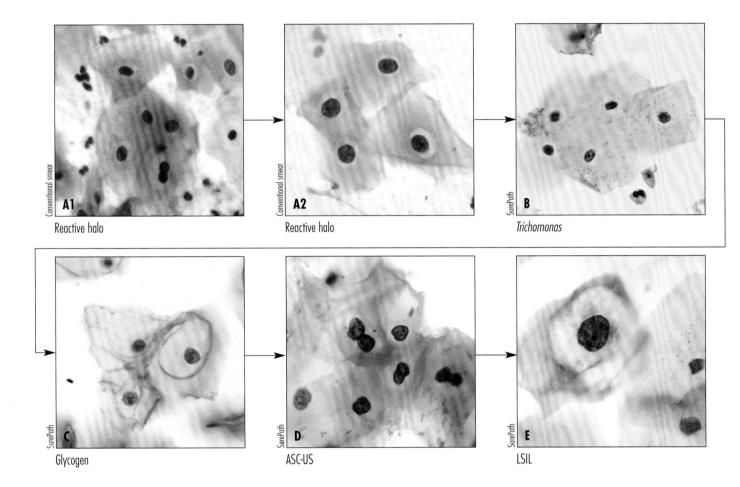

A1 — Conventional smear — Reactive halo

A2 — Conventional smear — Reactive halo

B — SurePath — *Trichomonas*

C — SurePath — Glycogen

D — SurePath — ASC-US

E — SurePath — LSIL

Figure 7-18. Mature large squamous cells: Benign to LSIL.

The morphologic spectrum in mature squamous cells is defined by changes in the nuclei, from small and round in superficial and intermediate cells to large and irregular in LSIL. There is significant variability in nuclear size, which was defined early on by cytomorphologists such as Patten (1978). Detailed measurements of nuclear areas showed that normal intermediate nuclei range from 28 to 50 µm^2 and benign squamous metaplastic cell nuclei range from 39 to 63 µm^2. The nuclei of classic mild dysplasia (LSIL) are the largest seen in squamous cells but show even more variation in size, ranging from 146 to 210 µm^2. These measurements were used to define the criteria for abnormal nuclear size and became the basis for the commonly used approach of comparing the area of the normal intermediate cell nucleus to other cells present in the Pap specimen. As a standard, however, these sizes may show considerable variation from patient to patient, especially in older women or in the background of inflammation. Individual Pap slides may show either little or alternatively significant variation in nuclear size, and, when large nuclei are seen, it is important to determine if they lie within the spectrum of size seen in the rest of the specimen or indeed represent an abnormal outlier more appropriately classified as an epithelial cell abnormality. Figure 7-18 demonstrates the spectrum of nuclear size seen in mature squamous cells. This spectrum begins with superficial squamous nuclei (A), continues with intermediate nuclei (B), and ranges up through reactive change (C), perimenopausal change (D), ASC-US (E), and finally to LSIL (F).

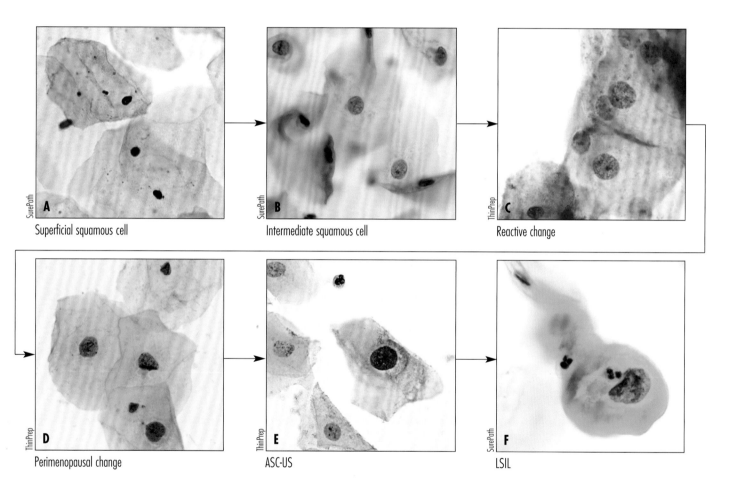

A — Superficial squamous cell

B — Intermediate squamous cell

C — Reactive change

D — Perimenopausal change

E — ASC-US

F — LSIL

Figure 7-19. Single small squamous cells: Benign to HSIL.

The morphologic spectrum of small squamous cells begins with parabasal-like cells and extends though squamous metaplastic cells, ASC-H, ending with HSIL. Within this spectrum, the differential diagnosis is generally between reactive cellular changes involving squamous metaplasia and high-grade dysplasia. Individually, these types of cells have been described in chapters 4 and 5. At the benign end, the cells are small and immature with round regular nuclei and an intermediate N:C ratio (A). The cells in this image most often represent a combination of reserve (arrow) and parabasal or early squamous metaplastic cells. More mature metaplastic and parabasal cells will show lower N:C ratios and slightly larger nuclei with a more polygonal cytoplasmic configuration (B). These are from a postpartum patient. Atypical changes to these cells develop with increasing N:C ratios and significant nuclear membrane irregularities. There will also be increasing variation in nuclear sizes and shapes. These changes may be difficult to classify as either benign (C) or atypical (D). If atypical, they would fit in the Bethesda classification of ASC-H. At the dysplastic end of the spectrum, the nuclear abnormalities become diagnostic of HSIL, with high N:C ratios, nuclear hyperchromasia, coarse nuclear chromatin, and nuclear membrane notching (E). These findings are also illustrated in chapter 5 (Figures 5-12 and 5-13).

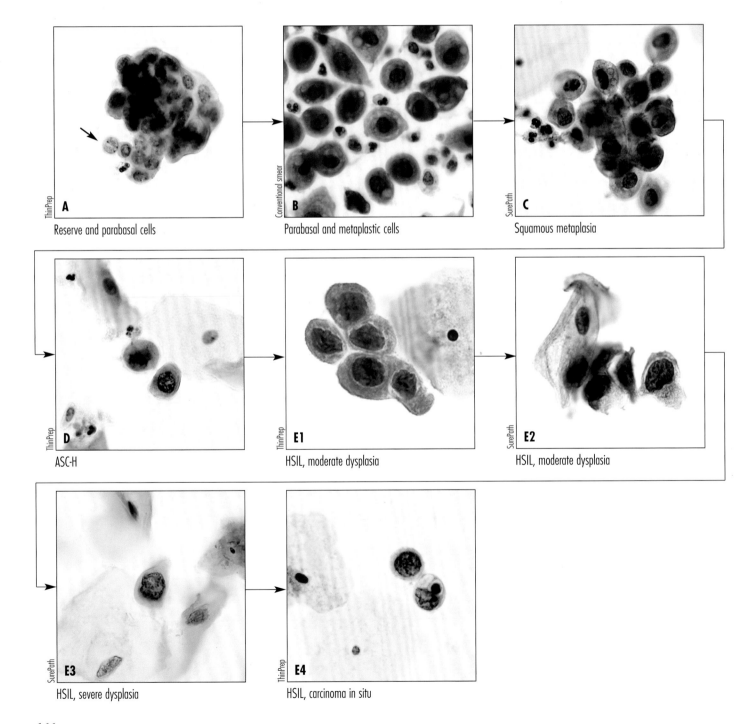

A — Reserve and parabasal cells

B — Parabasal and metaplastic cells

C — Squamous metaplasia

D — ASC-H

E1 — HSIL, moderate dysplasia

E2 — HSIL, moderate dysplasia

E3 — HSIL, severe dysplasia

E4 — HSIL, carcinoma in situ

Figure 7-20. Hyperchromatic crowded groups: Benign to HSIL.

As mentioned previously in this chapter and in detail in chapter 5, the cells of HSIL often present as hyperchromatic crowded groups, which are three-dimensional, thick, cellular clusters of dysplastic squamous cells. These groups may represent full-thickness fragments from the surface epithelium or cohesive groups removed from endocervical crypts. They are more commonly seen with the advent of modern sampling devices and may present a difficult diagnostic challenge due to the thickness and hyperchromaticity of the cells. In HSIL, the cells making up a hyperchromatic crowded group will demonstrate significant anisonucleosis and nuclear membrane irregularity, which is best appreciated at the edges of the clusters. Mitotic figures and apoptotic bodies are common. Also as noted previously (Figure 7-19), there is a spectrum of change in single immature squamous cells that ranges from benign to severely dysplastic (NILM to HSIL). This spectrum is also seen in hyperchromatic crowded groups, beginning with benign clusters of metaplastic cells (A), evolving into atypical groups that would fall into the ASC-H category (B), and finally ending with diagnostic HSIL (C). Throughout this progression, the hyperchromasia and N:C ratios increase, nuclear membranes become more irregular, and nuclear size can become quite variable.

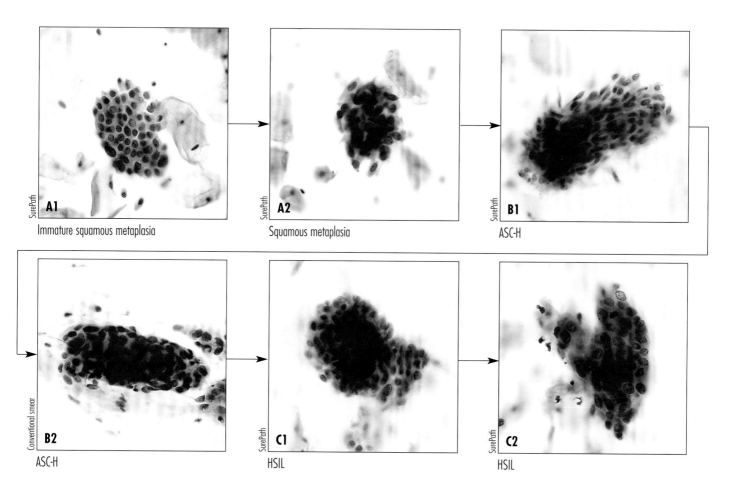

A1 — SurePath
Immature squamous metaplasia

A2 — SurePath
Squamous metaplasia

B1 — SurePath
ASC-H

B2 — Conventional smear
ASC-H

C1 — SurePath
HSIL

C2 — SurePath
HSIL

Figure 7-21. Abnormally keratinized cells: Benign to carcinoma.

The normal cervical/vaginal mucosa is nonkeratinizing, with three cell layers composed of basal cells at the base, intermediate squamous cells in the middle, and a surface layer of superficial squamous cells. Under certain reactive, hormonal, or, occasionally, neoplastic conditions, the mucosa may become keratinizing, with three additional layers: a surface with anucleated squamous cells, a parakeratotic layer, and an underlying granular layer. The morphologic spectrum in keratinizing squamous cells is related to cells derived from this abnormally keratinized surface layer. Anucleated squamous cells appear as hyperkeratosis on Pap specimens (A). As noted above, these are most often related to a benign underlying condition, and the presence of a few anucleated squamous cells does not warrant mention in the report (see Figure 4-3).

Hyperkeratosis may be accompanied by parakeratosis, or small keratinizing cells resembling miniature superficial cells (B). Typical parakeratosis is also considered to be benign (see Figure 4-7). Parakeratotic cells may develop greater nuclear size and shape variation with increasing N:C ratios. These changes are abnormal and fall into the category of ASC-US (C) or ASC-H (D), depending on the level of suspicion for LSIL or HSIL. The type of hyperkeratosis may also vary as the degree of abnormality increases from essentially normal superficial cells lacking nuclei (A) to more bizarre anucleated forms. When these more bizarre forms are present, there should be a careful search for abnormal nucleated cells. At the upper end of the spectrum of keratinization is the markedly abnormal keratinizing cells, both nucleated and anucleated, associated with either HSIL (E) or keratinizing squamous cell carcinoma (F).

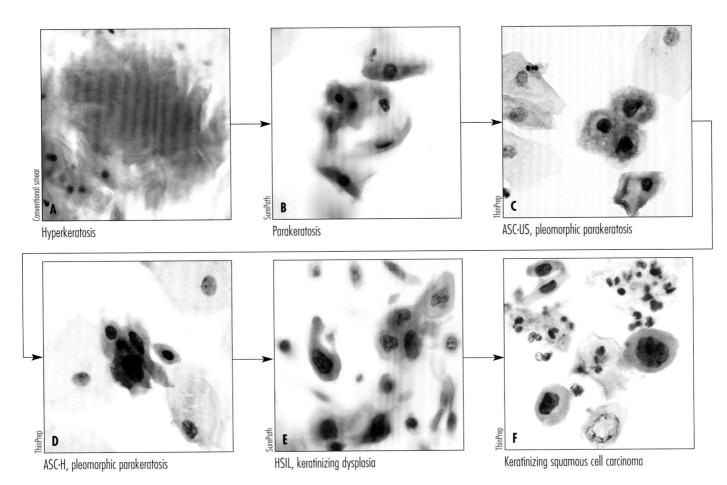

Conventional smear

A

Hyperkeratosis

SurePath

B

Parakeratosis

ThinPrep

C

ASC-US, pleomorphic parakeratosis

ThinPrep

D

ASC-H, pleomorphic parakeratosis

SurePath

E

HSIL, keratinizing dysplasia

ThinPrep

F

Keratinizing squamous cell carcinoma

Figure 7-22. Cells with nucleoli: Reactive to carcinoma.

Prominent nucleoli may be present in squamous cells ranging from benign lesions with reactive changes to invasive carcinoma. This is an interesting morphologic spectrum because it, for the most part, skips over intraepithelial squamous dysplasia, as the cells of SIL tend to have no or inconspicuous nucleoli (with the notable exception of HSIL involving endocervical gland crypts). Benign squamous cells with nucleoli are generally derived from a reactive/reparative process. These cells tend to form two-dimensional streaming sheets composed of cohesive cells. The nuclei tend to have single prominent nucleoli and may demonstrate an occasional normal mitotic figure. Classic repair may be seen in an inflammatory background, but necrosis is not common (A). Occasionally, these cells start to loose cohesion, form thicker groups, or demonstrate significant nuclear abnormalities (B). These findings are in the morphologic gray zone between benign repair and invasive carcinoma and should be flagged as atypical (see Figure 5-6). At the malignant end of the spectrum, the cells loose cohesion, malignant nuclear changes become apparent (see Figure 5-21), abnormal mitoses may be seen, and a background tumor diathesis is commonly present (C).

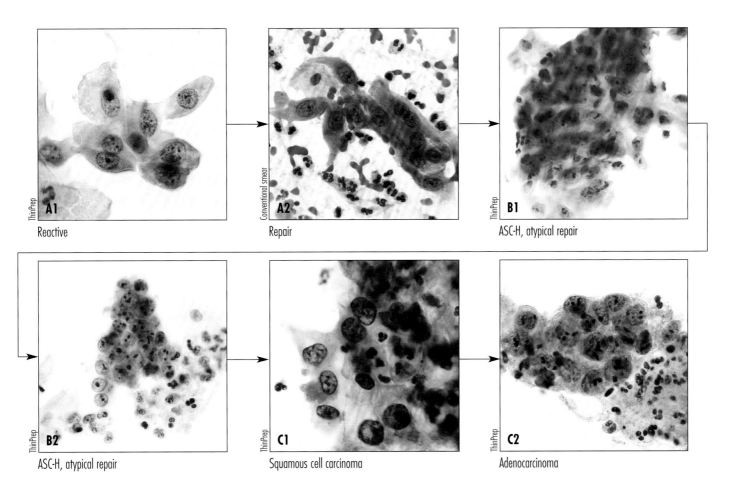

A1 — Reactive (ThinPrep)

A2 — Repair (Conventional smear)

B1 — ASC-H, atypical repair (ThinPrep)

B2 — ASC-H, atypical repair (ThinPrep)

C1 — Squamous cell carcinoma (ThinPrep)

C2 — Adenocarcinoma (ThinPrep)

Morphologic Glandular Spectrums

Figure 7-23. Endocervical cells: Benign to malignant, architecture.

The architectural spectrum of endocervical cells ranges from flat cellular groups with evenly spaced nuclei and distinct cell borders in benign endocervical cells to progressively more crowded nuclei that become overlapped, palisaded, and polarized in AIS. These changes are seen beginning with benign endocervical cells with an orderly honeycomb architecture (A) and continue with benign reactive endocervical cells with some nuclear overlap (B). Atypical endocervical cells with palisading and stratifica-

tion suggesting AIS are next (C), and cells diagnostic of AIS (D). Finally, some cases of AIS can begin to show features suspicious for invasive adenocarcinoma, with significant pleomorphism of size and shape and poorly organized architecture (E). Another architectural change is increasing nuclear disarray within the cell groups, associated with a variable amount of cytoplasm and thickness within the cell groups, and finally arriving at the marked disarray and discohesion associated with invasive adenocarcinoma. Early changes include loss of polarization (F), advancing to marked disarray with overlapping (G), and ending at the malignant end of the spectrum, where the architectural changes are diagnostic of adenocarcinoma (H).

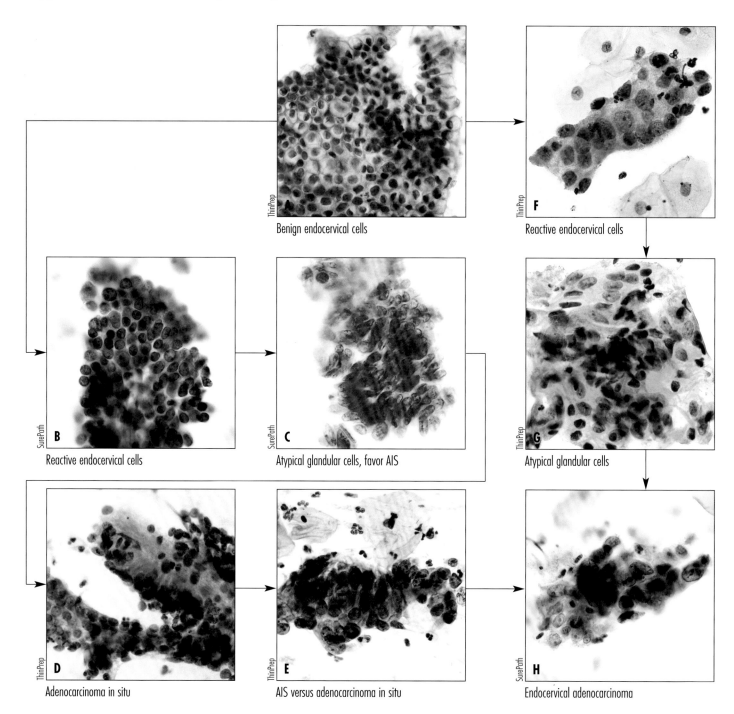

Benign endocervical cells

Reactive endocervical cells (F)

Reactive endocervical cells (B)

Atypical glandular cells, favor AIS (C)

Atypical glandular cells (G)

Adenocarcinoma in situ (D)

AIS versus adenocarcinoma in situ (E)

Endocervical adenocarcinoma (H)

Figure 7-24. Endocervical cells: Benign to malignant, nuclear features.

Benign endocervical cell nuclei are small, with round to slightly oval contours. In the spectrum of benign endocervical cells to AIS, progressive nuclear elongation and hyperchromasia with a fine to moderately coarse chromatin pattern are seen. These features progress through reactive endocervical gland changes (A2), endocervical polyp (B), atypical endocervical cells (C), and AIS (D). The transition between the tightly compacted, hyperchromatic, elongate nuclei of AIS and the angular vesicular nuclei of adenocarcinoma is presented in E. The spectrum of nuclear changes from benign to adenocarcinoma can also demonstrate nuclear enlargement with vesicular chromatin and prominent nucleoli. Relatively smooth nuclear contours are present with reactive endocervical cells (A3), and this feature progresses through repair (F) and ends with invasive carcinoma. Within this spectrum, the nuclei start to exhibit irregular nuclear contours and variable nuclear size differences (G), which becomes more apparent in endocervical adenocarcinoma (H).

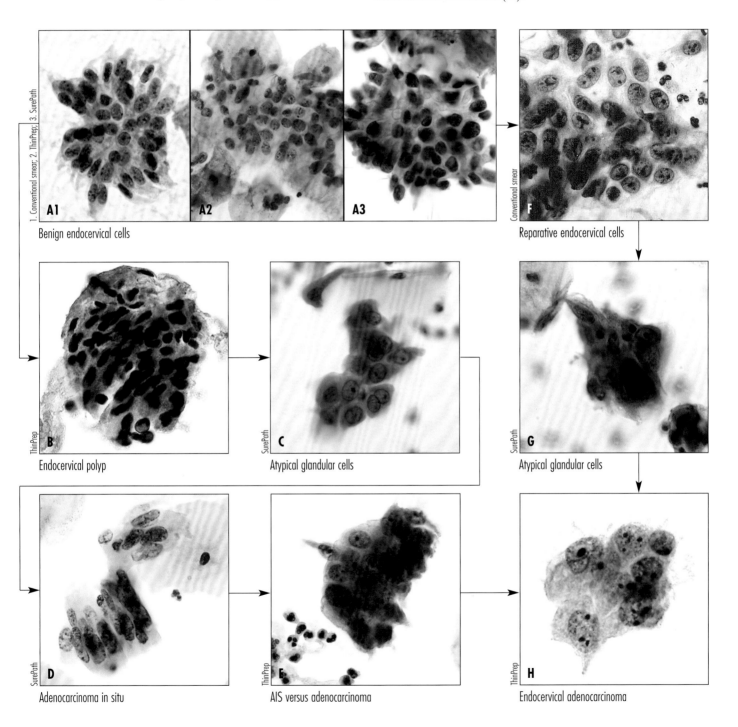

1. Conventional smear; 2. ThinPrep; 3. SurePath

A1 **A2** **A3**
Benign endocervical cells

Conventional smear
F
Reparative endocervical cells

ThinPrep
B
Endocervical polyp

SurePath
C
Atypical glandular cells

SurePath
G
Atypical glandular cells

SurePath
D
Adenocarcinoma in situ

ThinPrep
E
AIS versus adenocarcinoma

ThinPrep
H
Endocervical adenocarcinoma

Figure 7-25. Endometrial cells: Benign to malignant.

The spectrum of endometrial cells in cervical specimens include the benign shedding pattern, which can range from very small cells in small clusters (A1), to small cells with larger complex cell groups (A2), to slightly larger cells in loose clusters (A3). Stromal cells with more abundant cytoplasm (likely hormonal influence) may also be seen (B). The shedding clusters of menstrual endometrium (C) are biphasic, with collapsed stromal cores wrapped by syncytial-appearing epithelial cells. Reactive endometrial cellular changes associated with IUD effect (D) are indistinguishable from atypical endometrial cells (E). Likewise, endometrial hyperplasia (F) can be indistinguishable from well-differentiated endometrial adenocarcinoma. Poorly differentiated endometrial adenocarcinoma (G) is more readily distinguished from hyperplasia but may be difficult to distinguish from endocervical adenocarcinoma.

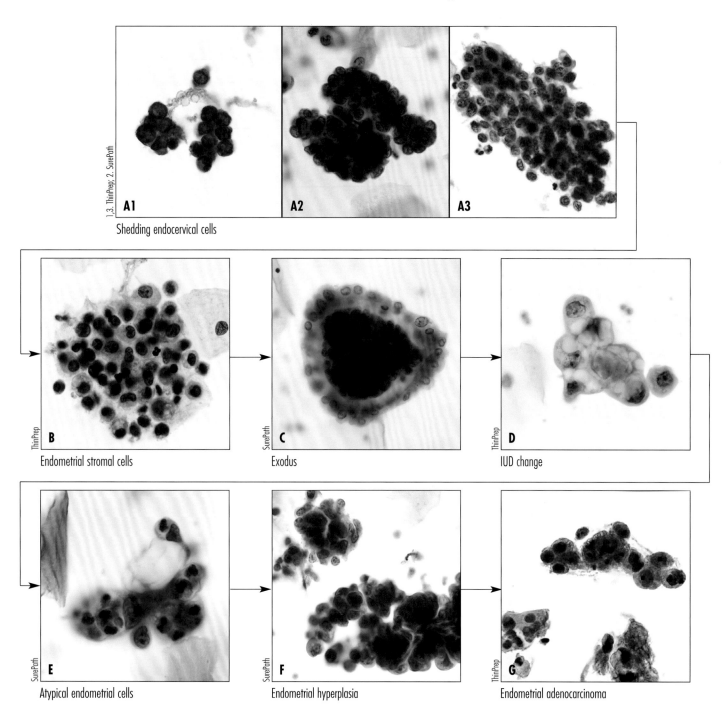

Shedding endocervical cells

Endometrial stromal cells

Exodus

IUD change

Atypical endometrial cells

Endometrial hyperplasia

Endometrial adenocarcinoma

Figure 7-26. Tubal metaplasia: Spectrum of morphologic features.

Tubal metaplasia can present with many morphologic appearances, depending on the preparation type and the degree of preservation within the cytology specimen. Conventional preparations will produce flatter, more open cell groups in which the nuclear features, cilia, and terminal may be more readily appreciated (A1). Liquid-based preparations allow the cell groups to round up and become more three-dimensional (A2). Tubal metaplasia is often easy to recognize in cytology specimens because of the presence of cilia or terminal bars (A3). However, mechani-

cal disruption of the cell groups by sampling and smearing may disrupt or remove the cilia (B). When degenerative changes are superimposed on these types of cell groups, they may take on the appearance of atypical glandular cells (C). Tubal metaplasia that originates from the upper endocervical canal typically demonstrates higher N:C ratios (tuboendometrioid metaplasia). These groups demonstrate significant crowding and hyperchromasia on Pap specimens (D). Finally, some cases of tubal metaplasia may demonstrate nuclear elongation, hyperchromasia, and nuclear palisading. This overlap can very closely mimic AIS (E).

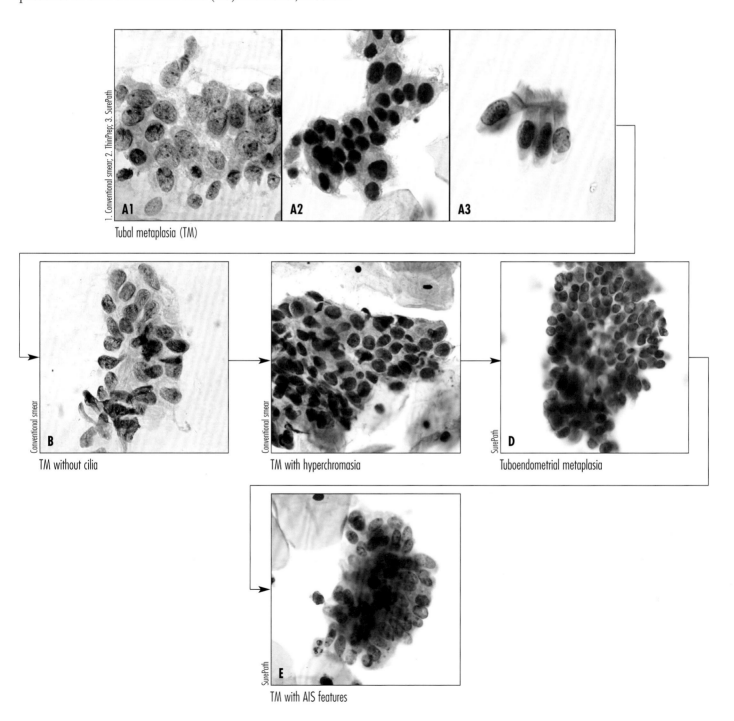

Tubal metaplasia (TM)

TM without cilia

TM with hyperchromasia

Tuboendometrial metaplasia

TM with AIS features

Figure 7-27. Endocervical adenocarcinoma in situ: Spectrum of morphologic features.

The cell groups of adenocarcinoma in situ may not always demonstrate classic features. Some groups may retain cytoplasmic mucin (A). Additional features that may lend a "reactive" endocervical cell appearance include slightly more open chromatin pattern with small visible chromocenters (B), or more abundant cytoplasm reducing the degree of nuclear crowding (C). The abnormal acinar arrangements, nuclear shape, and three-dimensional appearance help to identify these groups as abnormal.

The endometrioid variant of AIS has smaller nuclei (8 to 10 μm^2) and typically scant cytoplasm, bringing directly sampled LUS into the differential diagnosis (D). Close inspection will reveal significant nuclear hyperchromasia and architectural arrangements that support a diagnosis of AIS. The intestinal variant of AIS contains true goblet cells and resembles colonic adenocarcinoma (E).

Some cases of AIS may include cellular groups that have more rounded or angulated nuclei or chromatin granules that are coarser and larger than are typically present in AIS (F). These are nuclear features that are more commonly noted in squamous carcinoma in situ (CIS). While the nuclear polarization and acinar arrangements may help to confirm a glandular nature for the abnormal groups, these same architectural features can occasionally be seen in CIS involving endocervical glands. Finally, some AIS lesions are characterized by marked pleomorphism, including nuclear size variation, angulation, and visible nucleoli (G).

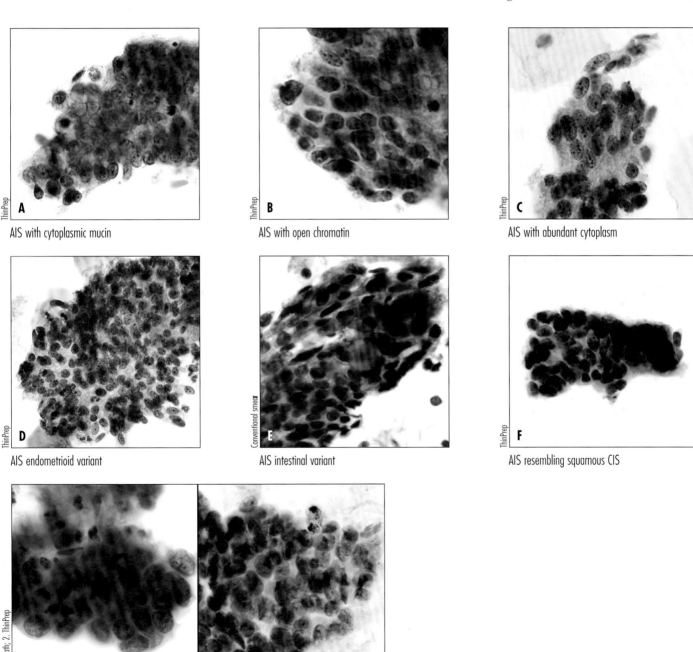

AIS with cytoplasmic mucin

AIS with open chromatin

AIS with abundant cytoplasm

AIS endometrioid variant

AIS intestinal variant

AIS resembling squamous CIS

AIS with nuclear pleomorphism

Figure 7-28. Endometrial adenocarcinoma: Spectrum of morphologic features.

Endometrial adenocarcinomas are graded from low grade (FIGO Grade 1) to intermediate grade (FIGO Grade 2) and high grade (FIGO Grade 3 endometrioid, serous and clear cell carcinoma). Low-grade endometrial adenocarcinomas are most commonly of the endometrioid type and exhibit small cells with scant cytoplasm (A) or occasionally intra-

cytoplasmic neutrophils (B). These tumors are often indistinguishable from endometrial hyperplasia or shedding endometrium (Figure 7-25). Intermediate-grade endometrioid tumors show progressive nuclear and cellular enlargement with nuclear atypia (C). High-grade endometrial adenocarcinomas can be of the endometrioid type, sometimes with squamous differentiation (D), or they can be of the clear cell (E) or serous (F) types.

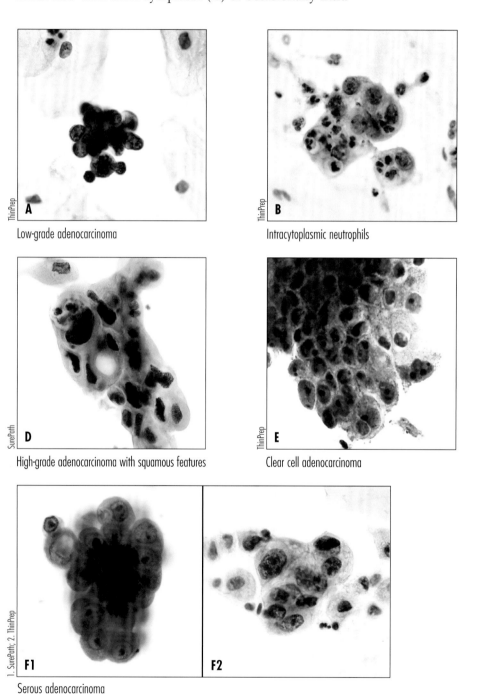

Low-grade adenocarcinoma

Intracytoplasmic neutrophils

Intermediate-grade adenocarcinoma

High-grade adenocarcinoma with squamous features

Clear cell adenocarcinoma

Serous adenocarcinoma

Bibliography

Chen TC. Proposed diagnostic flow chart for cervical smears. *Diagn Cytopathol.* 2004;30(3):212-215.

Patten SF. Diagnostic *Cytopathology of the Uterine Cervix. Monographs in Clinical Cytology.* 2nd ed. New York: S Karger; 1978.

Solomon D, Nayar R, eds. *The Bethesda System for Reporting Cervical Cytology. Definitions, Criteria, and Explanatory Notes.* 2nd ed. New York: Springer; 2004

Wright TC Jr, Massad LS, Dunton CJ, Spitzer M, Wilkinson EJ, Solomon D; 2006 American Society for Colposcopy and Cervical Pathology-sponsored Consensus Conference. 2006 consensus guidelines for the management of women with abnormal cervical cancer screening tests. *Am J Obstet Gynecol.* 2007;197(4):346-355.

Anal Cytology

Teresa Marie Darragh, MD

Introduction

Anal cytology, or anal-rectal cytology (ARC), may be used to screen for human papillomavirus (HPV)-related changes of the anal canal in a manner analogous to the cervical Pap test; it was included as part of the 2001 Bethesda System.[1] The similarities between cervical and anal cytology are numerous and far outweigh their differences. Anal cytology is reported using Bethesda terminology, modified only to body site.

The knowledge we have gained from cervical screening over the last half century can be applied to anal cancer screening.[2,3] Although anal cancer screening guidelines have not yet been formally adopted, studies have shown that anal cytologic screening, in conjunction with a digital rectal examination, is a useful tool, particularly in individuals most at risk for developing anal cancer: men who have sex with men; and all individuals with HIV disease, regardless of gender or sexual orientation.[4-7]

Sampling

The goal of ARC is to sample the entire anal canal, from the colonic mucosa of the rectal vault to the keratinized squamous mucosa at the anal verge. At rest, the mucosa of this region is opposed due to the resting tension of the anal sphincters. Anatomically, the anal canal contains a region of squamous metaplasia analogous to the transformation zone of the uterine cervix. This region is located proximal to the dentate line and merges with the glandular mucosa of the distal rectum. Similar to the leading edge of the cervical transformation zone, this region of immature squamous metaplastic cells is thought to be particularly susceptible to the oncogenic influences of high-risk HPV types.

Typically, the cellular sample for ARC is collected using a water-moistened Dacron swab. The swab is inserted into the distal rectum and then withdrawn in a cone-shaped arc, while applying lateral pressure. The swab is then rinsed in fixative for liquid-based cytology or smeared directly on a glass slide.

Morphology

As in cervical cytology, superficial and intermediate squamous cells and squamous metaplastic cells are seen. Rectal columnar cells are the ARC counterpart of endocervical glandular cells. Anucleate squamous cells are a normal component and arise from sampling of the keratinized, distal portion of the anal canal (Figures 8-1 through 8-3).

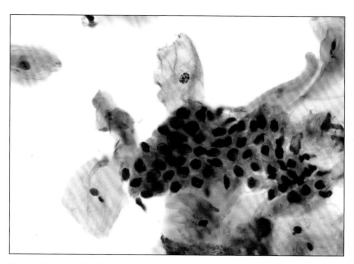

Figure 8-1. Rectal columnar cells and benign nucleated squamous cells. (Anal cytology, ThinPrep, high power.)

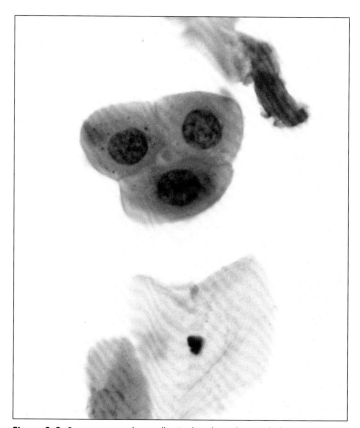

Figure 8-2. Squamous metaplastic cells. (Anal cytology, ThinPrep, high power.)

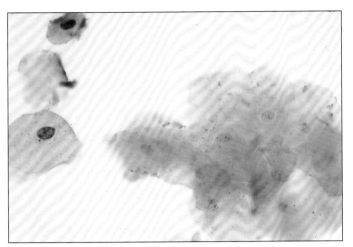

Figure 8-3. Anucleated squamous cells. (Anal cytology, ThinPrep, high power.)

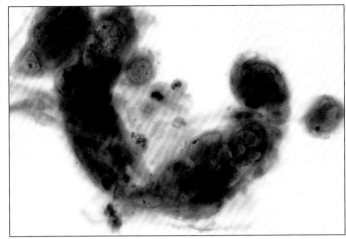

Figure 8-4. Herpes simplex virus infection. (Anal cytology, ThinPrep, high power.)

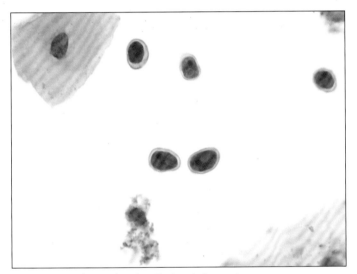

Figure 8-5. Ameba. (Anal cytology, ThinPrep, high power.)

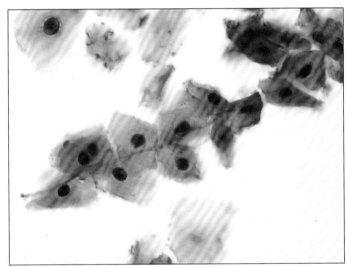

Figure 8-6. *Candida.* (Anal cytology, ThinPrep, high power.)

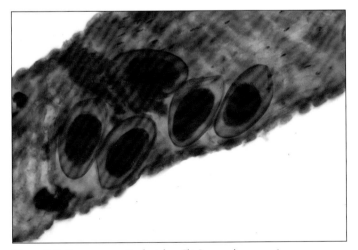

Figure 8-7. Pinworm eggs. (Anal cytology, ThinPrep, medium power.)

According to the Bethesda 2001 atlas, an adequate ARC consists of at least 2000 to 3000 nucleated squamous cells. This is equivalent to 1 to 2 nucleated squamous cells per high-power field (hpf) for ThinPrep preparations and 3 to 6 nucleated squamous cells/hpf for SurePath preparations.

A variety of organisms can also be encountered in ARC, some causing local disease similar to that seen in gynecologic cytology, while others are unique to the gastrointestinal tract. These organisms include viruses, protozoa, fungi, and helminthes (Figures 8-4 through 8-7).

HPV-Related Lesions of the Anal Canal

Morphologically, low-grade and high-grade lesions of the anal canal are very similar to their counterparts seen on gynecologic cytology. Given the juxtaposition of keratinized and nonkeratinized squamous mucosa in the anal canal, keratinized lesions are more commonly encountered on ARC than on cervical Paps. In addition, degenerative

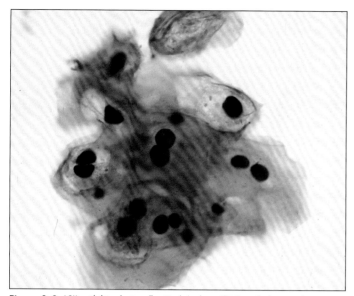

Figure 8-8. LSIL with binucleate cells. (Anal cytology, ThinPrep, high power.)

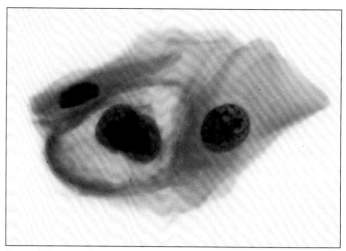

Figure 8-9. LSIL with HPV-cytopathic effect. (Anal cytology, ThinPrep, high power.)

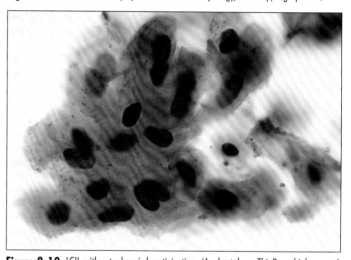

Figure 8-10. LSIL with cytoplasmic keratinization. (Anal cytology, ThinPrep, high power.)

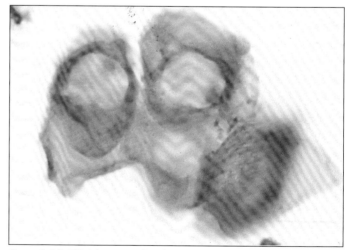

Figure 8-11. LSIL "ghosts." (Anal cytology, ThinPrep, high power.)

changes (eg, karyorrhexis) are frequently seen, especially in low-grade lesions.

Low-grade squamous intraepithelial lesion (LSIL) is characterized by some degree of nuclear abnormality in a cell with cytoplasmic maturation. The nuclear abnormalities include enlargement, nuclear chromatin alterations, nuclear contour irregularities, and binucleation and multinucleation (Figure 8-8). The classic cytoplasmic changes of perinuclear halos or koilocytosis are frequently seen in cells without evidence of marked cytoplasmic keratinization (Figure 8-9). Cytoplasmic halos may not be a prominent feature of LSIL when cytoplasmic keratinization is abundant (Figure 8-10). In addition, "empty halos" or LSIL "ghosts"—LSIL cells whose nucleus has degenerated—are frequently encountered on ARC (Figure 8-11).

As in gynecologic cytology, high-grade squamous intraepithelial lesion (HSIL) is characterized by cells with abnormal nuclei and high nuclear to cytoplasmic ratios (Figures 8-12 through 8-14). On ARC, HSIL can be seen as either individual dysplastic cells or clusters of dysplastic cells, frequently with metaplastic cytoplasm. In the high-risk population screened with ARC, a mixture of LSIL and HSIL in the same sample is common.

Management

The use of anal cytology as a screening test for anal intraepithelial lesions and cancer is still fairly new, and it is not yet clear how often it should be done or if it actually reduces the risk of anal cancer. Some experts recommend that the test be repeated yearly in HIV-positive men who have sex with men, and every 2 to 3 years if the men are HIV negative.[4,5] Patients with abnormal results should be referred for high-resolution anoscopy (the equivalent of cervical colposcopy) and biopsy. It is not clear whether or not reflex

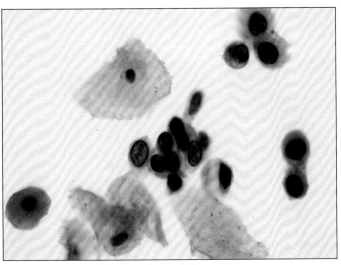

Figure 8-12. HSIL. (Anal cytology, ThinPrep, high power.)

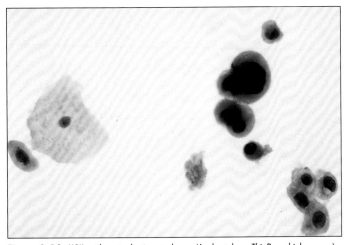

Figure 8-13. HSIL with metaplastic cytoplasm. (Anal cytology, ThinPrep, high power.)

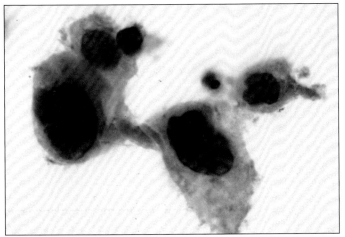

Figure 8-14. HSIL with prominent nuclear enlargement and nuclear contour irregularities. (Anal cytology, ThinPrep, high power.)

HPV testing for an anal cytology with atypical squamous cells of undetermined significance (ASC-US) is a useful adjunct, since the target populations for anal cancer screening have a high prevalence of HPV infection. Helpful information on this emerging topic of anal cancer screening can be found at the following websites: University of California, San Francisco, anal cancer information, www.analcancerinfo.ucsf.edu; the American Cancer Society, www.cancer.org; and the Centers for Disease Control and Prevention, www.cdc.gov.

References

1. Solomon D., Nayar R. *The Bethesda System for Reporting Cervical Cytology. Definitions, Criteria and Explanatory Notes.* 2nd ed. New York: Springer-Verlag; 2004.
2. Palefsky JM, Holly EA, Hogeboom CJ, Berry JM, Jay N, Darragh TM. Anal cytology as a screening tool for anal squamous intraepithelial lesions. *J Acquir Immune Defic Syndr Hum Retrovirol.* 1997;14:415-422.
3. Darragh TM. Anal cytology for anal cancer screening: is it time yet? *Diagn Cytopathol.* 2004;30(6):371-374.
4. Goldie SJ, Kuntz KM, Weinstein MC, Freedberg KA, Welton ML, Palefsky JM. The clinical effectiveness and cost-effectiveness of screening for anal squamous intraepithelial lesions in homosexual and bisexual HIV-positive men. *JAMA.* 1999;281:1822-1829.
5. Goldie SJ, Kuntz KM, Weinstein MC, Freedberg KA, Palefsky JM. Cost-effectiveness of screening for anal squamous intraepithelial lesions and anal cancer in human immunodeficiency virus-negative homosexual and bisexual men. *Am J Med.* 2000;108:634-641.
6. Piketty C, Darragh TM, Heard I, et al. High prevalence of anal squamous intraepithelial lesions in HIV-positive men despite use of highly active antiretroviral therapy. *Sex Transm Dis.* 2004;31(2):96-99.
7. Durante AJ, Williams AB, Da Costa M, Darragh TM, Khoshnood K, Palefsky JM. Incidence of anal cytologic abnormalities in a cohort of human immunodeficiency virus-infected women. *Cancer Epidemiol Biomarkers Prev.* 2003;12(7):638-642.

Management of Women with Abnormal Papanicolaou Tests

Ann T. Moriarty, MD
Karen M. Clary, MD

Introduction

Following the cervical cytology terminology changes made in the 2001 Bethesda Conference,[1] the American Society of Colposcopy and Cervical Pathology (ASCCP) Consensus Conference was convened in September of 2001. Using a web-based discussion format similar to that used in the 2001 Bethesda System deliberations, the ASCCP conference developed management algorithms for the newly designated Bethesda System categories of abnormal cervical cytology findings.[2] Five years later, the 2006 ASCCP Consensus Conference reconvened and modified the initial 2001 guidelines, based upon the scientific data which had been accumulated during the intervening years.[3] Several of the new management algorithms are published here with permission, including the follow-up for patients with biopsy-confirmed cervical intraepithelial neoplasia (CIN).[4] The major changes in follow-up and management of women with abnormal cervical cytology revolve around the recommendations for special clinical circumstances, including women who are age 20 years or younger, postmenopausal, pregnant, or immunosuppressed.

Atypical Squamous Cells

There are significantly different management guidelines, depending on whether a woman has atypical squamous cells of undetermined significance (ASC-US) or atypical squamous cells, cannot exclude high-grade intraepithelial lesion (ASC-H).

Atypical Squamous Cells of Undetermined Significance

Safe and effective (acceptable) methods for managing patients with ASC-US include (1) a program of repeat cervical cytology testing (two Pap tests at 6-month intervals), (2) colposcopy, or (3) DNA testing for high-risk human papillomavirus (HPV) types. Disadvantages to repeat cytology include lower sensitivity for detecting CIN II/III, necessitating repeat testing, multiple patient visits, and possible delays in the diagnosis of significant disease. Disadvantages to colposcopy include expense and the potential for overdiagnosis and overtreatment. The *preferred* management for patients with ASC-US detected with liquid-based Pap test specimens, or Pap tests with a co-collected specimen, is to perform oncogenic or high-risk HPV (hrHPV) DNA testing. In many laboratories, this is now a routine protocol, with hrHPV testing being performed in a reflex manner with all ASC-US Pap tests ("reflex testing"). A positive hrHPV result necessitates col-

poscopy; a negative hrHPV result allows for repeat cytological screening at 12 months (Figure 9-1). Women with ASC-US Pap test results who are hrHPV positive have the same risk of having CIN II/III as those with cytologic results of low-grade squamous intraepithelial lesion (LSIL) and are managed in an identical fashion.[5] If no lesion is identified at colposcopy, and the colposcopic examination is satisfactory, repeat hrHPV testing at 12 months postcolposcopy is acceptable; repeat hrHPV testing should not be done before a 12-month interval. Repeat Pap tests at 6 and 12 months are also an acceptable alternate postcolposcopy follow-up for women with hrHPV-positive ASC-US with no lesion detected at an adequate colposcopy. Any unsatisfactory colposcopy or "negative" colposcopy (a colposcopic examination that does not identify visible abnormalities) should be accompanied by endocervical sampling. Endocervical sampling is also acceptable when a lesion is detected at the transformation zone.

When repeat cytology is used as a follow-up for an initial ASC-US Pap test, cytological testing should be used at 6-month and 12-month intervals until a result of negative for squamous intraepithelial lesion or malignancy (NILM) is obtained. If either follow-up Pap test reveals an abnormality of ASC-US or greater, a colposcopic examination is required.

When colposcopy is performed as a follow-up for an ASC-US Pap test result (with either a positive hrHPV result, without hrHPV testing triage, or for a repeat cytologic examination of ASC-US or greater), women with biopsy-proven CIN should be managed according to the appropriate 2006 ASCCP consensus guideline for the management of cervical intraepithelial neoplasia.[4] For those women who have an initial Pap test interpretation of ASC-US and a negative satisfactory colposcopy, repeat Pap testing at 12 months is recommended.

ASC-US in Special Populations

In adolescent women (20 years and younger), the prevalence of acute hrHPV infection is high; the cumulative rate of infection is 71% in women 18 to 22 years old.[5] The risk for high-grade squamous intraepithelial lesion (HSIL) and invasive carcinoma is low in this adolescent population. Additionally, consecutive HPV infections of different high-risk types may masquerade as persistent hrHPV infection in this population. Using hrHPV for colposcopic referral in this population would result in frequent colposcopic examinations for transient infections, with resultant possible overtreatment, leading to potential and unnecessary com-

181

Management of Women with Atypical Squamous Cells of Undetermined Significance (ASC-US)

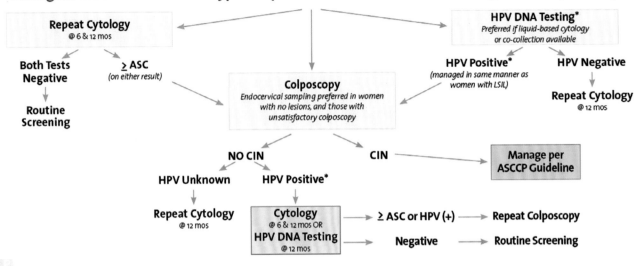

* Test only for high-risk (oncogenic) types of HPV

Figure 9-1. Management of women with atypical squamous cells of undetermined significance (ASC-US).

Reprinted from *The Journal of Lower Genital Tract Disease* Vol. 11 Issue 4, with permission of ASCCP © American Society for Colposcopy and Cervical Pathology 2007. No copies of the algorithms may be made without the prior consent of ASCCP.

Management of Adolescent Women with Either Atypical Squamous Cells of Undetermined Significance (ASC-US) or Low-grade Squamous Intraepithelial Lesion (LSIL)

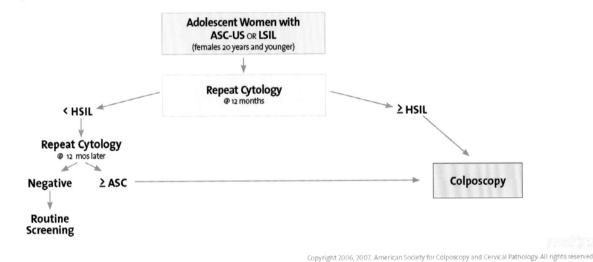

Figure 9-2. Management of adolescent women with either atypical squamous cells of undetermined significance (ASC-US) or low-grade squamous intraepithelial lesion (LSIL).

Reprinted from *The Journal of Lower Genital Tract Disease* Vol. 11 Issue 4, with permission of ASCCP © American Society for Colposcopy and Cervical Pathology 2007. No copies of the algorithms may be made without the prior consent of ASCCP.

plications. Adolescents with ASC-US interpretations on Pap tests should have repeat cytology at 12 months (Figure 9-2). Young women with HSIL on repeat cytology at 12 months should be referred for colposcopy. After 24 months, young women with persistent ASC-US or greater should be referred to colposcopy. For women age 20 years and younger, hrHPV reflex testing or colposcopy is *unacceptable* as a follow-up for an initial ASC-US Pap test. ASCCP guidelines go so far as to indicate, "If HPV testing is inadvertently performed, the results should not influence management."[3] Pregnant women older than 20 years, post-

menopausal women, and immunosuppressed women with ASC-US are managed in the same manner as the general population, with the exception that pregnant women with ASC-US should never undergo endocervical sampling, and it is acceptable to defer the initial colposcopy until 6 weeks postpartum.

Atypical Squamous Cells, Cannot Exclude High-Grade Intraepithelial Lesion

Because of the higher likelihood of histologic follow-up with CIN II/III and the presence of hrHPV in patients with

Management of Women with Atypical Squamous Cells: Cannot Exclude High-grade SIL (ASC - H)

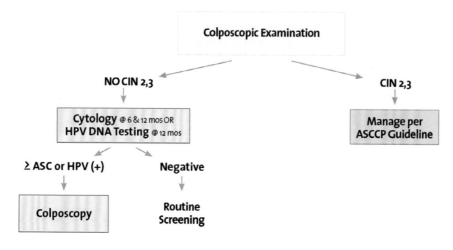

Figure 9-3. Management of women with atypical squamous cells: cannot exclude high-grade SIL (ASC-H).

Management of Women with Low-grade Squamous Intraepithelial Lesion (LSIL) *

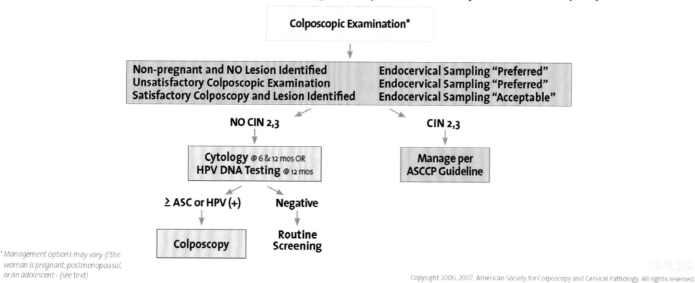

Management options may vary if the woman is pregnant, postmenopausal, or an adolescent - (see text)

Figure 9-4. Management of women with low-grade squamous intraepithelial lesion (LSIL).

ASC-H, colposcopy is recommended for initial management. Reflex hrHPV testing is not recommended for cases interpreted as ASC-H. When CIN II/III is not identified at colposcopy, follow-up with hrHPV testing at 12 months *or* cytology at 6 and 12 months is acceptable. Repeat colposcopy is recommended for those with recurring ASC-US or greater abnormality on repeat cytology or hrHPV detected at 12 months. If hrHPV is not detected at 12 months, or two consecutive Pap tests are interpreted as negative for intraepithelial lesion or malignancy (NILM), the patient can be returned to a routine screening program (Figure 9-3).

Low-Grade Squamous Intraepithelial Lesion

Women with LSIL have the same risk for the presence of CIN II and CIN III as women with hrHPV-positive ASC-US and are therefore managed in a similar fashion. Colposcopy is the first step for women in the general population with LSIL. Colposcopy with endocervical sampling is preferred for unsatisfactory colposcopy or in cases when no lesion is identified at the time of colposcopy. Endocervical sampling is also acceptable for those patients with a visible lesion in the transformation zone (Figure 9-4). For adolescents, instead of immediate colposcopy,

Management of Women with High-grade Squamous Intraepithelial Lesion (HSIL) *

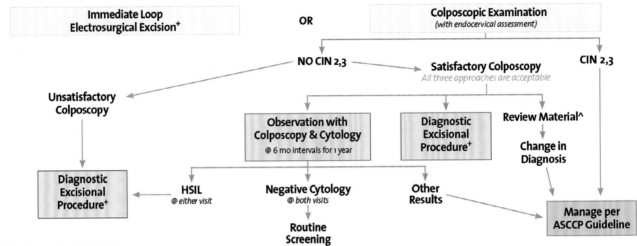

Figure 9-5. Management of women with high-grade squamous intraepithelial lesion (HSIL).

Reprinted from *The Journal of Lower Genital Tract Disease* Vol. 11 Issue 4, with permission of ASCCP © American Society for Colposcopy and Cervical Pathology 2007. No copies of the algorithms may be made without the prior consent of ASCCP.

repeat cytology at 12 months is recommended. Only if HSIL is present on the repeat Pap test should the adolescent patient undergo colposcopy. At the 24-month follow-up, an adolescent with ASC-US or greater abnormality should trigger colposcopy. High-risk HPV testing for triage is *unacceptable* for adolescents with LSIL and for the general population. Postmenopausal women with LSIL may be managed with reflex hrHPV testing, repeat cytology at 6 months or 12 months, or colposcopy. If the hrHPV test is negative and no lesion is visible colposcopically in the postmenopausal patient, repeat cytology at 12 months should be performed. If the hrHPV test is positive or repeat cytology is ASC-US or greater, colposcopy is recommended. The patient should return to regular screening if two consecutive Pap tests are interpreted as NILM. Pregnant women who are older than 20 years should have colposcopy for an LSIL Pap test interpretation. No endocervical sampling should be performed, and multiple colposcopies are unacceptable. Deferring colposcopy until 6 weeks postpartum is acceptable. Postpartum colposcopy should be performed if no lesion is detected at initial colposcopy.

High-Grade Squamous Intraepithelial Lesion

Women with a cytologic result of HSIL are at significant risk for CIN II/III or invasive carcinoma, and should undergo colposcopy with biopsy confirmation and endocervical assessment. An immediate loop electrosurgical excision (LEEP) is also acceptable (Figure 9-5). However, because of the increased risk of preterm delivery, low-birth-weight infants, and premature membrane rupture, LEEP excision as a primary treatment should be weighed against the future fertility desired by the patient. Use of hrHPV testing is *unacceptable* as a triage method to colposcopic examination in patients having cytologic interpretations of HSIL.

HSIL in Adolescents

In adolescents, immediate LEEP is *unacceptable*; colposcopy is recommended (Figure 9-6). If histologic CIN II/III is detected at colposcopy, the adolescent patient can be managed with 24 months of observation using colposcopy and cytology, assuming that adequate colposcopic examinations are obtained. When histologic CIN II is present, observation is recommended. When histologic CIN III is present or when colposcopy is unsatisfactory, treatment is recommended. Observation for 24 months is preferred, using colposcopy and cytology every 6 months when no CIN II or III is identified in an adolescent with an initial Pap test result of HSIL. If two consecutive NILM Pap tests are obtained during 24 months of observation, the patient is returned to regular screening intervals.

HSIL in Pregnancy

For pregnant patients with HSIL on Pap tests, colposcopic follow-up should be performed by colposcopists experienced in the nuances of cervical changes seen during pregnancy. Biopsy of the lesions is acceptable, but endocervical sampling is unacceptable. Repeat postpartum colposcopy at 6 weeks is recommended for those pregnant patients when HSIL is found on initial Pap test, but for whom CIN II or III is not identified during colposcopy. Unless invasive carcinoma is identified, excisional treatment is not recommended during pregnancy.

Atypical Glandular Cells, Including Adenocarcinoma In Situ

Atypical glandular cells (AGC) is an uncommon cytologic interpretation (College of American Pathologists benchmark data indicates that the 95 percentile reporting rate is less than 1.4% for all preparation types[6]), and the signifi-

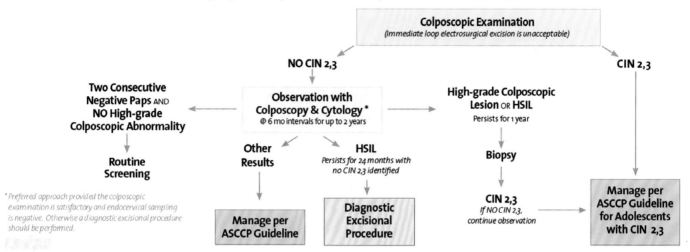

Figure 9-6. Management of adolescent women (20 years and younger) with high-grade squamous intraepithelial lesion (HSIL).

Reprinted from *The Journal of Lower Genital Tract Disease* Vol. 11 Issue 4, with permission of ASCCP © American Society for Colposcopy and Cervical Pathology 2007. No copies of the algorithms may be made without the prior consent of ASCCP.

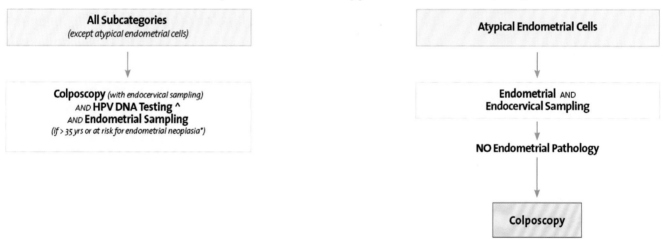

Figure 9-7. Initial workup of women with atypical glandular cells (AGC).

Reprinted from *The Journal of Lower Genital Tract Disease* Vol. 11 Issue 4, with permission of ASCCP © American Society for Colposcopy and Cervical Pathology 2007. No copies of the algorithms may be made without the prior consent of ASCCP.

cant lesions associated with this result are age dependent. Squamous abnormalities are more often seen in younger patients with a Pap test demonstrating AGC, and older women more often have endometrial lesions associated with AGC. High-risk HPV testing alone or repeat cytology are not sensitive enough and are *unacceptable* for the initial evaluation of AGC. Except for pregnant patients, all women with AGC and adenocarcinoma in situ (AIS) should have colposcopy and endocervical sampling. If not previously performed, at the time of colposcopy, hrHPV testing is preferred for women with AGC. In women age 35 or older, endometrial sampling is recommended in addi-

tion to colposcopy and endocervical sampling. Endometrial sampling should also be performed in patients younger than 35 who have clinical factors that suggest an increased risk for developing endometrial cancer (unexplained vaginal bleeding or chronic anovulation) (Figure 9-7). A negative colposcopy should be followed by repeat Pap testing and hrHPV testing at 12 months if the colposcopic hrHPV test was negative, and at 6 months if the hrHPV obtained at the time of colposcopy was positive. For negative Pap tests and negative hrHPV postcolposcopy, routine screening can be implemented. If the initial Pap test is AIS or AGC, favors neoplasia, and no inva-

Subsequent Management of Women with Atypical Glandular Cells (AGC)

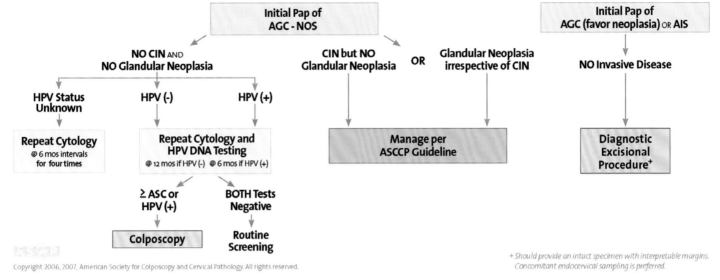

Figure 9-8. Subsequent management of women with atypical glandular cells (AGC).

+ Should provide an intact specimen with interpretable margins. Concomitant endocervical sampling is preferred.

Reprinted from *The Journal of Lower Genital Tract Disease* Vol. 11 Issue 4, with permission of ASCCP © American Society for Colposcopy and Cervical Pathology 2007. No copies of the algorithms may be made without the prior consent of ASCCP.

sive disease is detected at colposcopy with endocervical sampling, a diagnostic excisional procedure is appropriate (Figure 9-8).

Exfoliated Endometrial Cells in Women Age 40 Years and Older
General Category: Other

Once considered in the category "epithelial cell abnormalities" of the glandular group, exfoliated endometrial cells present on a Pap test are now designated as neither an epithelial cell abnormality nor a negative Pap test. They are now in the general category of "other." Because there is no convincing evidence that finding endometrial cells in a woman out of cycle or after menopause is reliably associated with significant endometrial pathology, inclusion in the abnormal category was not justified. The Bethesda System recommends reporting endometrial cells only in women age 40 and older, with inclusion of an educational note in the report recommending that the clinical care provider correlate the presence of endometrial cells with the patient's risk factors for endometrial cancer or pathology.

When benign-appearing endometrial cells are reported in women age 40 or older, and the patient is still having cyclic menses, no follow-up is necessary. However, if the patient is postmenopausal, endometrial assessment is recommended.[7]

Benign Endocervical Cells Following Hysterectomy

No follow-up is necessary in this population of patients. This glandular metaplasia may be seen as a response to surgery, radiation, chemotherapy, or with fallopian tube prolapse or adenosis.[8]

Unsatisfactory Pap Test or Pap Tests with Quality Indicators Identified

The 2001 Bethesda System introduced a binary system for reporting adequacy: Pap tests are reported as either "satisfactory" or "unsatisfactory." The category of "satisfactory but limited by..." a variety of conditions, seen in the earlier iteration of the Bethesda System, was retired. Instead, those Pap tests that are suboptimal are identified by the use of "quality indicators" following the statement of specimen adequacy. An ASCCP management guideline has been established for adequacy and quality indicators.[9]

For Pap tests with no endocervical/transformation zone, the preferred management is a repeat Pap test in 12 months. Possible reasons to consider an earlier repeat Pap test include a previous squamous epithelial cell abnormality in a patient without three previous consecutive negative Pap tests, a previous Pap test with a glandular abnormality, a positive hrHPV test in the previous 12 months, inability to visualize the cervix or sample the endocervical canal, immunosuppression, or a patient who is not participating in a regular screening program. If the patient is pregnant, lack of endocervical/transformation zone should prompt a repeat Pap test after delivery.

For women with a negative Pap test with quality indicators identifying partially obscuring inflammation, blood, air-drying, or other material, a repeat Pap test in 12 months is the preferred management. The same factors mentioned above may trigger an earlier repeat. If the situation applies to a pregnant patient, the Pap test should be repeated postpartum.

For women with an unsatisfactory Pap test, the ASCCP task force recommends a repeat Pap test within a 2- to 4-month period. If the Pap test is unsatisfactory due to inflammation, or infectious organisms are identified on an unsatisfactory Pap test, treatment prior to repeat Pap tests should be considered. With repeated unsatisfactory Pap tests, additional clinical evaluation, colposcopy, and biopsies may be appropriate.

Adjunctive HPV DNA Testing Used as a Screening Test

High-risk HPV testing as an adjunct to the Pap test is approved for use in patients older than 30 years as an option allowing a prolonged screening interval for those women who are negative for both tests. The pooled sensitivity of this combination is much higher than Pap tests alone; most importantly, the negative predictive value of the combined test is 99%.[10] If both tests are negative, they should not be performed more frequently than every 3 years. If the hrHPV test is positive, but the cytologic interpretation is NILM, both tests should be repeated at 12 months; if the hrHPV test is persistently positive, colposcopy is recommended.

There is no role for low-risk HPV testing in screening for cervical cancer; testing for nononcogenic HPV for cervical cancer screening and follow-up for cervical abnormalities is *unacceptable*.

Cytology alone continues to be acceptable in women older than 30 years.

Summary

The most recent ASCCP guidelines reflect a national and international consensus for patient management based upon the understanding of cervical neoplasia, its relationship to HPV, and its natural history. The evidence-based ASCCP guidelines are management guidelines providing caregivers a choice of acceptable plans for patient management that include allowances for local resources. The 2006 ASCCP guidelines reflect a growing understanding of the natural prevalence and biology of HPV, tempered with the concern for the possibility of overtreatment of women. Clinical judgment must direct the application of guidelines to a specific patient; guidelines that will apply to every patient's need cannot be developed. Prevention of cervical cancer rests upon a woman's access to widespread screening and her subsequent treatment and follow-up.

References

1. Solomon D, Nayar R. *The Bethesda System for Reporting Cervical Cytology. Definitions, Criteria and Explanatory Notes.* 2nd ed. New York: Springer-Verlag; 2004.
2. Wright TC, Cox JT, Massad LS, Twiggs LB, Wilkinson EJ. 2001 consensus guidelines for the management of women with cervical cytological abnormalities. *JAMA.* 2002;287:2120-2129.
3. Wright TC, Massad LS, Dunton CJ, Spitzer M, Wilkinson EJ, Solomon D; for the 2006 ASCCP-sponsored Consensus Conference. 2006 consensus guidelines for the management of women with abnormal cervical screening tests. *J Low Genit Tract Dis.* 2007;11:210-222.
4. Wright TC, Massad LS, Dunton CJ, Spitzer M, Wilkinson EJ, Solomon D; for the 2006 ASCCP-sponsored Consensus Conference. 2006 consensus guidelines for the management of women with cervical intraepithelial neoplasia or adenocarcinoma in situ. *J Low Genit Tract Dis.* 2007;11:223-239.
5. Sherman ME, Solomon D, Schiffman M. Qualification of ASC-US: a comparison of equivocal LSIL and equivocal HSIL cervical cytology in the ASC-US LSIL Triage Study. *Am J Clin Pathol.* 2001;116:386-394.
6. Commission on Laboratory Accreditation. Laboratory Accreditation Program. *Cytopathology Checklist.* Northfield, Ill: College of American Pathologists; 2007. Available at: http://www.cap.org/apps/docs/laboratory_accreditation/checklists/cytopathology_sep07.pdf. Accessed May 25, 2008.
7. Greenspan DL, Cardillo M, Davey DD, Heller DS, Moriarty AT. Endometrial cells and cervical cytology: a review of cytological features and clinical assessment. *J Low Genit Tract Dis.* 2006;10:111-122.
8. Tambouret R, Pitman MB, Bell DA. Benign glandular cells in posthysterectomy vaginal smears. *Acta Cytol.* 1998;42:1403-1408.
9. Davey DD, Austin RM, Birdsong G, et al. ASCCP Patient Management Guidelines: Pap Test Specimen Adequacy and Quality Indicators. *J Lower Genit Tract Dis.* 2002:195-199.
10. Cuzick J, Clavel C, Petry KU, et al. Overview of the European and North American studies on HPV in primary cancer screening. *Int J Cancer.* 2006;119:1095-1101.

Vaccine Against Human Papillomavirus: Current State of the Art

Marianne Prey, MD
Mary R. Schwartz, MD

Why Develop Vaccines?

The global impact of vaccines on the health of the world's population is remarkable. The World Health Organization (WHO) and UNICEF estimate that childhood vaccines alone prevent 3 million deaths and 750,000 cases of blindness every year. In the future, vaccines are expected to have a significant impact on the reduction of cancers caused by infectious organisms. Nearly 16% of all cancers worldwide are due to hepatitis B and C, *Helicobacter pylori*, and human papillomavirus (HPV). In the 20 years since the advent of the hepatitis B vaccine, the incidence of hepatocellular carcinoma has dropped in areas of the world where that cancer was very common. Researchers are actively working on the development of an *H pylori* vaccine for peptic ulcer disease and gastric carcinoma. Following very successful clinical trials, the United States Food and Drug Administration (FDA) approval of the first vaccine against HPV—and hence cervical cancer—has recently taken place.

Why Develop a Vaccine Against Human Papillomavirus?

Cervical cancer is a worldwide public health problem. It is the seventh most frequent cancer in the world and the second most common cancer among women worldwide. Globally, there are almost 500,000 new cases per year and an estimated 274,000 deaths from this disease. The geographic areas with no organized screening programs and subsequently the highest rates of cervical cancer include sub-Saharan Africa, Melanesia, Latin America, the Caribbean, South Central Asia, and Southeast Asia. These areas account for 20% of the global burden of disease and 83% of the deaths from cervical cancer.[1]

Despite the fact that organized screening programs in developed countries have reduced the incidence of cervical cancer by 75%, it is estimated that in 2006 there were 9710 new cases of cervical cancer, and 3700 women died from the disease in the United States.[2] This is due to a combination of HPV infection and insufficient screening in subsets of the population, especially minorities who are immigrants. The annual incidence (new cases) of HPV anal-genital infection in the US is 5.5 million, and the overall prevalence in the population is 20 million cases. Most of these infections are cleared by humeral immunity before the virus has a chance to become established within the squamous cells. Even so, 1.3 million women will develop a productive infection or low-grade squamous intraepithelial lesion (LSIL), and 400,000 women will develop a preneoplasia (dysplasia) or high-grade squamous intraepithelial lesion (HSIL) each year. Several years ago it was estimated that $6 billion is spent each year in the US to diagnose and treat just the low-grade lesions identified on Pap testing.[3]

Persistent infection with high-risk types of HPV is an obligate step in the progressive transformation from normal cervical epithelium to invasive cervical cancer. Molecular studies using polymerase chain reaction have shown that high-risk HPV types collectively account for 99.9% of cervical cancers.[4] HPV types 16 and 18 cause approximately 70% of cervical cancers and its precursors (SIL). These two types of HPV are more common in cancers than their prevalence in the population suggests. The odds ratio of having cervical cancer with persistent HPV 16 is 434 and with persistent HPV 18 is 248. Because of this strong association, WHO classifies all high-risk HPV types as human carcinogens. By comparison, the relative risk of lung cancer in a white male smoker in the US is only 8.[5] In addition, HPV types 16 and 18 cause 70% of anal cancers in men who have sex with men and 70% of squamous lesions of the penis.[2]

Infection with other types of HPV is associated with the development of other nonmalignant disease processes as well. HPV types 6 and 11 cause more than 90% of genital condyloma in men and women. In Europe, the incidence of genital condyloma has increased by 500% over the past 30 years.[6] Although condylomas are not associated with progression to cancer, the treatment is painful and, with a 30% recurrence rate overall, management can be costly. Types 6 and 11 are also associated with recurrent respiratory papillomatosis, which is a potentially life-threatening pediatric disease of the larynx and trachea. It is postulated that HPV is transmitted from an infected mother to the baby during birth.

These links between certain types of HPV and anogenital cancers and other benign disease processes are the impetus for the development of prophylactic and therapeutic vaccines. Since as many as 70% of sexually active women acquire one or more HPV infections in a lifetime, it is hoped that HPV vaccines can prevent (prophylactic) and eradicate (therapeutic) these highly prevalent disease processes.

Factors to Consider in the Development of a Vaccine

The immune responses that protect against HPV infection and subsequent HPV-related diseases are not completely understood. The immunogenicity of HPV involves presentation of viral capsid antigens to the immune system. The first generation of prophylactic vaccines is based upon the production of neutralizing antibodies against the L1 viral capsid protein. Vaccine production utilizes this protein in the form of virus-like particles (VLP), the components of which are produced biosynthetically and self-assemble into structures that resemble the viral protein envelope. VLPs do not contain the viral genome and hence do not contain the potentially harmful viral genes; therefore, VLPs are not infectious and are safe to use in a vaccine for healthy subjects.[7,8] Furthermore, VLPs induce a strong humeral immune response—stronger than that produced by a natural infection with HPV.

An important issue in the development of an HPV vaccine is the number of types of HPV that are to be included as immunogens. Because HPV types 16 and 18 account for the majority of cancers as well as most HSILs, incremental improvement in cancer prevention is not greatly affected by including L1 VLPs for additional high-risk types of HPV. However, since there is significant morbidity and cost associated with the treatment of genital condylomas, and HPV types 6 and 11 cause more than 90% of these lesions, it is reasonable to include VLPs of these types in a vaccine.

Studies to prove efficacy of HPV vaccines must demonstrate that the risk for anal-genital cancers is reduced in the vaccinated population, that the risk for developing precursor lesions for these cancers is reduced, and that the risk for persistent HPV infection is reduced. If the vaccine also includes HPV 6 and 11 L1 VLPs, studies must also show that the risk for developing genital condylomas is reduced.

Since using cancers as an endpoint in vaccine effectiveness is neither feasible nor ethical, the clinical trial endpoint must include the presence or absence of HPV 16 or 18. Demonstration of efficacy for HPV type-related cervical intraepithelial neoplasia 2/3 (CIN II/III) (HSIL) is also required for vaccine licensure. Clinical trials must also demonstrate immunogenicity that is not only protective, but also has longevity that is sufficient to avoid a negative impact on compliance by requiring frequent additional doses. Overall patient tolerance for the method of vaccine administration and side effects must also be acceptable, again to ensure maximum patient compliance.

HPV Vaccine Production and Clinical Trials

Vaccine development follows a specific stepwise progression. Invariably there is an animal model that precedes investigation in humans. When a vaccine demonstrates good results in animal models, it is further tested in three phases in humans before it is approved by the FDA and is available for large-scale implementation.

Phase I trials are the first human tests of a vaccine, usually taking 8 to 12 months to complete. The main goal is evaluation of safety and, to a lesser extent, analysis of the immune response evoked by the vaccine. Phase II trials involve a larger number of volunteers, usually a mixture of

low-risk and higher-risk individuals from the population where Phase III (vaccine efficacy) trials will eventually be conducted. Phase II trials generate additional safety data as well as information for refining the dosage and immunization schedule, and are sometimes large enough to yield preliminary indications of efficacy. These trials generally take 18 to 24 months.

Phase III trials are the large-scale definitive tests of whether a vaccine is effective in preventing disease. Successful demonstration of efficacy in a Phase III trial can lead to an application for FDA or other regulatory agency approval. Phase III trials of vaccines are generally expected to require a minimum of 3 years for enrollment, immunizations, and assessment of efficacy.

Multiple Phase I and Phase II clinical trials have demonstrated the safety and immunogenicity of HPV 11, 16, and 18 vaccines.[7-13] A number of routes of vaccine administration have been studied, including parenteral (intramuscular), oral, intranasal, and intravaginal.[14] To date, the clinical Phase I, II, and III trials have all used a series of three intramuscular immunizations, given at day 1, month 2, and month 6. The vaccines have been well tolerated and shown to be highly immunogenic. In general, the adverse effects in the HPV vaccine groups have been similar to those in the placebo group. The most common adverse effect is pain at the injection site, which was slightly higher in the HPV vaccine group in some of the studies. No serious vaccine-related adverse events have been reported.

Data from the Merck & Co, Inc (Whitehouse Station, New Jersey) Phase III trial included 15,796 females, age 16 to 26 years, who were followed for up to 4 years in the previously reported and above described studies. During the study period, none of the vaccinated patients developed CIN II/III and cervical adenocarcinoma in situ (AIS), or genital condylomas. On the basis of this demonstrated efficacy, the Merck vaccine, Gardasil®, was approved by the FDA in 2006.[15]

Gardasil is a quadrivalent vaccine containing epitopes against HPV types 6, 11, 16, and 18. The vaccine is indicated for use in girls and women age 9 to 26 years. Contraindications include hypersensitivity to any of the active substances of the vaccine, and it is not recommended for use during pregnancy. Ideally, the vaccine should be administered before the onset of sexual activity. However, it is recommended that females who are sexually active should still be vaccinated since it is unlikely that an individual would have been previously infected with all four of the HPV types included in the vaccine; hence, some protection would still be expected.

A second prophylactic vaccine, Cervarix®, manufactured by GlaxoSmithKline (Middlesex, United Kingdom), was approved for use in the European Union and Australia in 2007 and is currently undergoing FDA review. In contrast to Gardasil, Cervarix is protective against high-risk HPV types 16 and 18, and incorporates a different immune adjuvant, which may be responsible for greater immune responses and potential protection against closely related HPV types, such as 45, 51, and 52. Phase III trials have shown 100% efficacy against CIN II/III caused by HPV types 16 and 18.[16]

Unknowns and Challenges

There are still unknowns about the vaccines despite the great success with current clinical trials. Preliminary evidence suggests that neutralizing antibodies raised against VLPs for viral types 16 and 18 may be cross-reactive for other oncogenic HPV types, potentially increasing the efficacy of the vaccine.[16] More extensive study of cross-reactive antibody production is needed. In addition, the duration of the effective immune response is not well known at present. Several trials have shown that following the prescribed dosage schedule, the current vaccines result in an antibody titer response that is 100-fold that of natural infections. Follow-up from these trials now exceeds 5 years, and efficacy is still at 100% for CIN. It is not known if continued protection will require a booster vaccine after longer periods. A recent report showed that there is an anamnestic response in women who were seropositive for the vaccine HPV types prior to administration of the vaccine.[17] Unfortunately, HPV serologic tests are not yet robust enough for routine clinical application. This means that there is no easy way to test for natural immunity before administering the vaccine or for testing antibody response post vaccination. Studies do, however, show that vaccine efficacy is minimal in women already having been infected with the HPV types included in the vaccine.

Therapeutic vaccines that will effect prevalent HPV infection and associated neoplasia are much less developed than are the prophylactic vaccines discussed above. Based on HPV biology, such vaccines would need to use epitopes retained in transformed cells, most likely the gene products of E6 and E7, in distinction to the capsid antigens found in the infective stages. In order to have effects against already transformed host epithelial cells, therapeutic vaccines will require cellular immune responses to be elicited. A number of studies have been published using E6 and E7 epitopes with variable success. While the specifics of antigen delivery are beyond the scope of this review, methods utilized to data have included viral vectors such as Vaccinia, small peptides, proteins, bare or encapsulated DNA, and direct inoculation of antigen into autologous dendritic cells. For further information on methods of antigen presentation, the reader is referred to the excellent review article by Schreckenberger and Kaufmann.[18] Needless to say, although results to date using therapeutic vaccines have shown promise, further development and study will be required with all such modalities.

FDA approval of a vaccine does not mean that there will be immediate widespread acceptance and implementation. There are five recognized steps for introduction of a vaccine. The first step is FDA approval for safety and efficacy. The second step is review by the Centers for Disease Control and Prevention (CDC) Advisory Committee on Immunization Practices. The third step is deciding if the vaccine will be paid for through the Vaccines for Children program and

Section 317 funding, both of which are US federal programs for the uninsured and underinsured. The fourth step is for professional medical societies to review the clinical trial data and stipulations of FDA approval and to formulate their own recommendations for use of the vaccine by their respective memberships. The fifth step for successful introduction of a vaccine is for advocacy groups to educate, encourage vaccination, and seek funding. Interestingly, over 30 countries have now approved the vaccine for use in their populations at the time of this writing, and many of the steps to implementation have already been passed. In 2006, the CDC Advisory Committee on Immunization Practices (ACIP) unanimously voted to recommend vaccination in 11- to 26-year-old women, with the 9- to 10-year age group added at the individual physician's discretion. The Committee recommendation noted that prior Pap or HPV testing was not necessary prior to vaccination, and that individuals could receive the vaccine regardless of a prior positive HPV or abnormal Pap test. In addition, Gardasil was added to the CDC's Vaccines for Children Contract, meaning that the vaccine would be made available to girls and women, age 9 to 18 years, who are Medicaid eligible, uninsured or underinsured, or are Native American. An additional initiative by Merck will make the vaccine available to women 19 years of age or greater who are uninsured or unable to pay by themselves.[19-22]

The last step to vaccine implementation, education, will have to include overcoming the stigma of vaccination for a sexually transmitted infection. The message for physicians, patients, and parents of patients must be that HPV infection is simply an indicator of sexual activity, with a lifetime risk of acquiring the infection of greater than 70%. Physicians will have to explain to parents and patients that administration of the vaccine does not condone promiscuous behavior, does not have any protective effect for other sexually transmitted infections, and does not eliminate all risk of cervical cancer.

A combined strategy of vaccination for primary prevention and cervical cytology screening for secondary prevention will be the means to further reduce cervical cancer. In time, screening methods and guidelines may change to coincide with the onset of high-grade disease, rather than the onset of sexual activity, and be geared toward detection of abnormalities in a low-prevalence environment.[23]

Several investigative mathematical models show that the addition of an HPV 16/18 vaccine to current cervical cancer screening in the United States is cost effective, even at the current high price of the three-dose regimen (approximately $300). A program that combines a vaccine that is at least 70% effective, vaccination at 12 years of age, and screening every 3 years beginning at age 25 provides a 92% decrease in cervical cancer incidence and costs approximately $50,000 per quality-adjusted life year.

Will health care payers in the US support vaccination to prevent cervical cancer when it has such a relatively low prevalence and death rate? Experience with other recently introduced vaccines indicates that an HPV vaccine will be supported. Merck press releases indicate that approximately 94% of all private insurers currently provide some benefit for HPV vaccine administration; however, it is not clear at this point whether the amount of coverage is complete compared with the cost of the vaccine and its administration.

The Future

The FDA approval of Gardasil and the European/Australian approvals for Cervarix came much faster than originally predicted because the Phase III trials demonstrated such profound efficacy for the prevention of CIN II/III, with minimal side effects. Implementation of both of these vaccines has the ability to significantly reduce cervical cancer in both screened and unscreened populations. Studies will continue for years to determine the lasting effect of the neutralizing antibodies and to determine if a booster vaccine will be needed. In addition, clinical trials in heterosexual and homosexual men are also underway to study the effect of vaccination on HPV disease in men. In addition, studies are indicated to address the issue of vaccination in preadolescent boys and the effect of "herd immunity" in enhancing the overall effect of cervical cancer prevention in women. In the midst of rapid vaccine development, the medical community must not lose sight of the fact that patients will not benefit from this scientific progress unless they present to a health care provider who offers and provides appropriate counseling regarding cervical cytology screening and HPV vaccination.

References

1. Parkin DM, Bray F, Ferlay J, Pisani P. Global cancer statistics, 2002. *CA Cancer J Clin.* 2005;55:74-108.
2. Jemal A, Siegel R, Ward E, et al. Cancer statistics, 2006. *CA Cancer J Clin.* 2006;56:106-130.
3. Goldie SJ, Kohli M, Grima D, et al. Projected clinical benefits and cost-effectiveness of a human papillomavirus 16/18 vaccine. *J Natl Cancer Inst.* 2004;96:604-615.
4. Waalboomers JM, Jacobs MV, Manos MM, et al. Human papillomavirus is a necessary cause of invasive cervical cancer worldwide. *J Pathol.* 1999;189:12-19.
5. *Educate the Educators: HPV and the New HPV Vaccines Program.* Hagerstown, MD: ASCCP; 2006.
6. Sexually transmitted infections quarterly report: anogenital warts and HSV infection in England and Wales. *CDR Weekly.* 2001;11(35). Available at: http://www.hpa.org.uk/cdr/archives/archive01/news01_1.htm. Accessed April 14, 2008.
7. Ault KA, Giuliano AR, Edwards RP, et al. A phase I study to evaluate a human papillomavirus (HPV) type 18 L1 VLP vaccine. *Vaccine.* 2004;22:3004-3005.
8. Fife KH, Wheeler CM, Koutsky LA, et al. Dose-ranging studies of the safety and immunogenicity of human papillomavirus type 11 and type 16 virus-like particle candidate vaccines in young healthy women. *Vaccine.* 2004;22:2943-2952.
9. Villa LL, Costa RL, Petta CA, et al. Prophylactic quadrivalent human papillomavirus (type 6, 11, 16, and 18) L1 virus-like particle vaccine in young women: a randomized double-blind placebo-controlled multicenter phase II efficacy trial. *Lancet.* 2005;6:271-278.
10. Brown DR, Bryan JT, Schroeder JM, et al. Neutralization of human papillomavirus type 11 (HPV-11) by serum from women vaccinated with yeast-derived HPV-11 L1 virus-like particles: correlation with competitive radioimmunoassay titer. *J Infect Dis.* 2001;184:1183-1186.
11. Evans TG, Bonnez W, Rose RC, et al. A phase I study of a recombinant viruslike particle against human papillomavirus type 11 in healthy adult volunteers. *J Infect Dis.* 2001;183:1485-1493.
12. Harro CD, Pang YY, Roden RB, et al. Safety and immunogenicity trial in adult volunteers of a human papillomavirus 16 L1 virus-like particle vaccine. *J Natl Cancer Inst.* 2001; 93:284-292.
13. Fife KH, Wheeler CM, Koutsky LA, et al. Dose ranging studies of the safety and immunogenicity of human papillomavirus Type 11 and Type 16 virus-like particle candidate vaccines in young healthy women. *Vaccine.* 2004;22:2943-2952.
14. Nardelli-Haefliger D, Lurati F, Wirthner D, et al. Immune responses induced by lower airway mucosal immunisation with a human papillomavirus type 16 virus-like vaccine. *Vaccine.* 2005;23:3634-3641.
15. *Patient Information about Gardasil.* Whitehouse Station, NJ: Merck & Co, Inc; 2007. Available at: http://www.merck.com/product/usa/pi_circulars/g/gardasil/gardasil_ppi.pdf. Accessed January 18, 2008.
16. Harper DM, Franco EL, Wheeler CM, et al. Sustained efficacy up to 4.5 years of a bivalent L1 virus-like particle vaccine against human papillomavirus types 16 and 18: follow-up from a randomized control trial. *Lancet.* 2006;367:1247-1255.
17. Villa LL, Ault KA, Giuliano AR, et al. Immunologic responses following administration of a vaccine targeting human papillomavirus types 6, 11, 16, and 18. *Vaccine.* 2006;24:5571-5583.
18. Schreckenberger C, Kaufmann AM. Vaccination strategies for the treatment and prevention of cervical cancer. *Curr Opin Oncol.* 2004;16:485-491.
19. Gonik B. Strategies for fostering HPV vaccine acceptance. *Infect Dis Obstet Gynecol.* 2006;2006 Suppl:36797.
20. Rolling out HPV vaccines worldwide [editorial]. *Lancet.* 2006;367:2034.
21. Should HPV vaccine be mandatory for all adolescents? [editorial]. *Lancet.* 2006;368:1212.
22. Merck press release. November 1, 2006. Whitehouse Station, NJ: Merck & Co, Inc; 2006. Available at: http://www.merck.com/newsroom/press_releases/product/2006_1101.html. Accessed January 12, 2007.
23. Schiffman M. Integration of human papillomavirus vaccination, cytology, and human papillomavirus testing. *Cancer.* 2007;111:145-153.

New Technology in Gynecologic Cytology

Joel S. Bentz, MD

Terence J. Colgan, MD

Rodolfo Laucirica, MD

Cytology Automation

New technologies have been developed to improve short-comings in the conventional Papanicolaou (Pap) test, and to expand on the scope of methodologies used in the cervical neoplasia screening process. The technologies introduced to date have included liquid-based cytology; computer-assisted, automated, Pap test slide screening; and adjunctive testing of these samples for the causative agent of cervical carcinoma, human papillomavirus (HPV). These technological advancements have improved accuracy and efficiency in cytologic screening for cervical carcinoma and have allowed more cost-effective management of patients.

The first part of this chapter will introduce the reader to the new technologies available, highlighting the important clinical features and how they can be implemented into the cytology laboratory. Each summary for these liquid-based cytology and screening devices will include a review of specimen collection and storage, principles of specimen processing, intended use, and clinical performance. The differences among the various types of new technologies also will be highlighted. Adjunctive testing and biomarkers will be discussed in the latter part of the chapter.

Liquid-Based Cytology

Early attempts at automated instrumentation of Pap tests started with the optimization of the cellular material on the slide, with the goal of utilization of cytology material with imaging devices. However, it was quickly realized that improving the quality of the slide preparation also led to general improvements in cervical cytology accuracy and productivity. With the switch to liquid-based cytology, enhanced quality was attributed to better cervical sampling and improved ability to interpret the slides. Liquid-based cytology slides have uniform and thorough fixation, homogenized and cleaner specimens, and uniform, well-segmented, thin-layer distribution of cellular material.[1,2]

To obtain a liquid-based cytology specimen, the sample is collected in the conventional manner, but the use of optimal sampling devices (cervical broom or endocervical brush/plastic spatula combination) is required. Rather than making a smear on a glass slide from this material, the collection device is either rinsed in or detached and placed into a vial of preservative fluid. Through this collection method, the cellular sample is immediately fixed, and a large proportion of cells are recovered from the collection device. A uniform thin-layer slide preparation is then produced using one of the instruments (The ThinPrep® Pap Test, SurePath™ Pap test, and MonoPrep®) that are currently approved by the US Food and Drug Administration (FDA). The changes in practice when converting from conventional Pap smear preparations to liquid-based preparations are highlighted in Table 11-1.

Advantages of Liquid-Based Cytology

In comparison to conventional Pap smear preparations, liquid-based cytology presents representative cellular material from the specimen in a more consistent and well-preserved fashion, with minimal cellular crowding and overlapping, and reduction of interfering debris, blood, inflammation, and processing artifacts. The advantages and disadvantages of conventional preparations and liquid-based cytology are presented in Table 11-2.

Compared to conventional Pap smear preparation methods, the FDA-approved liquid-based cytology instruments have been shown to, on average, increase the detection rates for squamous intraepithelial lesions and glandular lesions, and have demonstrated superior adequacy rates.[3-9] In addition, the cellular material that remains in the vial following slide processing permits adjunctive "out-of-the vial" molecular testing for high-risk HPV, other sexually transmitted diseases, and, potentially, oncologic biomarkers associated with cervical carcinoma and high-grade precursor lesions. Finally, these liquid-based cytology systems now permit the use of FDA-approved companion automated screening devices that enhance slide screening accuracy and improve laboratory productivity.

Differences in Liquid-Based Cytology Cellular Presentation

Although the cytomorphology of liquid-based cytology preparations has many general similarities with that of conventional Pap smears, there are morphologic differences that must be appreciated in order to achieve optimal results. The FDA requires preinitiation training of new users (coordinated by the manufacturers) prior to the introduction of these technologies into the laboratory.

For example, groups of endocervical and squamous metaplastic cells often tend to "round up" and present as tight three-dimensional clusters of cells, a characteristic that can lead to overinterpretation of such hyperchromatic crowded groupings as dysplasia or even carcinoma. Overall, cells from conventional smears tend to appear larger than their liquid-based counterparts because cells are spread out on a slide in conventional smears, whereas they tend to shrink in the liquid medium. The dispersed

Table 11-1. Differences in Collection, Processing, and Evaluation: Conventional Smear Versus Liquid-Based Cytology

Technique	Conventional Smear	Liquid-Based Cytology
Sampling device	Wooden spatula, cytobrush	Plastic spatula, cytobrush, cervical broom
Sample taking	No changes	Careful attention to number and direction of rotations with sampling device
Fixation	Manual spray fixation; delayed dry fixation	Immediate and homogeneous fixation in a solution of fixative (methanol or ethanol)
Transportation	Small slide tray sent in mail, etc	Vials with fixative require special shipping instructions, etc
Laboratory preparation	Ready for staining	Semiautomated instrument preparation; need manual handling before preparation (SurePath) and staining (ThinPrep)
Staining	No changes	Standardized cell deposit; uniform staining
Screening	Uneven distribution of cellular material, fixing artifacts, 300,000 cells to screen	Need morphology training; uniform distribution; fewer cells to screen (60,000-75,000)

Table 11-2. Advantages and Disadvantages of Conventional Smear and Liquid-Based Cytology for Cervical Cancer Screening

Methodology	Advantages	Disadvantages
Conventional Pap test	The "gold standard" for 50 years Comfortable with the method Ready for staining when arrives in lab Inexpensive; can be run on automated screener (BD FocalPoint Slide Profiler)	>80% of the cellular material is lost after collection 300,000 cells screened ("needle in haystack") Uneven distribution of cellular material, fixation artifacts, unsatisfactory smears
Liquid-based cytology	Virtually all cellular material collected is recovered Ease of use for "smear taker" Limited obscuring material, fewer unsatisfactory slides Even distribution of cells, clean background, fewer artifacts Fewer but well-preserved cells to examine Ease of examination, screening time may be reduced Extra slides can be made, material available for cell blocks and immunocytochemical/DNA molecular probe Specific CPT code(s) available for liquid-based cytology (88142,88143) Mated automated screening devices available (FocalPoint, ThinPrep Imaging System)	"New technology" causes insecurity Training of clinicians, lab techs, cytotechs, and pathologists is necessary Increased workload in prep lab, monotony in preparing slides Fixatives used (shipping, disposal); some are hazardous Requires vigilance, greater intensity of screening Increased costs (prep lab labor and disposables)

character of diagnostic cells in hypocellular high-grade squamous intraepithelial lesion (HSIL) cases may be challenging despite the cleaner background and fewer obscuring artifacts. The specimen adequacy criteria are similar for liquid-based cytology slides as for conventional smears, but the cellularity criteria for adequacy differs, as per the 2001 Bethesda System. In addition, there are subtle morphologic differences between ThinPrep, SurePath, and MonoPrep specimens, primarily due to the differences in fixative (methanol versus ethanol) and in slide preparatory

Table 11-3. General Cytological Features of Liquid-Based Cytology and the Conventional Smear

Features	ThinPrep	SurePath	MonoPrep	Conventional Smear
Background Clean RBCs Neutrophils Necrosis	 Yes Reduced Reduced Persists/reduced/clumped	 Yes Reduced Reduced Persists/reduced/clumped	 Yes Reduced Reduced Persists/reduced/clumped	 No Present/obscures Present/obscures Diffuse/obscures
Cellularity	Adequate	Adequate	Adequate	Adequate
Cell preservation	Good	Good	Good	Variable
Cell distribution	Uniform; one plane	Uniform; different planes	Uniform	Uniform to uneven
Cell size	Smaller	Smaller	Smaller	Larger
Architecture	Preserved	Preserved	Preserved	Preserved
Cytomorphology	Preserved	Preserved	Preserved	Preserved
Endocervical cells Quantity Quality	 Reduced Clumped to monodispersed	 Reduced Clumped to monodispersed	 Reduced Clumped to monodispersed	 Diffuse
Artifacts	None	None	None	Usually
Slide evaluation	Easier	Easy to difficult	Easier	Easy to difficult
Reproducibility	Present	Present	Present	Present/even/not present dependent on the individual specimen
Ancillary studies	Possible	Possible	Possible	Usually not

technique (Table 11-3). The differences in morphology and adequacy determination between conventional Pap smears and the various liquid-based types are discussed in other chapters of this text.

Liquid-Based Cytology Preparatory and Interpretive Training

Laboratories implementing new technologies are required by federal regulations to follow the manufacturer's instructions and recommendations, which include training of personnel. Given the differences in cellular presentation, this personnel training includes technology and interpretive training as mandated by the FDA. A "train-the-trainer" system is typically used.[10] A cytotechnologist and pathologist from the laboratory are initially trained by the manufacturer and are responsible for training the remaining members of the laboratory staff. The FDA requires that training for the examination of liquid-based cytology specimens be done under the supervision of an authorized person and be followed by a proficiency examination.

Subsequent to formal training, cytologists have referred to a continued learning curve, which can last for weeks to months. It is generally recommended that, during the introductory phase of implementation, "split samples" be analyzed, with conventional specimens made first followed by liquid-based preparations from the residual material. This procedure allows for "side-by-side" comparisons to be made to facilitate the transition from interpreting conventional smears to interpreting liquid-based specimens. Laboratories using this verification method have generally processed between 100 and 500 such cases prior to full liquid-based-cytology-only sample processing. The quality and success of individual performance with these preparations is directly proportional to the quality and quantity of training given. Continuing education and re-education are emphasized in order to maintain optimal slide quality and interpretive skills.

The ThinPrep Pap Test

The ThinPrep Pap Test (Hologic, Inc, Bedford, Massachusetts) incorporates a conventionally collected cervico-vaginal sample into a vial of liquid fixative, followed by controlled membrane filtration of the cellular material and transfer to a glass slide (Table 11-4). The system consists of the PreservCyt® fixative media (Figure 11-1) for sample col-

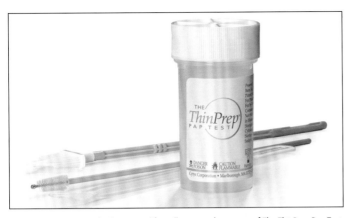

Figure 11-1. PreservCyt fixative vial for collection and transport of The ThinPrep Pap Test. (Courtesy of Hologic, Inc. and affiliates.)

Table 11-4. Components of The ThinPrep Pap Test

Component	Function
ThinPrep 2000/3000 processors	Semiautomated/automated slide preparation
PreservCyt	Sample collection and preservative vial
ThinPrep microscope slides	20-mm cell deposit
Collection device	Broom, brush, or plastic spatula
TransCyt filter	Filter vial contents (disposable)

lection, combined with the ThinPrep 2000 or ThinPrep 3000 slide processors (Figure 11-2).

ThinPrep Specimen Collection and Storage. The cervical sample is collected using either a broom-type device or the combination of a plastic spatula and endocervical brush. A wooden spatula should not be used with The ThinPrep Pap Test due to cell trapping, resulting in decreased cellular recovery. The collection device is then rinsed in a vial of PreservCyt. The PreservCyt fixative contains methanol and should be stored and disposed of in accordance with local, state, and federal regulations. The PreservCyt liquid media has a cellular sample stability of 6 weeks at room temperature (15 to 30°C) or refrigerated (2 to 10°C), and the residua can be retained for additional testing. The preservative fluid without cells has a shelf life of 36 months from date of manufacture.

ThinPrep Specimen Processing. The vial containing the specimen is placed into the ThinPrep 2000 benchtop instrument (Figure 11-2), along with a disposable membrane filter cartridge (TransCyt filter) attached to a plastic cylinder. The ThinPrep 2000 model is a single-load device. The instrument immerses the filter and cylinder into the preservative vial, which rotates to homogenize the cell sample, enough to separate loosely joined material and disperse mucus, blood, and nondiagnostic debris. A vacu-

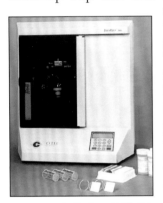

Figure 11-2. ThinPrep 2000 Slide Processor. Also shown are the TransCyt plastic disposable filters, microscope slides, and PreservCyt vials. (Courtesy of Hologic, Inc. and affiliates.)

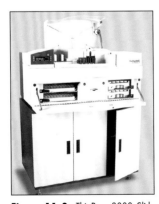

Figure 11-3. ThinPrep 3000 Slide Processor. Up to 80 ThinPrep samples can be run per cycle, with unattended operation. (Courtesy of Hologic, Inc. and affiliates.)

um is then applied across the filter, resulting in collection of cells on the filter. The pressure differential across the filter is constantly monitored by the device, and as increased numbers of cells are collected on the filter, the flow across the filter diminishes, ensuring appropriate cellularity on the final slide. The filter is then removed from the vial, inverted, and touched to a glass slide to transfer cells in a circular area measuring 20 mm in diameter. The overall process yields uniform cell deposits with a mean cell content of 50,000 to 75,000 cells. The slide preparation is then immediately immersed into an alcohol fixative and is ready for the laboratory's routine staining procedure.

ThinPrep slides are stained off-line, coverslipped, and evaluated by trained laboratory personnel using criteria similar to the conventional Pap smear. The use of a disposable filter prevents sample-to-sample contamination. Some laboratories reprocess "unsatisfactory for evaluation" cases (usually bloody specimens) with a CytoLyt® solution and glacial acetic acid wash, which was FDA approved in 2006. Throughput is approximately 25 samples per hour or up to 50,000 samples per year with a single 8-hour shift.

The ThinPrep 3000 Processor is designed for high-volume cytology laboratories (Figure 11-3). The processing methodology for each individual vial/slide combination is identical to that of the ThinPrep 2000. The ThinPrep 3000 can process 80 PreservCyt vials in one cycle, in an unattended fashion, taking approximately 2.0 to 2.5 hours per run. In an 8-hour shift, three runs can theoretically be accomplished. Throughput is approximately 30 slides per hour or up to 60,000 samples per year utilizing a single 8-hour shift.

ThinPrep Pap Test Intended Use. The ThinPrep system is intended as a replacement for conventional Pap smears for use in screening for the presence of atypical cells, cervical cancer or its precursor lesions (low-grade squamous intraepithelial lesions [LSIL], HSIL), and other cytologic categories as defined by the Bethesda System.[11]

ThinPrep Clinical Performance. In clinical trials, The ThinPrep Pap Test was shown to be significantly more effective than the conventional Pap smear for the detection of LSIL and more severe lesions (LSIL+) in a variety of patient populations.[12] Data from a multisite clinical outcome trial, in which ThinPrep specimens were collected prospectively and compared against a historical control cohort, indicated a 59.7% increase in the detection of HSIL and more severe lesions (HSIL+).[13] More recently, the FDA

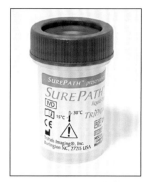

Figure 11-4. SurePath fixative vial for the SurePath Pap test. (Courtesy and © Becton, Dickinson and Company.)

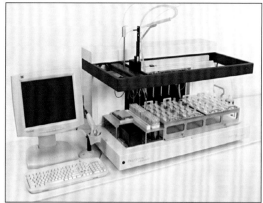

Figure 11-5. BD PrepStain Slide Processor. (Courtesy and © Becton, Dickinson and Company.)

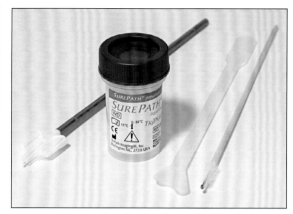

Figure 11-6. SurePath vial with collection devices with detachable heads. (Courtesy and © Becton, Dickinson and Company.)

has approved labeling that references multiple peer-reviewed publications that report improved ability of The ThinPrep Pap Test to detect glandular disease as compared to the conventional Pap smear.[14-16] In addition, specimen quality (adequacy) is significantly improved over that of conventional preparations in a variety of patient populations.

SurePath Pap Test

The BD SurePath Pap test (Becton, Dickenson and Company, Franklin Lakes, New Jersey) consists of the SurePath fixative media (Figure 11-4) for sample collection combined with the BD PrepStain™ Slide Processor (Figure 11-5). Formerly, SurePath was known as AutoCyte® PREP and CytoRich®, and literature citations to both of these are equivalent to SurePath (Table 11-5).

SurePath Specimen Collection and Storage. Similar to the ThinPrep system, the SurePath Pap test uses a process that standardizes cell collection with either a single-pass broom-type collection device (eg, Cervex-Brush®, Cervex-Brush Combi [Rovers, Oss, The Netherlands]) or a combination of a plastic spatula and endocervical brush (eg, Cytobrush® Plus GT and Pap Perfect® Plastic Spatula [Cooper Surgical, Trumbull, Connecticut]) (Figure 11-6). Each of these collection devices is equipped with a detachable head. Following sample collection, the tip of the collection device is separated from the handle stem and dropped into SurePath preservative fluid, avoiding any loss of cellular material.[17] Nondetachable collection

devices or wooden spatulas should not be used with the SurePath Pap test due to cell trapping resulting in decreased cell recovery.

The preservative contains an aqueous solution of denatured ethanol fixative, which is essentially nonhazardous for disposal purposes but can be flammable at very high temperatures. The SurePath liquid media has a cellular sample stability of 4 weeks at room temperature (15 to 30°C) and 6 months refrigerated (2 to 10°C), and the residua can be retained for additional testing. The preservative fluid vial without cells has a shelf life of 36 months from date of manufacture.

SurePath Specimen Processing. SurePath slide production begins with an enrichment process, which combines a variety of steps, including homogenization of the sample, and gravity dispersion and density gradient centrifugation to prepare a processed cell pellet to be placed on the PrepStain Slide Processor. The PrepMate™ is a benchtop accessory that batches and automates the process of homogenization and dispensing the specimen onto the density gradient reagent (Figure 11-7). The PrepStain instrument then completes the process with automated pipetting for gravity sedimentation to produce a thin-layer slide preparation, followed by batched automated Pap staining.

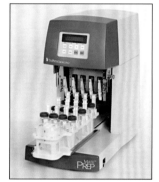

Figure 11-7. PrepMate benchtop accessory for automated syringing, mixing, and loading specimen onto density gradient, reagent-filled centrifuge tubes. (Courtesy and © Becton, Dickinson and Company.)

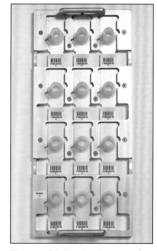

Figure 11-8. PrepStain settling chambers atop the coated microscope slides. (Courtesy and © Becton, Dickinson and Company.)

Table 11-5. Components of the SurePath Pap Test

Component	Function
PrepStain Slide Processor	Automated slide preparation approved by the FDA for gynecologic specimens
SurePath preservative fluid	Sample collection and preservative vial
SurePath coated microscope slides	13-mm cell deposit
Collection device	Broom, brush or plastic spatula
PrepMate	Batched, automated sample dispenser

As many as 48 samples are preprocessed in batches prior to loading onto the PrepStain device, which then completes the cell deposit and automated Papanicolaou staining process. An aliquot of the preprocessed cell pellet material is transferred to a settling column placed on top of a glass slide (Figure 11-8), which is adhesive coated in order to "grab" cells in a uniform cell disc formation, 13 mm in diameter, thus controlling the final slide cellularity. Batch processing allows 92 slides per hour without staining, 48 slides per hour with staining.

SurePath Intended Use. The PrepStain System is a liquid-based thin-layer cell-preparation process that produces SurePath slides, which are intended as replacements for conventional gynecologic Pap smears, for use in the screening and detection of cervical cancer, precancerous lesions, atypical cells, and all other cytologic categories as defined by the Bethesda System.[18] Since its approval, additional data submitted to the FDA allowed the claim of a 64.4% increase in detection of HSIL+ lesions using SurePath.[19]

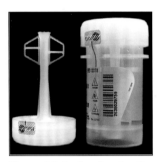

Figure 11-9. MonoPrep Pap Test Specimen Transport Solution. The built-in stir bar is shown under the lid. (Courtesy of MonoGen, Inc.)

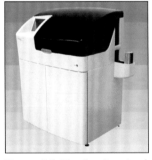

Figure 11-10. MonoPrep Liquid-Based Preparation Processor. (Courtesy of MonoGen, Inc.)

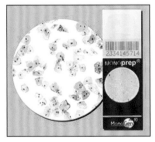

Figure 11-12. MonoPrep Pap Test slide. (Courtesy of Monogen, Inc.)

The SurePath method is associated with significantly fewer unsatisfactory and "limited" ("satisfactory but limited by" [SBLB]) slides.

SurePath Clinical Performance. From clinical trial data, the FDA has recognized via the labeling process that the SurePath Pap test provides an increased detection of HSIL+ and a significant reduction of unsatisfactory specimens in comparison to conventional Pap smears.[20-22]

MonoPrep Pap Test*

With the MonoPrep Pap (MonoGen, Inc, Lincolnshire, Illinois), slides are produced using the MonoPrep Processor, which is the primary component of the integrated system and automates the preparation of cellular specimens (Table 11-6). The system consists of the MonoPrep fixative media (Figure 11-9) for sample collection combined with the MonoPrep Processor (Figure 11-10).

MonoPrep Specimen Collection and Storage. The MonoPrep Pap test process begins with collecting ectocervical and endocervical specimens using the provided collection devices and MonoPrep Specimen Transport Solution

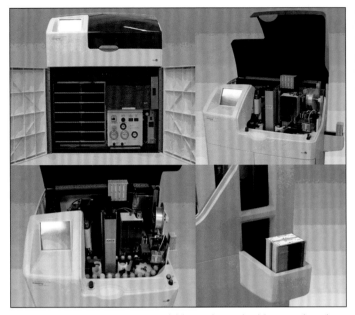

Figure 11-11. MonoPrep Processor, with lid opened. Note the slide output chute (lower right). (Courtesy of MonoGen, Inc.)

preservative fluid. The clinician transfers the specimen to the MonoPrep vial by rinsing the collection devices in the preservative fluid vial.

The vial has an integrated vial stirrer, and the vial internal ribs work together to mix the specimen and disperse mucus, clumps, and aggregates. The homogenized specimen is then aspirated or "drawn up" the stirrer, and a representative sample is captured on a disposable filter. The filter is pressed against the slide to transfer the cells.

The MonoPrep preservative uses a methanol-isopropanol fixative, which should be stored and disposed of in accordance with local, state, and federal regulations. The MonoPrep Pap Test Specimen Transport Solution has a cellular sample stability of 12 months at room temperature (15 to 30°C) after collection. The preservative fluid vial without cells has a shelf life of 12 months from date of manufacture.

MonoPrep Specimen Processing. The MonoPrep instrument accessions, processes, samples, and then prepares the slide (Figure 11-11). Initially, the MonoPrep Liquid-Based Preparation Processor automatically extracts a representative sample from a liquid-based specimen and transfers a thin layer of cells to a glass slide using disposable filters. The sample is deposited within a 20-mm circle on the bar-coded MonoPrep slides (Figure 11-12). The lab-

Table 11-6. Components of the MonoPrep Pap Test

Component	Function
MonoPrep Liquid-Based Preparation Processor	Automated slide preparation
MonoPrep Specimen Transport Solution	Sample collection and preservative vial
MonoPrep microscope slide	20-mm cell deposit
Collection device	Broom, brush or plastic spatula

oratory stains and evaluates MonoPrep slides in accordance with its customary practice, after training. The MonoPrep Processor processes 40 slides per hour, or 320 samples in an 8-hour shift, and is capable of fully automated, unattended operation. One instrument can process approximately 160,000 samples per year.

MonoPrep Intended Use. The MonoPrep Pap test is intended for use in collecting and preparing cervico-vaginal cytology specimens for Pap-stain based screening for cervical cancer, its precursor lesions and other cytologic categories and conditions defined by the 2001 Bethesda System.[23] The MonoPrep Pap Test produces slides that are intended to replace conventionally prepared Pap smear slides.

MonoPrep Clinical Performance. Compared with conventional Pap smears, the MonoPrep Pap test showed statistically increased adjudicated abnormalities at diagnostic thresholds of atypical squamous cells of undetermined significance or greater (ASC-US+), atypical squamous cells, cannot exclude HSIL (ASC-H)/atypical glandular cells (AGC)+, and LSIL+; and nonsignificant increases for HSIL+ and cancer.[24] The specificities of conventional Pap smear and MonoPrep Pap diagnoses were essentially identical. There was a 58% decrease in unsatisfactory cases with MonoPrep as compared with the conventional Pap smear, and MonoPrep slides demonstrated no difference in the adequacy of the endocervical/transformation zone component.

Points to Consider

Compared to the conventional Pap smear, liquid-based cytology appears to provide equivalent or greater sensitivity for detection of SIL and glandular lesions, but at an increased cost to the laboratory. On the other hand, the increased test sensitivity allows for more effective screening, which could offset the increased cost. Clinicians and laboratories should use cervical cytology screening methods that are most appropriate for their patient population and clinical practice (Table 11-7). The clinical laboratory faced with the challenge of selecting a liquid-based cytology product must consider all the factors, including quality, staffing, pricing, reimbursement, liability, productivity, growth, and local competition. These decisions must be continually re-evaluated as technologies evolve and as clinical studies provide scientific data on cost-effective strategies to further reduce morbidity and mortality from cervical cancer.

Automated Screening Instruments

Automated cytology screening devices are instruments that combine robotics, automated microscopy, image capture with high-speed image analysis, and computer algorithms or neural networks to determine the significance of analyzed morphologic findings. This process aids in the determination of whether or not a cervical cytology test needs additional evaluation by a human screener. With 50,000 to 300,000 cells per slide, presented in a highly variable fashion, with potentially large numbers of artifacts present, accurate processing may require capturing and processing over 15,000 images per slide. These devices may be operated by a laboratory assistant and offer the convenience of unattended operation.

One-third of cervical cytology false-negatives are caused by screening and interpretive errors in which abnormal cells present on slides are incorrectly classified. Automated screening instruments address these key sources of error and cost, such as observer fatigue and visual habituation, variability in screening techniques, high complexity of cell morphology presentations, and rarity of abnormal cells. This process can help cytotechnologists focus their efforts on fields of view (specific areas on slides) having highest probability of abnormality, or on particular high risk slides (as determined by the device) truly requiring human review.

Currently there are two FDA-approved systems marketed in the United States for automated screening of cervical cytology specimens, the BD FocalPoint™ Slide Profiler and the ThinPrep Imaging System (Table 11-8).

FocalPoint Slide Profiler**

The BD FocalPoint Slide Profiler is an automated primary screening system that ranks and sorts cervical cytology slides according to their likelihood of being abnormal. This triage method places slides into distinct groups (no further review, review, and quality control [QC] review) using a high-speed video microscope, image interpretation software, and a computer to image, capture, and analyze images on cervical cytology slides.

The forerunner of the FocalPoint system was the AutoPap® 300 QC System (NeoPath Inc, Redmond, Washington), which was FDA approved for automated QC rescreening of negative conventional smears. In this format, the AutoPap would screen negative conventional Pap smears following the manual review process, and identify a cohort of slides that were most likely to harbor missed abnormal cells for focused manual QC rescreening.[25] This QC system was incorporated into the FocalPoint primary screener function. SurePath slides have additionally been inte-

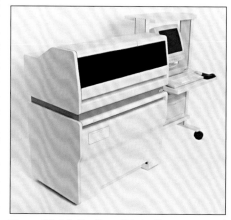

Figure 11-13. FocalPoint Slide Profiler. (Courtesy and © Becton, Dickinson and Company.)

grated into the FocalPoint system, and now the system is FDA approved for primary screening of both conventional Pap smears and PrepStain processed slides, but not ThinPrep slides. (Figure 11-13).

Table 11-7. Comparison of FDA-Approved Liquid-Based Cytology Systems

Product Component	SurePath	ThinPrep	MonoPrep
Sampling technique	Head of collection device detached, dropped into vial	Broom/spatula/brush rinsed in vial	Broom/spatula/brush rinsed in vial
Sampling device	Rovers Cervex-Brush, Cervex-Brush Combi *or* Plastic spatula + endocervical cytobrush	Wallach papette or plastic spatula + endocervical cytobrush	Cervical broom *or* Plastic spatula + endocervical cytobrush
Preservative fluid	SurePath: ethanol (36-month expiration); vial with cells is stable 4 weeks at room temperature, 6 months if refrigerated	PreservCyt: methanol (36-month expiration); vial with cells is stable 6 weeks, room temperature or refrigerated	MonoPrep Specimen Transport Solution: methanol (12-month expiration); vial with cells is stable 12 months, room temperature or refrigerated
Technology	Density gradient centrifugation and gravity sedimentation	Controlled vacuum membrane filtration and cell transfer	Filtration and cell transfer
Staining	Automated	Off-line	Off-line
Size of cell deposit	13 mm	20 mm	20 mm
Intended use FDA labeling	"As a replacement for the conventional Pap smear..." "superior HSIL detection"	"As a replacement for the conventional Pap smear..." "significantly more effective than the conventional Pap smear" "superior HSIL detection" "detection of glandular disease"	"As a replacement for the conventional Pap smear..."
Device	PrepStain Slide Processor	ThinPrep 2000 Processor	MonoPrep Processor
Preparation time	48 tests/hour	25-30 tests/hour	40 tests/hour
Screening time	Same or less	Same	Same
Cost for disposables (approx)	Varies (<$10.00)	Varies (<$10.00)	Varies (<$10.00)
Cost for processor (approx)	$50,000	$50,000	Unknown
Out-of-the-vial molecular testing (FDA approved)	No: self-validate	Yes: HPV, CT/NG	No: self-validate

Intended Use of FocalPoint. The FocalPoint Slide Profiler is an automated device intended for use in the initial screening of cervical cytology slides. The FocalPoint system identifies up to 25% of successfully processed slides as requiring no further review by human screeners. This population consists of the lowest scoring slides and hence slides having the lowest probability of containing abnormal cells. The FocalPoint system also identifies at least 15% of all successfully processed slides for a second QC manual review. This population consists of the highest scoring slides remaining after removal of positive cases on manual screening of the review population. The device is intended to be used on both conventionally prepared and PrepStain prepared cervical cytology slides. For both preparation methods, the device is intended to detect slides with evidence of squamous carcinoma and adenocarcinoma and their usual precursor conditions; it is not intended to be used on slides designated by the laboratory as high risk. High-risk slides are those for which a primary health care provider has requested special handling of a case for a specified concern, or where the clinical laboratory, through its own procedures, has identified a need for an additional screening of the case. These cervical cytology slides must move to the usual laboratory slide review process.[26]

Description of FocalPoint. The FocalPoint Slide Profiler prioritizes and sorts slides based on likelihood of abnormality to help reduce false-negatives during the screening process. FocalPoint uses algorithms to assign a score (0.0 to

Table 11-8. History of FDA Approval of Automated Cytology Screening Instrumentation

Year	Device	Function	Improvement
1995	AutoPap (NeoPath)	Quality control re-screening of negative conventional smears	Reduced screening false-negatives
1998	FocalPoint (TriPath)	Primary screening of conventional Pap smears	Reduced screening false-negatives; increased productivity
2001	FocalPoint (TriPath)	Primary screening of SurePath Liquid Based Pap Test	Reduced sampling and screening false-negatives; increased productivity
2003	ThinPrep Imaging System (Cytyc)	Primary screening of The ThinPrep Pap Test	Reduced sampling and screening false-negatives; increased productivity

Table 11-9. Advantages and Disadvantages of the BD FocalPoint Slide Profiler

Advantages	Disadvantages
Compatible with both SurePath and conventional Pap smears	Not compatible with The ThinPrep Pap Test; not compatible with all staining techniques
Reduces number of slides needing manual screening; improved productivity	Performance characteristics for reactive changes, atrophy, and endometrial cells have not been established
Increased disease detection; reduced false-negatives	Not approved for use in a high-risk patient population
Unattended operation	All slides selected for review must have a full manual screen. Cytotechnologists focus on slides most needing review. Increased cost per slide

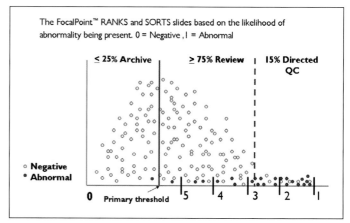

Figure 11-14. FocalPoint ranking and sorting of slides. (Courtesy and © Becton, Dickinson and Company.)

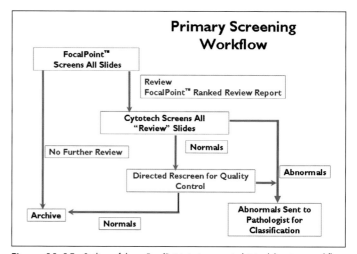

Figure 11-15. Outline of how FocalPoint is incorporated into laboratory workflow. (Courtesy and © Becton, Dickinson and Company.)

1.0) to each slide based on the probability of abnormality. This information is used to classify slides into "Review" and "No Further Review (NFR)" groups and then to rank Review slides into five quintiles (1= highest risk, 5=lowest risk), helping cytologists to understand the risk inherent in each slide (Figure 11-14). NFR cases do not require a manual screening by a cytotechnologist and, with the exception of high-risk cases, can be reported as negative and archived, without human review. The remaining 75% of slides are classified as Review and require manual screening. In addition, FocalPoint identifies at least 15% of successfully processed slides for a second QC manual review.

These slides must be screened a second time if the first manual screen was negative (Figure 11-15).

The FocalPoint provides an assessment of the squamous cellularity of the specimen during its scan. As a safety issue, specimens with low squamous cellularity will not be classified in the No Further Review category.

Trained cytology laboratory personnel operating under the direct supervision of a qualified cytology supervisor or laboratory manager/director load properly accessioned, bar-coded, clean and stained slides (8 slides per tray) onto the FocalPoint. The instrument input and output hoppers can be loaded with up to 180 slides in a 24-hour period, or 288 slides for 30 hours of continuous operation. The FocalPoint instrument is housed and maintained within the individual laboratory and requires regular maintenance and cleaning. Advantages and disadvantages of the FocalPoint are shown in Table 11-9.

Performance of FocalPoint Slide Profiler Using Conventional Smears. In trials conducted by the manufacturer, the FocalPoint identified a greater (statistically significant) number of cancerous and precancerous lesions than current manual practice.[27] The FocalPoint-assisted arm of the study was superior to the current practice arm

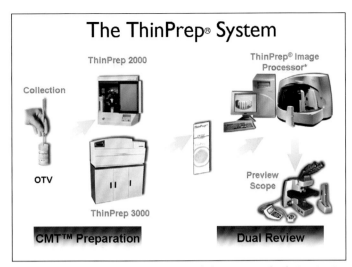

Figure 11-16. The ThinPrep Imaging System, which incorporates The ThinPrep Pap Test with companion automated screener. (Courtesy of Hologic, Inc. and affiliates.)

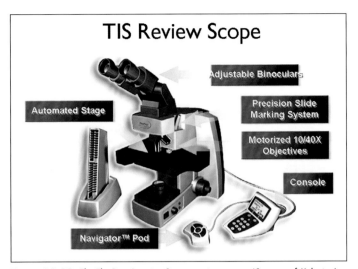

Figure 11-18. The ThinPrep Imaging System review scope. (Courtesy of Hologic, Inc. and affiliates.)

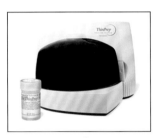

Figure 11-17. ThinPrep Imaging System processor. (Courtesy of Hologic, Inc. and affiliates.)

for the identification of abnormal slides at the level of ASC-US, LSIL, and LSIL+ lesions. However, due to small numbers of high-grade lesions, although performing slightly better than the current practice arm, FocalPoint was only statistically equivalent to current practice for HSIL.[28]

Performance of FocalPoint Slide Profiler Using SurePath Liquid-Based Cytology. The FDA approved SurePath slides to be screened on the FocalPoint Slide Profiler. According to clinical trial data, FocalPoint effectively places preparations with abnormal cells into the review population. A manufacturer-sponsored clinical trial showed that it could do this more effectively than could current manual practice.[26]

The ThinPrep Imaging System

The ThinPrep Imaging System (Hologic Inc) is a automated primary screener that combines imaging technology with interactive human visual inspection of each ThinPrep 2000/3000 processed slide (Figure 11-16). The ThinPrep Imaging System consists of two components: an image processor and a review scope. The image processor (Figure 11-17) assists in the primary screening of ThinPrep Pap tests through the provision of slide coordinates of abnormal fields of view (FOV) for subsequent microscope review by cytotechnologists on the review scope (Figure 11-18).

Intended Use of the ThinPrep Imaging System. The ThinPrep Imaging System uses computer imaging technology to assist in screening ThinPrep slides for the presence of atypical cells, cervical neoplasia and its precursor lesions (LSIL, HSIL), and carcinoma, as well as all other cytologic criteria as defined by the Bethesda System.[29]

Description of the ThinPrep Imaging System. Slides used with this system must first be prepared on a ThinPrep

2000 or 3000 Processor and stained. In order to scan ThinPrep slides accurately, a consistent, nonhematoxylin nuclear stain is required, using a synthetic nuclear dye ("ThinPrep Stain") to permit quantitative measurements of nuclear DNA content.

The image processor acquires and processes data from the ThinPrep slides to identify diagnostically relevant cells or cell groups based on an imaging algorithm (Optical Cellular Selection) that considers cellular features and nuclear darkness. During slide imaging, the alphanumeric slide accession identifier is recorded, and the x and y coordinates of 22 FOV containing cells of diagnostic interest are stored in the computer database. The computer also coordinates the communication of information between the image processor and the review scope.

After image processing, slides are distributed to cytotechnologists for review with the review scope. The review scope is a standard cytology microscope equipped with an automated stage to facilitate locating the 22 FOV containing the cells of diagnostic interest. Slides are individually loaded onto the review scope stage, the alphanumeric slide accession identifier is automatically scanned, and the stored coordinates representing the FOV for that slide are electronically downloaded from the computer to the review scope. The cytotechnologist then uses a keypad to step through each of the fields of view. If the cytotechnologist identifies any of these fields as containing abnormal objects, the field(s) may be marked electronically for further review (Figure 11-19). The cytotechnologist determines specimen adequacy and the presence of infections during the review of the 22 FOV. At the conclusion of the slide review, electronically marked objects are automati-

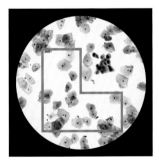

Figure 11-19. ThinPrep Imaging System. Example of a field of view with electronic "L" dotting cells of interest. (Courtesy of Hologic, Inc. and affiliates.)

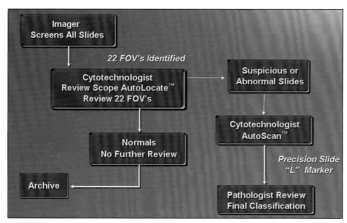

Figure 11-20. Outline of how the ThinPrep Imaging System is incorporated into laboratory workflow.

Table 11-10. Advantages and Disadvantages of the ThinPrep Imaging System

Advantages	Disadvantages
Small size of system	Not compatible with traditional Pap staining method
Motorized microscope stage limits; ergonomic concerns for cytotechnologists	Not compatible with conventional Pap smears or SurePath liquid-based Pap test
Fewer fields of view to review; increased productivity	All slides selected for review must be manually screened
Standardized Pap stain	Synthetic Pap stain requires adjustment
Increased disease detection; fewer false-negatives	Increased cost per slide

cally ink-marked. Any coordinates representing marked locations along with a slide completion status are then electronically transmitted back to the computer for storage.

If the cytotechnologist identifies an abnormality in any of the 22 FOV, they must revert to a full manual slide review. Alternately, the cytotechnologist can determine that the slide is negative after the 22 FOV review and sign the case out. Through the FOV screening and triage process, the amount of time required to screen a negative ThinPrep slide is reduced. Pathologists review dotted ThinPrep slides using a standard microscope in the usual fashion. ThinPrep Imaging System laboratory workflow is illustrated in Figure 11-20.

The benchtop image processor can be loaded with 250 ThinPrep slides for analysis (25 slides per "magazine") for an annual throughput of approximately 100,000 slides. Continuous loading onto the image processor is possible. With each slide imaging taking about 4 minutes, up to 360 slides can be processed in 24 hours. Advantages and disadvantages of the ThinPrep Imaging System are shown in Table 11-10.

Performance of the ThinPrep Imaging System. A clinical trial sponsored by the manufacturer showed a statistically significant improvement in sensitivity for ASC-US+ slides, equivalent sensitivity for LSIL+ and HSIL+ slides, and statistically significant improvement in specificity for HSIL+ compared to the manual screening arm.[30] The adjudicated results for ASC-US+ showed a 39% reduction in false-negative slides using the ThinPrep Imaging System.

The workload limit for the ThinPrep Imaging System has been established at 200 slides in no less than an 8-hour workday for 22 FOV triage only. For slides triaged to full manual screening, the workload limit remains at a maximum of 100 slides in an 8-hour workday (or lower as dictated by any more stringent local regulations). Any combination of FOV-only and full manual reviews must be integrated to not exceed either limit.

Points to Consider

A variety of factors affect the implementation and successful outcome of adopting any new or more expensive tech-

Table 11-11. Points to Consider Before Implementing New Technologies in the Cytology Laboratory

Pap test volume

Number of pathologists, cytotechnologists, and laboratory technicians

Perceived expectations of performance

Labor costs and availability

Payer mix (Medicare, private insurer, HMO, etc)

Physical laboratory facilities

Cost-benefit justification

Direct and indirect costs per billed test

Federal, state, and laboratory workload policies

Clinician acceptance and education

Adaptability to new preparatory workflow and morphology (liquid-based cytology)

nology in a specific laboratory setting (Table 11-11). Among the factors to consider are significant laboratory variations in (1) reasons for adopting the technology, along with preconceived expectations of performance; (2) direct and indirect costs, especially those related to high-volume discounts for reagents and disposables; (3) physical laboratory facilities; (4) Pap test volumes; (5) labor cost and availability; (6) federal, state, and individual laboratory policies regarding workload regulations or "guidelines"; (7) flexibility in adapting to new preparatory workflow and modified cytomorphology; (8) extent of cooperation with clinical sites and thoroughness of clinician education; (9) number of cytotechnologists, pathologists, and laboratory technicians; and (10) reimbursement (payer mix, Medicare, physician versus laboratory billing).

Other factors involved in making this decision include specific test performance (including specimen collection issues), costs (including secretarial, preparatory, evaluation, and reporting issues), compatibility with other instrumentation/current laboratory practice, differences in manual screening (including morphology issues), availability of out-of-the-vial testing, demand for a specific test from clients/clinicians/patients, and, unfortunately, persistence and effectiveness of vendor marketing activities. Presence or absence of adequate reimbursement will likely be more of an issue in determining whether or not liquid-based testing occurs at all, rather than an issue in terms of which liquid-based test to choose—both use the same CPT codes, so they are reimbursed at the same rate. However, differences in costs can certainly make a specific level of reimbursement more adequate for one product than for another.

The main difference in the costs of these two preparations is in the disposable testing kits, and these costs can add up and be significant. Increased screening efficiency may or may not occur in individual laboratories. However, if increases in screening numbers do occur, this could have a significant impact on staffing and costs of screening per billed test. When assessing these preparations, if increased screening efficiency is an expectation, the cost analysis would need to be modified accordingly to determine screening costs and how they affect overall feasibility for the particular laboratory situation.

The motivation for implementing automated screening of liquid-based preparations is similar to that for performing liquid-based testing in general, added to the motivation for automated screening of liquid-based cytology and/or conventional Pap smears, with the caveat that, as both tests address different problems related to false-negative results, their effects should at least partially combine to provide a synergistic effect with greater sensitivity (or other factor) than either test used alone. Additionally, increased reimbursement levels for integrated liquid-based testing /automated screening, and the addition of potential efficiencies with automated screening that may temper increased costs associated with this technology, could combine to make this testing modality the most financially feasible of all.

New Instrumentation in the Cytopathology Laboratory

The cytology laboratory has traditionally performed a small variety of tests employing manual processes. Instruments that were put into use (eg, centrifuges, stainers, coverslipper) were rarely checked to assure they were operating properly before implementation into clinical practice. The advent of new technologies in cervicovaginal cytology has led to the increased use of instrumentation and complex test methods in cytopathology. The increasing use of molecular methods in cytopathology further adds to the changing needs for validation.

Similar to the rest of the clinical laboratory, the cytopathology laboratory must assure that testing performed is accurate and consistent, and is in compliance with regulatory and accreditation programs, such as the Clinical Laboratory Improvement Amendments of 1988 (CLIA '88), the College of American Pathologists (CAP) Laboratory Accreditation Program (LAP), and Joint Commission standards. Even if the instrument or test is FDA approved, it must undergo a verification study prior to implementation.

The CAP LAP Cytopathology Checklist standard CYP.05257 reads as follows: "Is there documentation of adherence to the manufacturer's recommended protocol(s) for implementation and validation of new instruments?" The appended note reads: Before implementing use of new gynecologic liquid-based methods and instruments, automated preparations, and automated screening instruments, the laboratory must validate and document the functioning of the instrument *in its own specific laboratory environment,* including the capability of the instrument to replace existing procedure(s), if applicable. If the manufacturer does not provide validation and instrument monitoring recommendations, the laboratory must document the specific validation procedure used.

There are further standards that are now included in the CAP Cytopathology Checklist, including CYP.05260, "Is there documentation of ongoing monitoring of instrument maintenance and function for all devices"; and CYP.05264, "Is there documentation of appropriate technical and interpretative training for each of the instruments used?"

Many manufacturers provide assistance by establishing guidelines for the validation of their instruments; however, the absence of a formal protocol does not create an exemption for an instrument. Often, the clinical laboratory section of a general laboratory can provide assistance with establishing a protocol if the cytology laboratory lacks experience and knowledge in this area. The CAP Laboratory General Checklist standard includes GEN.42020, "Has the laboratory verified or established documented analytic accuracy and precision for each test"?

Any event that may alter the previously established function of the instrument also requires revalidation. This includes major repair of the instrument, especially if the repair requires shipping the instrument to an off-site location. The Joint Commission also establishes similar requirements for instrument validation. Failure to establish and verify method performance prior to reporting patient test results is one of the most frequently cited deficiencies from data based on Joint Commission laboratory surveys.

It is important to develop a procedure that provides guidance for the management of work when any cytology laboratory instrument fails. The CAP LAP Cytopathology Checklist standard CYP.05285, a Phase II standard, reads, "Is there a documented procedure for handling workload during instrument failure and/or downtime?" It includes this note: "This procedure must address: (a) final processing and resulting of any cases/specimens that are within the instrument at the time of failure, and (b) alternative procedures to be used during instrument downtime." Although this procedure may appear to be common sense, it is important that it be clearly and thoroughly documented. Furthermore, though this standard was originally developed to address issues relating to newly introduced instrumentation associated with automated Pap test screening, including instruments used in the production of Pap test slides as well as the automated computer-assisted evaluation, it should also be applied to other instruments in use within the cytology laboratory, including the laboratory information system.

Finally, if the instrument has been cleared or approved by the FDA, *the laboratory must document and report adverse events (eg, failures).* A user facility must report to the device manufacturer and the FDA whenever the facility has information that reasonably suggests a device has or may have caused or contributed to a patient's death. If a facility has information that reasonably suggests a device has or may have caused or contributed to a patient's serious injury, it must report this information to the device manufacturer. In most circumstances, the cytology laboratory should document and report these instrument events (eg, failures) to the manufacturer (not the FDA). Specifically, the FDA states: "User facilities must establish and maintain MDR [medical device report] event files. MDR event files are written or electronic files maintained by the user facility. They must be prominently identified as such and filed to facilitate timely access. MDR files must contain:

- information in the possession of the user facility or references to information related to the event. This includes all documentation of the reporting decisions and decision-making process; and
- copies of all completed MDR forms and other information submitted to FDA, distributors, and manufacturers.

Records related to an adverse event, whether reported or not, must be kept for two (2) years from the date of the event. A user facility must permit FDA employees to have access, at all reasonable times, to all required records for copying and verification." Finally, the FDA encourages that user facilities use form 3500A to report to the manufacturer, since this form provides for more detail about the event and the device.

Even if the laboratory has already performed the initial validation process on a previously installed instrument, a new instrument of the same type must still undergo validation. It is appropriate to use the same protocol used to validate the original instrument.

Conclusions

Many of the shortcomings in the effort to rid the world of cervical cancer are related to nonexistent or inadequate Pap test screening. False-negative Pap tests play a lesser but still significant role in up to about 40% of failures to detect cervical cancer and its precursor lesions, with sampling and detection errors contributing in a ratio of about two to

one. Inadequate management or follow-up of abnormal tests may play a role in around 10% of failures.

The rapid growth of new technologies in Pap smear testing—at least of automated screening—would appear to be a natural part of the evolution of Papanicolaou testing. While attempts to begin automating the task of screening cervical smears can be found as early as the 1950s, it hasn't been until the last 10 to 15 years that imaging and image processing technology have become sophisticated enough (and inexpensive enough) to make clinically useful screening systems possible.

External forces also have driven the development of automated screening. Not long after attention was focused on the shortcomings of the Pap test, intense pressure was brought to bear on the cytology laboratories from the public, regulatory agencies, and the legal profession to do something about "so many" Pap smears being misinterpreted. Despite efforts from the cytology community, device manufacturers, armed with the strength of a frightened public, gained enough momentum to move forward.

Another force driving this technology is that the capability of laboratories to continue to screen volumes of Pap smears and deal with increasing regulatory demands is likely to become more limited. With the advent of primary automated screening, new technologies could significantly take pressure off overburdened laboratories. Finally, advent of new technologies will allow cytotechnologists to spend more time focusing on more difficult cases, which are more likely to be abnormal, rather than spending extra time on Pap tests that have a high probability of being negative. This concept is especially important in the post–HPV-vaccine era, when disease prevalence is predicted to decrease, making screening procedures inherently less sensitive. Automated instrumentation will improve the laboratory's ability to maintain adequate levels of sensitivity by prioritizing only high-probability slides and/or fields for manual review.

Adjunctive Testing of Gynecologic Cytology Specimens

With the advent of liquid-based cytology in cervicovaginal screening, cervical cells are now collected and maintained in a liquid preservative, leaving residual cells that were never available following the making of a conventional Pap smear. HPV DNA testing was the first "out-of-the-vial" test assay validated for clinical use with gynecologic liquid-based cytology samples. Because of the availability of so many preserved cells in the residual material, the opportunity has been opened for the performance of other tests. With the explosion of nucleic-acid-based methods, tests are being developed that can be added on to the routine cervical cytology sample. Table 11-12 lists in vitro molecular diagnostic products that have been used for out-of-the-vial testing from gynecologic liquid-based cytology samples. Some have been cleared or approved by the FDA for diagnostic use. Such tests are classified as "medical devices." More information is available at the website for

Table 11-12. Examples of In Vitro Molecular Diagnostic Assays that are Used for Out-of-the-Vial Testing from Liquid-Based Cytology Samples

Analyte	Sample	Method	Regulatory Status
Human papillomavirus	ThinPrep SurePath MonoPrep	Hybrid Capture 2	FDA approved (PMA) No; CLIA validation No; CLIA validation
Chlamydia/gonorrhea	ThinPrep SurePath MonoPrep	AMPLICOR or APTIMA	FDA cleared (510k) No; CLIA validation No; CLIA validation
Herpes simplex virus	Cervicovaginal liquid-based cytology	Polymerase chain reaction	No; CLIA validation
Group B streptococci	Cervicovaginal liquid-based cytology	Amplification	No; CLIA validation
Trichomonas vaginalis	Cervicovaginal liquid-based cytology	Hybridization	No; CLIA validation
Cystic fibrosis	Cervicovaginal liquid-based cytology	Polymerase chain reaction	No; CLIA validation

FDA's Office of In Vitro Diagnostic (OIVD) Evaluation and Safety (www.fda.gov/cdrh/oivd/index.html).

Human Papillomavirus

DNA testing for the oncogenic high-risk types of HPV is approved by the FDA for use in cervical cancer screening. The cervical sample in PreservCyt has been approved for testing for the oncogenic high-risk types of HPV using the Digene® HPV Test with Hybrid Capture® 2 (hc2) technology (also known as the hc2 High-Risk HPV DNA Test" or as the DNAwithPap Test") (Qiagen, Venlo, The Netherlands). A study conducted by the National Cancer Institute concluded that high-risk HPV testing is a viable method for determining which patients with borderline Pap results (ASC-US) are at highest risk for developing cancer.[31] The hc2 High-Risk HPV DNA Test was also approved for primary cervical cancer screening, when used in conjunction with The ThinPrep Pap Test, for women older than age 30 years. For high-risk HPV testing, the laboratory can either use the residual cellular material in The ThinPrep Pap Test or collect a second sample and place it in a Qiagen Cervical Sampler container. Gynecologic specimens collected in PreservCyt may be held up to 3 months at 15 to 30°C or 59 to 86°F following collection and prior to processing for the HPV DNA assay.

The consensus guidelines of the American Society for Colposcopy and Cervical Pathology (ASCCP) recommend high-risk HPV testing as one of the triage options in the management of patients with an initial ASC-US Pap but is the preferred method when using liquid-based cytology.[32] For purposes of adjunctive testing from liquid-based cytology, removal of a 4-mL aliquot from The ThinPrep Pap Test PreservCyt vial prior to preparation of The ThinPrep Pap Test was FDA approved in 2005. This aliquot is only to be used to support performance of ancillary tests approved by the FDA on PreservCyt material.

At the time of publication, SurePath and MonoPrep have not been FDA approved for ancillary out-of-the-vial testing for high-risk HPV. Laboratories wishing to use these preparations for such testing must perform analytical and clinical validation studies as required for FDA "off-label" assays under CLIA '88 regulations and CAP LAP checklist standards.

Independent studies, not manufacturer sponsored, have shown excellent performance of high-risk HPV detection utilizing Qiagen's hc2 High-Risk HPV DNA Test with the SurePath vial.[33]

Clinical performance data on the Monogen liquid-based platform from a manufacturer-sponsored study of high-risk HPV (hc2 assay) demonstrates statistical equivalence with Qiagen Cervical Sampler Specimen Transport Medium results, absence of Quantity Not Sufficient (QNS) issues, and 6 months room temperature stability for cells in the vial.[34]

Chlamydia/Gonorrhea

In 2002, Hologic's Cytyc Corporation gained FDA approval for *Chlamydia trachomatis* (CT) and *Neisseria gonorrhea* (NG) testing directly from the ThinPrep PreservCyt collection vial, using Roche Diagnostics' COBAS® AMPLICOR and Gen-Probe's APTIMA Combo 2® CT/NG assay. The AMPLICOR package insert makes no claims regarding the use of The ThinPrep Pap Test in their assay; instructions for processing and testing PreservCyt specimens should be obtained from the ThinPrep package insert. This was later followed by approval of Gen-Probe's APTIMA Combo 2 CT/NG assay.[35-37] There are other CT/NG assays manufactured by Becton Dickinson (BD), Qiagen, and Gen-Probe, but gynecologic liquid-based cytology media are not an approved specimen source.

At the time of this writing, SurePath and MonoPrep have not been FDA-approved for ancillary out-of-the-vial testing for CT/NG. Laboratories wishing to use these preparations for such testing must perform analytical and clinical validation studies as required for FDA "off-label" assays under CLIA '88 regulations and CAP LAP checklist standards.

Culture is considered the reference method for CT/NG infection confirmation, and material collected into liquid-based cytology transport media is unsuitable for culture. CT/NG molecular tests are FDA approved for testing endocervical swab, male and female urethral swab, male and female voided urine, and cervical cell specimens collected in ThinPrep PreservCyt media. Independent studies, not manufacturer sponsored, have documented good performance using the SurePath media as an alternative specimen type for the APTIMA CT/NG assay.[38]

Laboratories performing nucleic acid testing must be aware of the risk of cross-contamination causing false-positives and follow meticulous methods to avoid cross-contamination if using liquid-based cytology specimens. Additional specimen handling procedures are required according to the ThinPrep package insert. Removal of a 4-mL aliquot from the PreservCyt vial prior to preparation of The ThinPrep Pap Test is approved by the FDA. PreservCyt is considered antimicrobial, but sterile technique must be carefully observed when handling specimens.

The use of CT/NG testing from liquid-based cytology media appears to be sensible. While not the most ideal sample source for CT/NG assays, the nature of out-of-the-vial testing with liquid-based cytology is convenient for patients and clinicians and avoids missed opportunities for screening. CT/NG infection is widespread in the population receiving Pap tests and is associated with significant morbidity. Recommended guidelines for screening involve young women who are already in screening programs for cervical carcinoma. CT/NG screening, like cervical cancer screening, is a screening test with false-positives and false-negatives. CT/NG testing out of the vial is not a culture, and practitioners must be educated about the causes of false-negative and false-positive tests.

Herpes Simplex Virus

Molecular detection of herpes simplex virus (HSV) is recognized as the reference standard for sensitive and specific diagnosis of HSV, especially for central nervous system infections. Testing for genital HSV-2 can be performed using nucleic acid methods and residua from liquid-based cytology vials. Most of this HSV testing is done via "home brew" assays and is not subject to FDA regulatory oversight. However, according to CLIA, usage of liquid-based cytology media requires careful in-house validation prior to starting patient testing. Close attention must be paid to avoid cross-contamination of the sample preparations.

Group B Streptococci

The Centers for Disease Control and Prevention (CDC), the American College of Obstetricians and Gynecologists (ACOG), and the American Academy of Pediatrics recommend the use of either risk assessment or screening for group B streptococci in pregnant women to identify candidates for intrapartum antimicrobial prophylaxis. Risk assessment is performed at the onset of labor, and the presence of fever, a prolonged interval between rupture of membranes and delivery, or imminent preterm delivery is considered indicative of the need for prophylaxis. Additionally, the CDC has recommended routine screening for vaginal streptococcus B for all women during pregnancy. This screening is performed between the 35th and 37th week of pregnancy. This bacterium can be cultured from rectal/vaginal swabs, but the liquid-based cytology media are bacteriostatic, and are an inappropriate sample source for group B streptococci cultures. Testing for group B streptococci can be done using nucleic acid testing and residua from liquid-based cytology vial, which is more rapid than culture methods. None of the liquid-based cytology media is mentioned as a specimen source for the 510(k)-cleared group B streptococci assay kits available from BD, Cephid, or Gen-Probe.

Trichomonas Vaginalis

Trichomonas vaginalis is the most common nonviral cause of vaginitis in the world. In the US, it is a nonreportable sexually transmitted infection and is estimated to cause at least 5 to 7 million infections annually. Infections with *T vaginalis* are frequently asymptomatic but may cause adverse health sequelae such as preterm labor, pelvic inflammatory disease, infertility, and an increase in HIV transmission.

Cervicovaginal cytology appears to be both insensitive and nonspecific for the diagnosis of *T. vaginalis*, and a sensitive molecular assay, such as the BD Affirm™ VPIII Microbial Identification Test, might be more suitable. Testing for *T vaginalis* could be done using nucleic acid testing and residua from liquid-based cytology vials. None of the liquid-based cytology media is mentioned as a specimen source for the *T vaginalis* assay.

Genetic Screening for Cystic Fibrosis

Cystic fibrosis is one the most common inherited diseases in the United States, affecting one infant out of every 3,000 live births. If both parents are carriers, then their child has a 25% chance of being born with cystic fibrosis, a 50% chance that the child will not have cystic fibrosis but will be a carrier, and a 25% chance the child will not be a carrier.

ACOG now recommends that OB-GYN physicians make DNA screening for cystic fibrosis available to all couples seeking preconception or prenatal care, and not just to those with a personal family history of carrying the cystic fibrosis gene, as was previously recommended. ACOG recommends a screening panel of 25 common cystic fibrosis mutations and associated polymorphisms. A polymerase chain reaction (PCR) assay is used to determine affected or carrier status of the most common cystic fibrosis mutations and associated polymorphisms. It detects >90% of cystic fibrosis mutations in the Northern European Caucasian populations; there may be higher or lower detection rates

Table 11-13. Examples of Biomarkers for Cervical Intraepithelial Neoplasia or Cancer

Target	Sample	Method	Regulatory Clearance
p16	Cervicovaginal liquid-based cytology	Immunocytochemistry	Analyte-specific reagent
ProEx C	Cervicovaginal liquid-based cytology	Immunocytochemistry	Analyte-specific reagent
DNA aneuploidy	Cervicovaginal liquid-based cytology	Fluorescence in situ hybridization	IUO / RUO
Cyclins	Cervicovaginal liquid-based cytology	Immunocytochemistry	IUO / RUO
Ki-67	Cervicovaginal liquid-based cytology	Immunocytochemistry	IUO / RUO
MYC	Cervicovaginal liquid-based cytology	Fluorescence in situ hybridization	IUO / RUO
Telomerase	Cervicovaginal liquid-based cytology	Immunocytochemistry	IUO / RUO
Epigenetic markers (eg, methylation)	Cervicovaginal liquid-based cytology	Polymerase chain reaction	IUO / RUO

Abbreviations: IUO, investigational use only; RUO, research use only.

for other ethnic groups. Liquid-based cytology residua can provide extracted DNA material to perform this assay.

Generally, a minimum volume from SurePrep or ThinPrep preparations is required for genomic DNA extraction.

Although not the most ideal sample source for cystic fibrosis genetic assays, out-of-the-vial testing with liquid-based cytology specimens is convenient for patients and clinicians and avoids missed opportunities for screening. Recommended guidelines for screening for cystic fibrosis involve young women of childbearing age, who are usually already in screening programs for cervical carcinoma.

Points to Consider

Although liquid-based cytology vials provide abundant cells for analysis, the vials are not an inexhaustible supply of nucleic acid. The collection of cells still depends on the clinician's procurement technique, the ability to transfer cells from the collection device to the media, and the extraction and transfer of the nucleic acid into the test system. First and foremost, cells must be collected in adequate amounts for screening for cancer and HPV, as this is the primary role for this collection vehicle. If laboratories routinely prealiquot specimens for other tests, the effectiveness of liquid-based cytology to detect cervical cancer might be hindered. The value of the additional tests must be weighed against the "dilution" of the cervical cytology specimen and its ability to detect cervical cancer.

Finally, laboratories performing nucleic acid testing must be aware of the risk of cross-contamination causing false-positives and follow meticulous methods to avoid cross-contamination if using liquid-based cytology specimens. The preservative component of most liquid-based cytology tests may be used as an alternative collection and transport medium for gynecologic specimens tested with these assays. However, additional specimen handling procedures are required. If not cleared or approved by the FDA, careful attention to in-house CLIA validation and CAP LAP checklist standards are necessary before patient testing.

Cervical Carcinoma Biomarkers

The use of biomarkers that are sensitive and specific for cervical dysplasia/carcinoma might help reduce the false-negative rate of gynecologic cytology, improve the cost-effectiveness in the management of abnormal cervical cytology, and increase the interobserver agreement for interpreting cervical lesions. Biomarkers could also potentially decrease false-positive rates, for instance, in differentiating the cellular changes associated with atrophy from preneoplastic cellular changes. Many ASC-US and LSIL cases are found to be CIN II/III or higher after tissue confirmation. Therefore, cervical cancer biomarkers could serve as predictors of such cases and could be used to identify which patients should receive more aggressive diagnostic interventions.

Recent studies utilizing gene expression profiling have identified a set of candidate biomarkers that are associated with high-grade lesions and carcinoma of the cervix.[39] These molecules fall into several categories, including those associated with the extracellular matrix and those involved in cell replication and proliferation. Many of these biomarkers represent "downstream" effects of infection of the cervix with oncogenic-types of HPV (Table 11-13).

For example, induction of cell proliferation (S-phase) in HSIL cells is initiated, in part, by the activity of the E6 and E7 proteins of HPV. HPV-associated E7 is known to bind the retinoblastoma gene protein and displace the transcriptional activator E2F from its complex, thus inducing the aberrant transcription of S-phase proteins, such as minichromosome maintenance protein 2 (MCM2) and topoisomerase IIα (TOP2A), responsible for DNA synthesis and cell proliferation.[40-43]

p16INK4a

p16INK4a is a tumor suppressor protein, the normal function of which is to prevent cells from dividing in the absence of an appropriate signal. The deletion or inactivation of p16INK4a contributes to tumor progression in many types of cancer, including cancers of the esophagus, head and neck, biliary tract, bladder, colon, breast, and lung, as well as lymphomas, leukemias, glioblastoma, and melanoma. In contrast, a majority of studies suggest that p16INK4a is overexpressed in cervical dysplasia/cancer. p16INK4a is upregulated in cervical lesions as a result of the inactivation of retinoblastoma gene protein by high-risk HPV gene product E7, and resultant activation of the transcription factor E2F, leading to p16INK4a paradoxical overexpression in cervical neoplasia (Figure 11-21).

Numerous immunochemical studies have been published on the expression of p16INK4a in cervical dysplasia/carcinoma using histological and/or cytological samples. Thin-layer slides are prepared from cervical liquid-based cytology specimens and treated with a pretreatment buffer for target retrieval. Brown nuclear and cytoplasmic staining is indicative of aberrant p16 overexpression. The vast majority of the studies support the idea that p16INK4a expression is increased in cervical dysplasia/carcinoma,[44-48] although some suggest that there is a subpopulation of HSIL and squamous cell carcinoma that follow a different path to tumor progression that results in a loss or decrease in p16INK4a expression.

A summary of representative studies of p16 expression in cervical cytologic liquid-based specimens showed positive p16 immunostaining in 11% NILM (negative for intraepithelial lesion or malignancy), 45% ASC-US, 46% LSIL, 96% HSIL, and 99% in carcinoma.[48] Only a small number of studies have analyzed the performance of p16 immunocytochemistry to detect high-grade lesions using liquid-based cervical cytology. The sensitivity and specificity of p16 for high-grade lesions was most recently reported to be 77% and 57%, respectively.[49]

Performance of p16 staining studies on liquid-based cytology specimens for either triage or screening should be interpreted carefully. The preanalytic phase, the reagents used, and the immunostaining procedures should be uniform and consistent. More important, interpretation of immunocytochemical findings must be standardized and validated carefully. Additional studies of p16 for triage or screening use in cervical cytology are needed.

BD ProEx C Reagents

BD ProEx™ C is a Class I immunohistochemical in vitro diagnostic used with standard immunocytochemistry techniques. It can be used to detect the presence of aberrant S-phase induction in liquid-based cervical cytology speci-

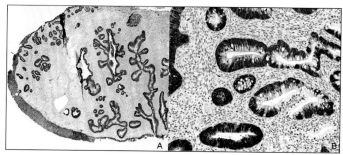

Figure 11-21. p16 immunohistochemistry expression in an abnormal cervical biopsy specimen. **A.** Low power showing diffuse p16 staining is present in both the dysplastic squamous epithelium and the glandular epithelium. **B.** Note the intense nuclear and cytoplasmic staining in the higher magnification of the glandular epithelium, which turned out to be adenocarcinoma in situ. (Courtesy of Dr. Galen Eversol.)

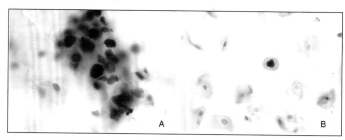

Figure 11-22. ProEx C stain on SurePath slide with hematoxylin counterstain. **A.** Group of HSIL cells with positive staining in a patient with biopsy-proven CIN II. **B.** Single positively staining HSIL cell with biopsy-proven CIN II (X60; courtesy of Dr. Rosemary Tambouret.)

mens.[50-52] ProEx C contains antibodies to MCM2 and TOP2A proteins. The minichromosome maintenance proteins function during DNA replication by loading the pre-replication complex onto DNA and also by unwinding DNA through helicase activity to permit DNA synthesis. TOP2A is responsible for the enzymatic unlinking of DNA strands during replication.

Thin-layer slides are prepared from liquid-based cytology specimens and treated with a pretreatment buffer for target retrieval. Brown nuclear staining is indicative of aberrant S-phase induction (Figure 11-22). In an initial report of staining in liquid-based cervical cytology slides, intense nuclear staining was noted in 0% NILM, 20% ASC-US, 50% LSIL, and 100% of HSIL slides.[51]

Preliminary manufacturer-sponsored studies have shown the performance of ProEx C detection of CIN II/III in cervical liquid-based cytology slides (SurePath) has a sensitivity of 85.3% and specificity of 71.7%,[52] and when used in conjunction with associated cytologic abnormality the sensitivity improved to 92% with a specificity of 84%.[53]

DNA Aneuploidy

Disturbances of the mitotic spindle apparatus are induced early by deregulated expression of high-risk HPV oncogenes, resulting in nondiploid nuclei (aneuploidy). Consequently, aneuploidy is characteristic for HPV-transformed lesions, even at precancerous stages. Different techniques exist to measure the DNA content of cervical squamous cells. Presently, the most promising technique appears to be using fluorescently labeled chromosomal enumeration probes and interphase fluorescence in situ hybridization (FISH) on liquid-based cytology slides.[54]

Cyclins

Cyclins are a large family of regulatory proteins with central functions in the coordination of the cell cycle. The expression of several cyclins has been analyzed in cervical cancer and precancer using immunohistochemistry or immunocytochemistry. Cyclin D has been shown to be overexpressed in LSIL. Cyclin E has been analyzed in liquid-based cytology slides and found to be associated with HPV abnormalities.

Ki-67

The increased proliferation of cervical epithelial cells induced by deregulated HPV oncogene expression is reflected in the activation of proliferation markers such as Ki67 (MIB-1). This protein is strongly expressed in CIN lesions. It can be detected by immunocytochemistry on liquid-based cytology slides. All except totally quiescent populations of cells will show some staining with Ki67. The importance of the marker is to identify increases in the number of cells positive in populations. In histologic sections, the location within the epithelium of positive-staining cells is of significance. In normal squamous epithelia, basal-level staining only is present. In dysplastic lesions, positive cells are noted at increasingly high levels in the epithelium, with increasing grades of dysplasia.

MYC

The oncogene MYC is frequently found amplified and overexpressed in cervical carcinoma. It has been found to be activated in precancerous lesions and might be used to assess dysplastic lesions. It can be detected by FISH probes performed on liquid-based cytology slides.

Telomerase

Telomeres are located at the outermost end of chromosomes. They function in chromosome protection, positioning, and replication. As mitotic clocks, they will shorten in a replication-dependent manner and are a trigger of cell senescence. The telomerase protein complex adds short repetitive DNA stretches to the chromosome ends. The gene encoding the RNA subunit of the complex, TER, is located on chromosome 3q and is frequently amplified in cervical lesions. Most CIN II/III lesions and a high proportion of CIN I lesions are composed of immortalized cell populations. Immunocytochemical staining for human telomerase reverse transcriptase (hTERT) on liquid-based cytology slides can detect expression and is associated with dysplasia and carcinoma; however, its actual utility is uncertain.

Epigenetic Markers

Methylation of CpG islands is an epigenetic modification of gene expression. In many cancers, tumor suppressor genes are found to be inactivated by methylation. This is true for cervical carcinoma and could be a potential biomarker of cervical neoplasia and carcinoma.

Points to Consider

In both primary screening and triage settings, novel biomarkers that allow monitoring of the previously described essential molecular events in histological or cytological specimens are likely to improve the detection of lesions that have a high risk of progression. Gynecologic samples collected by liquid-based cytology have not been FDA approved for use with these assays. If a laboratory uses these methods, internal laboratory CLIA validation should be performed, and rigorous methods to support analytic and clinical performance and accuracy must be implemented and documented.

Finally, performance of biomarkers on gynecologic liquid-based cytology specimens for either triage or screening should be interpreted carefully. The preanalytic phase, the reagents used, and the immunostaining procedures should be uniform and consistent. More importantly, interpretation of immunocytochemical findings must be standardized and validated carefully. Additional studies are necessary before these biomarkers can be considered for incorporation into routine practice.

FDA, Off-Label Use, and Validation Studies

The FDA considers clinical laboratory tests as Class I medical devices and, as such, reviews and approves tests and methodologies for "in vitro diagnostic use."[55] New technologies in gynecologic cytology, such as liquid-based methods, are included under this FDA review and approval. This also applies to other analytes that might be tested from liquid-based cytology media.

FDA "approval" refers to a test, reagent, or kit approved by the FDA for marketing under the premarket approval (PMA) process for new devices. It can take years before premarket approval is given, and the PMA process is often the most costly method of approval for the manufacturer. The label usually carries the designation "for in vitro diagnostic use." The kit and reagent must be used exactly as defined in the package insert, both procedurally and with regard to its indications for use. If any alterations from manufacturer-defined procedures are used, then the test with the alterations must be validated according to CLIA '88. These "off-label" uses should not be necessarily considered "investigational" or "experimental." Any FDA-approved or cleared test is still required to have verification performed by the laboratory prior to testing patients.

Some tests are marketed as FDA "cleared." FDA clearance refers to a test reagent or kit that is cleared for marketing under a 510(K) review. Generally, the FDA approval process is more stringent, targeting truly novel products. Products that are conceptually similar to those already on the market, or that represent improvements over existing products, can elect for FDA clearance under a 510(k). A 510(k) premarket notification must contain information about indications for use, safety and effectiveness, con-

Table 11-14. Examples of Laboratory Disclaimers Used on Reports

Test Labeling	Report Disclaimer
Analyte-specific reagent (ASR)	This test was developed and its performance characteristics determined by XYZ Laboratories. The US Food and Drug Administration has not approved or cleared this test; however, the FDA has determined that such clearance or approval is not necessary.
Research use only / Investigational use only (RUO/IUO)	This test was developed and its performance characteristics determined by XYZ Laboratories. The US Food and Drug Administration has not approved or cleared this test; however, FDA clearance or approval is not currently required for clinical use. The results are not intended to be used as the sole means for clinical diagnosis or patient management decisions.
DNA sequence mutation tests (eg, cystic fibrosis)	The performance characteristics of this test were determined by XYZ Laboratories. The US Food and Drug Administration has not approved or cleared this test; however, FDA clearance or approval is currently not required for clinical use. The results are not intended to be used as the sole means for clinical diagnosis or patient management decisions.
"Research Use" kit	This test uses a kit designated by the manufacturer as "for research use, not for clinical use." The performance characteristics of this test were determined by XYZ Laboratories. The US Food and Drug Administration has not approved or cleared this test. The results are not intended to be used as the sole means for clinical diagnosis or patient management decisions.
FDA-approved kits: Off-label use, laboratory validated	The manufacturer has not determined the efficacy of this test when performed on (insert specimen type) specimens. The performance characteristics of this test were determined by XYZ Laboratories.
FDA-approved test: Altered procedure or iindication for use, not laboratory validated	Test performed on (insert specimen type). The performance characteristics of this test have not been established.

traindications, warnings, precautions, adverse reactions, and special patient populations. Prescription devices are subject to additional labeling requirements.

If the test is a laboratory-developed test instead of an FDA-approved or cleared test, the laboratory is required to perform full validation as well as verification. Clinical diagnostic assays without FDA approval must meet the validation criteria of CLIA '88. CLIA regulations only require an analytical validation be performed for non-FDA-approved or cleared tests, but the CAP Laboratory Accreditation Program requires that both analytical as well as clinical validation be performed. This validation process can be accomplished in a variety of different ways. The laboratory must document how it determined that the new method produces accurate results; this can be based upon determining clinical sensitivity, clinical specificity, positive predictive value, and negative predictive value. Many laboratories will encounter difficulties with verification of some assays due to lack of samples available for testing (consider using calibration, quality control, or proficiency testing material); molecular assays that often measure a different target; and molecular assays that are more sensitive than the current "gold standard." Finally, CLIA regulations state what must be done but don't give any specifics on *how* it must be done.

In general, the laboratory must verify that the method produces the correct result (test reliability). This can be accomplished by a variety of methods, such as testing ref-

erence materials, comparing test results with a reference method that has been shown to provide clinically valid results, comparing split sample results, and comparing test samples with patient samples that have known results. During the process, the laboratory must document how day-to-day, run-to-run, within-a-run, and operator variance are evaluated.

According to the FDA, analyte-specific reagents (ASRs) are antibodies, specific receptor proteins, ligands, nucleic acid sequences, and similar reagents that, through specific binding or chemical reactions with substances in a specimen, are intended for use in a diagnostic application for identification and quantification of an individual chemical substance or ligand in biological specimens.[56] These reagents enable laboratories to use commercial products that would otherwise not be available for the benefit of patients; however, the FDA has not reviewed the safety or efficacy of the product. They are limited to sale and distribution to high-complexity laboratories with persons qualified in test development.

Some laboratories use FDA-approved test kits, but with alterations. For example, a test, reagent, or kit that has been approved by the FDA is used with alterations in the manufacturer-defined procedures or indications for use (eg, an FDA-approved kit used off label with nonapproved sample type).

There are assays or tests that are labeled as "investigational use only" (IUO) or "research use only" (RUO). The

FDA has designated those in vitro diagnostic devices or reagents as IUO if its uses are intended to determine the safety of efficacy of a device for researchers.[57] The FDA has designated those in vitro diagnostic devices or reagents as RUO if its uses are not intended to determine the safety or efficacy of the device, and it is used to conduct tests for researchers. Both IOU and RUO diagnostic devices and reagents cannot be used for human clinical diagnosis unless the diagnosis is being confirmed by another medically established diagnostic product or procedure.

The laboratory should attach a result disclaimer for laboratory-developed tests using ASR, RUO, or IUO reagents or components; genetic tests; or FDA-approved test kits with alterations or changes in intended use (Table 11-14). Disclaimers are not required for FDA-approved or cleared test kits or reagents used according to the manufacturer instructions.

Points to Consider

The discovery that cervical carcinoma is induced by persistent infection by oncogenic HPV and subsequent advances in molecular genetics and biotechnology have provided physicians a new set of tools with which to detect cervical neoplastic disease. These assays may or may not come with product labeling that has been approved by the FDA. The FDA labeling addresses those uses for which the manufacturer has established the product's safety and efficacy.

In circumstances in which safety and efficacy have not been established, physicians must decide, based on a review of the medical data, whether to use the product in a manner not specified in the labeling. This decision should be guided by the physician's best judgment, in light of the medical literature and the physician's experience, regarding what is in the best interest of the patient. In terms of the FDA, such "unapproved" or, more precisely, "unlabeled" uses may be appropriate and rational in certain circumstances and may, in fact, reflect approaches to diagnosis that have been extensively reported in the medical literature.

References

1. Goodman A, Hutchinson M. Cell surplus on sampling devices after routine cervical cytologic smears: A study of residual cell populations. *J Reprod Med.* 1996;41:239-241.
2. Hutchinson M, Isenstein L, Goodman A, et al. Homogeneous sampling accounts for the increased diagnostic accuracy using the ThinPrep processor: subsampling-a problem with Pap smears. *Am J Clin Pathol.* 1994;101:215-219.
3. Klinkhamer P, Meerding W, Rosier P, Hanselaar A. Liquid-based cervical cytology: a review of the literature with methods of evidence-based medicine. *Cancer (Cancer Cytopathol).* 2003;99(5):263-271.
4. Linder J, Zahniser D. The ThinPrep Pap Test: a review of clinical studies. *Acta Cytol.* 1997;41:30-38.
5. Davey E, Barratt A, Irwig L, et al. Effect of study design and quality on unsatisfactory rates, cytology classifications, and accuracy in liquid-based versus conventional cervical cytology: a systematic review. *Lancet.* 2006;367:122-132.
6. Bernstein SJ, Sanchez-Ramos L, Ndubisi B. Liquid-based cervical cytologic smear study and conventional Papanicolaou smears: a metaanalysis of prospective studies comparing cytologic diagnosis and sample adequacy. *Am J Obstet Gynecol.* 2001;185:308-317.
7. Austin RM, Ramzy I. Increased detection of epithelial cell abnormalities by liquid-based gynecologic cytology preparations: a review of accumulated data. *Acta Cytol.* 1998;42:178-184.
8. Bentz JS. Liquid-based cytology for cervical cancer screening. *Exp Rev Mol Diagn.* 2005;5(6):857-871.
9. Obwegeser J, Schneider V. Thin-layer cervical cytology: a new meta-analysis. *Lancet.* 2006;367:88-89.
10. ASC Bulletin No. 8, December 1999.
11. ThinPrep Pap Test Package Insert. Marlborough, Mass: Cytyc Corp. 2001.
12. Lee KR, Ashfaq R, Birdsong GG, Corkill ME, McIntosh KM, Inhorn SL. Comparison of conventional Papanicolaou smears and a fluid-based, thin-layer system for cervical cancer screening. *Obstet Gynecol.* 1997;90:278-284.
13. ThinPrep Pap Test Package Insert: "The results from this study showed a detection rate of 511/20,917 for the conventional Pap smear versus 399/10,226 for the ThinPrep slides. For these clinical sites and these study populations, this indicates a 59.7% increase in detection of HSIL+ lesions for the ThinPrep specimens." Marlborough, Mass: Cytyc Corp.
14. Ashfaq R, Gibbons D, Vela C, Saboorian MH, Iliya F. ThinPrep Pap Test: accuracy for glandular disease. *Acta Cytol.* 1999;43:81-85.
15. Bai H, Sung CJ, Steinhoff MM. ThinPrep Pap Test promotes detection of glandular lesions of the endocervix. *Diagn Cytopathol.* 2000;23:19-22.
16. Hecht JL, Sheets EE, Lee KR. Atypical glandular cells of undetermined significance in conventional cervical/vaginal smear and thin-layer preparations. *Cancer Cytopathol.* 2002;96:1-4.
17. Bigras G, Rieder MA, Lambercy JM, et al. Keeping collecting device in liquid medium is mandatory to ensure optimized liquid-based cervical cytologic sampling. *J Low Genit Tract Dis.* 2003;7(3):168-174.
18. BD PrepStain Slide Processor Product Insert. Doc. No. 779-100002-03. Rev. B. Burlington, NC: BD-Diagnostic Systems, TriPath.
19. Marino JF, Fremont-Smith M. Direct-to-vial experience with AutoCyte PREP in a small New England regional cytology practice. *J Reprod Med.* 2001;Apr;46(4):353-358
20. Bishop JW. Comparison of the CytoRich system with conventional cervical cytology: preliminary data on 2,032 cases from a clinical trial site. *Acta Cytol.* 1997;41:15-23.
21. Bishop JW, Bigner SH, Colgan TJ, et al. Multicenter evaluation of AutoCyte PREP thin layers with matched conventional smears. *Acta Cytol.* 1998;42:189-197.
22. Bishop JW, Kaufman RH, Taylor DA. Multicenter comparison of manual and automated screening of AutoCyte gynecologic preparations. *Acta Cytol.* 1999;43:34-38.
23. MonoPrep Pap Test Package Insert. Lincolnshire, Ill: MonoGen, Inc.
24. Cibas ES, Alonzo TA, Austin RM, et al. The MonoPrep Pap test for the detection of cervical cancer and its precursors, part I: results of a multicenter clinical trial. *Am J Clin Pathol.* 2008;129:193-201.
25. Abulafia O, Sherer DM. Automated cervical cytology: meta-analysis of the performance of the AutoPap 300 QC System. *Ob Gyn Surv.* 1999;54:469-476.
26. FocalPoint Slide Profiler Package Insert. Burlington, NC: BD-Diagnostic Systems, Tripath.

27. Wilbur DC, Prey MU, Miller WM, Pawlick GF, Colgan TJ. The AutoPap System for primary screening in cervical cytology: comparing the results of a prospective, intended-use study with routine manual practice. *Acta Cytol.* 1998;42:214-220.

28. Wilbur DC, Prey MU, Miller WM, Pawlick GF, Colgan TJ, Taylor DD. Detection of high grade squamous intraepithelial lesions and tumors using the AutoPap system: results of a primary screening clinical trial. *Cancer Cytopathol.* 1999; 87:354-358.

29. ThinPrep Imaging System Operation Summary and Clinical Information, Part No. 86093-001. Marlborough, Mass: Cytyc Corporation.

30. Biscotti C, Dawson A, Dziura B, Galup L, Darragh T, Rahemtulla A, Wills-Frank L. Assisted primary screening using the automated ThinPrep Imaging System. *Am J Clin Pathol.* 2005;123(2):281-287.

31. Solomon D, Schiffman M, Tarone R. Comparison of three management strategies for patients with atypical squamous cells of undetermined significance: baseline results from a randomized trial. *J Natl Cancer Inst.* 2001;93:293-299.

32. Wright TC Jr, Massad LS, Dunton CJ, Spitzer M, Wilkinson EJ, Solomon D; 2006 American Society for Colposcopy and Cervical Pathology-sponsored Consensus Conference. 2006 consensus guidelines for the management of women with abnormal cervical cancer screening tests. *Am J Obstet Gynecol.* 2007 Oct;197(4):346-355.

33. Ko V, Tamboret RH, Kuebler DL, Black-Schaffer WS, Wilbur DC. Human papillomavirus testing using Hybrid Capture II with SurePath collection: initial evaluation and longitudinal data provide clinical validation for this method. *Cancer.* 2006;108:468-474.

34. Holladay B, Bolick D, Molina, JT, Alonzo TA, Gamerman GE. HC2 HPV testing with the MonoPrep Pap Test: clinical demonstration of performance and stability for HPV results, CIN2+ detection, and QNS elimination. *Cancer Cytopathol.* 2007;111(S5):384-385.

35. Bianchi A, Moret F, Desrues JM, et al. PreservCyt transport medium used for the ThinPrep Pap test is a suitable medium for detection of Chlamydia trachomatis by the COBAS Amplicor CT/NG test: results of a preliminary study and future implications. *J Clin Microbiol.* 2002;40(5):1749-1754.

36. Koumans EH, Black CM, Markowitz LA, et al. Comparison of methods for detection of Chlamydia trachomatis and Neisseria gonorrhoeae using commercially available nucleic acid amplification tests and a liquid Pap smear medium. *J Clin Microbiol.* 2003;41(4):1507-1511.

37. Chernesky M, Jang D, Portillo E, et al. Abilities of APTIMA, AMPLICOR, and ProbeTec assays to detect Chlamydia trachomatis and Neisseria gonorrhoeae in PreservCyt ThinPrep Liquid-based Pap samples. *J Clin Microbiol.* 2007;45(8):2355-2358.

38. Chernesky M, Freund GG, Hook E 3rd, Leone P, D'Ascoli P, Martens M. Detection of Chlamydia trachomatis and Neisseria gonorrhoeae infections in North American women by testing SurePath liquid-based Pap specimens in APTIMA assays. *J Clin Microbiol.* 2007;45(8):2434-2438.

39. Hildebrandt EF, Lee JR, Crosby JH, Ferris DG, Anderson MG. Liquid-based Pap smears as a source of RNA for gene expression analysis. *Appl Immunohistochem Mol Morphol.* 2003; 11(4):345-351.

40. Malinowski DP. Molecular diagnostic assays for cervical neoplasia: emerging markers for the detection of high-grade cervical disease. *Biotechniques.* 2005; 38:S17-S23.

41. Dallenbach-Hellweg G, Trunk MJ, von Knebel Doeberitz M. Traditional and new molecular methods for early detection of cervical cancer. *Arch Pathol Lab Med.* 2004;66(5):35-39.

42. Lin WM, Ashfaq R, Michalopulos EA, Maitra A, Gazdar AF, Muller CY. Molecular Papanicolaou tests in the twenty-first century: molecular analyses with fluid-based Papanicolaou technology. *Am J Obstet Gynecol.* 2000;183:39-45.

43. Wentzensen N, von Knebel Doeberitz M. Biomarkers in cervical cancer screening. *Dis Markers.* 2007;23:315-330.

44. Murphy N, Ring M, Heffron CC, et al. p16INK4A, CDC6, and MCM5: predictive biomarkers in cervical preinvasive neoplasia and cervical cancer. *J Clin Pathol.* 2005;58(5):525-534.

45. Holladay EB, Logan S, Arnold J, Knesel B, Smith GD. A comparison of the clinical utility of p16(INK4a) immunolocalization with the presence of human papillomavirus by hybrid capture 2 for the detection of cervical dysplasia/neoplasia. *Cancer.* 2006;108(6):451-461.

46. Akpolat I, Smith DA, Ramzy I, Chirala M, Mody DR. The utility of p16INK4a and Ki-67 staining on cell blocks prepared from residual thin-layer cervicovaginal material. *Cancer.* 2004;102(3):142-149.

47. Moore GD, Lear SC, Wills-Frank LA, Martin AW, Snyder JW, Helm CW. Differential expression of cdk inhibitors p16, p21cip1, p27kip1, and cyclin E in cervical cytological smears prepared by the ThinPrep method. *Diagn Cytopathol.* 2005;32(2):82-87.

48. Dehn D, Torkko KC, Shroyer KR. Human Papillomavirus testing and molecular markers of cervical dysplasia and carcinoma. *Cancer Cytopathol.* 2007;111:1-14.

49. Benevolo M, Vocaturo A, Mottolese M, et al. Clinical role of p16INK4a expression in liquid-based cervical cytology: correlation with HPV testing and histologic diagnosis. *Am J Clin Pathol.* 2008;129(4):606-612.

50. Shroyer K, Homer P, Heinz D, Singh M. Validation of a novel immunocytochemical assay for topoisomerase II-a and minichromosome maintenance protein 2 expression in cervical cytology. *Cancer Cytopathol.* 2006;108:324-330.

51. Kelly D, Kincaid E, Fansler Z, Rosenthal DL, Clark DP. Detection of cervical high-grade squamous intraepithelial lesions from cytologic samples using a novel immunocytochemical assay (ProEx C). *Cancer.* 2006;108(6):494-500.

52. Shi J, Liu H, Wilkerson M, et al. Evaluation of p16INK4a, minichromosome maintenance protein 2, DNA topoisomerase IIalpha, ProEX C, and p16INK4a/ProEX C in cervical squamous intraepithelial lesions. *Hum Pathol.* 2007;38(9):1335-1344.

53. Tambouret RH, Misdraji J, Wilbur DC. Longitudinal clinical valuation of a novel antibody cocktail for detection of high-grade squamous intraepithelial lesions on cervical cytology specimens. *Arch Pathol Lab Med.* 2008;132:918-925.

54. Sokolova I, Algeciras-Schimnich A, Song M, et al. Chromosomal biomarkers for detection of human papillomavirus associated genomic instability in epithelial cells of cervical cytology specimens. *J Mol Diagn.* 2007;9(5):604-611.

55. Code of Federal Regulation. Title 21 CFR Part 809. In Vitro Diagnostic Products for Human Use, Part 812 - Investigational Device Exemptions, and Part 864 - Hematology and Pathology Devices. October 2007.

56. Guidance for Industry and FDA Staff Commercially Distributed Analyte Specific Reagents (ASRs). Frequently Asked Questions. September 14, 2007. Available at: http://www.fda.gov/cber/guidelines.htm#asr. Accessed May 2008.

57. Commercialization of In Vitro Diagnostic Devices (IVD's) Labeled for Research Use Only or Investigational Use Only. Draft. January 5, 1998. Available at: http://www.fda.gov/cdrh/comp/ivddrfg.html. Accessed May 2008.

Notes Added in Press

* Monogen ceased commercial operations on October 7, 2008. The availability of the MonoPrep system as described in this monograph is therefore unknown at the time of publication.

** The BD FocalPoint GS Imaging System was approved by the US FDA in November of 2008. The device is for use with BD SurePath slides only. This System incorporates slide ranking and the Directed QC Technology™ present in the previous BD FocalPoint Slide Profiler with the ability to identify 10 fields of view (FOV) on each slide using an automated microscopy review station (Figure 11-23). FOVs are presented to the cytologist hierarchically, beginning with the highest-probability fields. If abnormality, potential abnormality, or issue with adequacy of the specimen is not present in the FOVs, the slide can be reliably called Negative without a full manual screening. Slides having potential abnormalities or adequacy issues detected require a full manual screening prior to reporting. In this device, all qualified slides receive at least an FOV review; there is no population indicated as "No Further Review." Slides in which scant squamous cellularity is detected are automatically "flagged" for a full manual screening, and no FOVs are generated. Quality control rescreening is performed on only high-scoring slides, analogous to the process utilized for the prior Slide Profiler product.

The FDA approval was based on data generated in a clinical trial comprised of over 12,000 slides. In the trial, the results of manual screening were directly compared to screening using the BD FocalPoint GS System. Data from the clinical trial show an increase of 19.6% in the sensitivity for the precise diagnosis of HSIL+ (with a

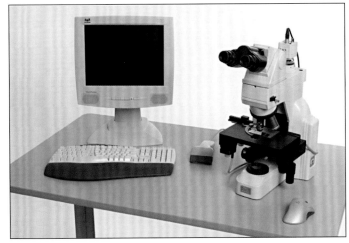

Figure 11-23. The BD FocalPoint GS Imaging System Review Station consists of a motorized microscope and computer console. The computer screen will display a still image taken from the FocalPoint Slide Profiler as well as a live image from the microscope. These images are to confirm the location of the field of view. The cytotechnologist can monitor the screening process as they progress from one FOV to the next. (Courtesy and © Becton, Dickinson and Company)

decline in specificity of 2.6%), an increase of 9.8% in the sensitivity for the precise diagnosis of LSIL+ (with a decline in specificity of 1.9%), and a decrease of 1.5% for the precise diagnosis of ASC-US+ (with an increase in specificity of 1.8%).

Workload limits have been set at 170 slides per 8-hour work period but include both FOV-only and full slide reviews in the calculation. There are no limitations on processing with the GS System related to high-risk or other types of slides.

Quality Improvement in the Cytopathology Laboratory

Theresa M. Voytek, MD
Margaret Havens Neal, MD
Christine Noga Booth, MD

General Laboratory Quality Assurance

This chapter is designed to give an overview of basic tenets of quality assurance in the cytopathology laboratory. For further information on this subject, please refer to the College of American Pathologists (CAP) manual, *Quality Management In Anatomic Pathology: Promoting Patient Safety Through Systems Improvement and Error Reduction*.[1]

In addition, review of the CAP Laboratory Accreditation Program Cytopathology Checklist can provide valuable assistance in guiding quality assurance programs. This checklist is available online at www.cap.org.[2]

Quality Improvement Program

A good quality improvement plan should be comprehensive in order to reflect all testing performed by the laboratory. The content of the plan is at the discretion of the individual laboratory. A comprehensive quality improvement plan should include:

- A description of quality indicators and how these are used to improve the quality of laboratory testing performed by the laboratory.
- Documentation of efforts to maintain and continually improve laboratory quality.
- Regular policy review and updating.
- Monitoring of individual and laboratory statistics.
- Action plans for quality-indicator thresholds that are exceeded.

Quality assurance should include all steps in the process:

- Specimen collection, labeling, requisition form, and delivery (preanalytical).
- Specimen preparation, staining, screening/interpretation, and reporting (analytical).
- Correlation with laboratory statistics, follow-up data, and tissue biopsy (postanalytical).

Components of a cytopathology laboratory quality improvement plan may include:

- Screening abnormal identification rates.
- Cytology-histology correlation.
- Hierarchical review, cytotechnologist-cytopathologist correlation.
- Retrospective reviews/rescreen data.
- Monitoring laboratory and individual interpretation rates (eg, atypical squamous cells of undetermined significance [ASC-US]/squamous intraepithelial lesion [SIL]).

- Monitoring cytology results with other independent measures (eg, ASC-US/human papillomavirus (HPV) + rates).
- Correlation with clinical history and follow-up data, monitors that are required by the Clinical Laboratory Improvement Amendments of 1988 (CLIA '88) or the CAP Laboratory Accreditation Program (LAP) inspection checklist.
- Group multihead microscopy consensus conferences for the review of difficult cases, refining of criteria, and group review of educational materials

All elements should have defined action thresholds and plans for corrective action if these thresholds are exceeded. To maintain a comprehensive, state-of-the-art quality assurance/improvement program and a high-quality laboratory, regular review of changes to CAP checklists and CLIA '88 regulations is recommended. CLIA updates can be found at http://www.phppo.cdc.gov/clia/regs/toc.aspx.[3]

Specimen Collection and Adequacy

General. The first step in cytopathology quality assurance is assessing specimen adequacy. Adequacy includes both specimen integrity and labeling.

Written instructions for the collection and submission of gynecologic samples should be available to all clinicians who send specimens to the laboratory. These can be either distributed as hard copies or available online, as long as clinicians have access to the necessary information.

The type of specimen received should be documented (eg, conventional Pap smear, ThinPrep, SurePath, MonoPrep®). The laboratory should have written criteria for rejecting specimens.

The laboratory should maintain a policy of notifying clinicians when their specimens are rejected. Examples of rejection criteria include unlabeled slides or specimens, broken slides, improperly collected specimens (eg, wrong/absent fixative), or specimens received without requisitions. Specimen rejection and clinician notification should be documented by the laboratory.

Specimens received without any label/identification should be discarded and recollected, or returned to the clinician for further identification, as per the laboratory policy. An example letter for clinician notification of specimen rejection is presented in Figure 12-1.

Requisition Forms. Requisition forms should contain the following information:
- Patient name
- Date of birth/age

Date:

Dear Dr. _____:

Re: _____ specimen submitted on your
patient _____.

This specimen could not be processed by the
laboratory due to:

____ Slides received broken and could not be repaired.

____ Slides/specimen received unlabeled.

____ Slides/specimen received without a requisition.
If the specimen is labeled/identified, it will be
processed when a completed requisition form is
received by the laboratory.

Figure 12-1. An example of a specimen rejection notification letter.

- Sex
- Date/time of specimen collection
- Specimen source
- Submitting clinician
- Relevant clinical information

Relevant clinical information for gynecologic specimens includes history of prior abnormal Pap, date of last menstrual period (LMP), hormone or other drug or radiation therapy, or pertinent surgery (eg, hysterectomy).

Slide Adequacy. Gynecologic specimens that are processed and screened are evaluated for cellular adequacy. The laboratory should have adequacy criteria defined in its procedure manual. Any slide having identifiable abnormal/atypical cells should never be reported as unsatisfactory despite the inadequate cellularity or other factor making the overall specimen less than optimal.

The adequacy criteria most widely utilized for gynecologic cytology specimens are those of the 2001 Bethesda System.[4] If other adequacy criteria are being routinely utilized in the laboratory, documentation of such should be included in the procedure manual.

Sample Preparation/Staining

All methods of sample preparation and staining should be described in the laboratory procedure manual (eg, conventional smear, liquid-based preparations). Automated preparation devices must be validated according to the manufacturer's protocol. If the manufacturer does not provide validation instructions, the validation procedure developed by the laboratory must be documented. Personnel should receive training in the use of all instrumentation. Documentation of the validation procedures and personnel training should be maintained for the life of the instrument. All gynecologic specimens should be stained with a Papanicolaou or modified Papanicolaou

stain. Stains should be checked daily for proper staining characteristics.

The laboratory should have procedures in place to prevent cross-contamination of specimens. Gynecologic specimens should be stained separately from non-gynecologic samples because of the risk of cross-contamination. All methods used by the laboratory should be documented in the procedure manual. Some examples include the following:

- Use at least two staining setups and, while using one, filter the other so that a clean set is always available.
- Document each time the stains are filtered or changed. This will keep track of the steps used to prevent cross-contamination and provide documentation during inspections.

Workload Limits

CLIA '88 allows a maximum primary manual screening workload of 100 slides per day, over no less than 8 hours. Some states have lower limits, and laboratories must adhere to the most restrictive limit in effect for their state. The 100 slide limit equates to a maximum screening rate of 12.5 slides per hour. The workload limit applies to both previously unscreened gynecological (gyn) and non-gynecological (non-gyn) slides. Slides manually rescreened for quality control are also included in this workload limit. Pathologists who function as primary screeners (of gyns, non-gyns, or both) are subject to the workload limit, and compliance must be documented. Cases prescreened by a cytotechnologist are not counted as part of the pathologist workload. All manually screened gyn slides count as whole slides, regardless of the preparation method. Non-gyn slides prepared by concentration methods that result in the sample covering one-half or less of the slide (such as ThinPrep, SurePath, or Cytospin®) may be counted as half slides. CLIA has made allowances for the ThinPrep Imaging System, which is a computer-assisted Pap screening device, allowing a maximum workload limit of up to 200 slides screened by the 22 fields of view (FOV) review process (see chapter 11). A caveat in this process is that if any slides are referred to a full manual screening, the 100 slide per 8 hours rule applies. Therefore, combinations of ThinPrep Imaging System FOV-only screening and full manual screening require interpolations of the 100 and 200 slide limit rules. Data from the two procedures may be kept as separate records to ensure compliance with the hourly maximal screening rate.

Workload limits must be based upon the number of hours spent screening slides, considering other duties performed by the cytotechnologists and part-time employees. Although CLIA '88 regulation sets the maximum workload allowed by law, the technical supervisor of each laboratory must set individual workload limits based upon the ability of each individual cytotechnologist. This individualized workload limit is not a productivity goal, but rather a maximum limit. The workload limit for each screener in the laboratory must be reassessed every 6 months by the cytology technical supervisor. CLIA regulations mandate that this assessment be based upon a minimum of 10% Pap

---

Cytotechnologist Workload Assessment

Name: _____

Period of Evaluation: _____

Based upon the following data, the cytotechnologist's maximum workload is set at _____ slides/day.

Date : _____

	Cytotechnologist Data	Laboratory Average
10% Rescreen Discrepancies		
Cytopath/Cytotech Discrepancies		
Statistical Comparisons		
% unsat		
% negative		
% abnormal		
ASC-US:SIL		
ASC-US:HPV+		
PT		
Competency Assessment		
Continuing Education Hours		

The definition of a discrepancy should be determined by the laboratory. Many laboratories consider discrepancies to be two-step variances in interpretation. Examples of two-step discrepancies include the following:

Cytotechnologist Interpretation	Pathologist Interpretation
Negative	LSIL+
ASC	HSIL+
LSIL	Carcinoma

Figure 12-2. An example of a screening workload 6-month assessment form.

rescreen data and cytotechnologist-cytopathologist correlation data. Other factors may also be helpful to consider when assessing workload limits, including cytotechnologist competency assessments, performance on proficiency tests and interlaboratory comparison programs, abnormal detection rates, and years of experience in the field. An example of a workload assessment form is provided in Figure 12-2.

Cytopathology Reporting

The cytopathology report should be clear and use standard descriptive terminology. CLIA regulations require the following elements in the report:
- Name and age or birth date of patient
- Accession number
- Name of physician or clinic
- Name of pathologist
- If applicable, name and address of testing laboratory date of report and test performed

Other desirable elements include:
- Date/time of specimen collection
- Date/time of receipt in laboratory
- Description of specimen
- Designation of automated screening device, if applicable
- Results of ancillary testing, if applicable (eg, HPV test results)

Reports must be signed by the cytotechnologist and/or pathologist responsible for the interpretation. Electronic signatures are acceptable, although the individual responsible for the case should personally review and release the report. Rare exceptions may be necessary, when the individual who reviewed the case is not available to release the report. When this occurs, the individual who releases the report should be clearly distinguished from the one who is responsible for the interpretation. The signature(s) associated with the interpretation should be only for those who have personally examined the slides. Although the practice of identifying the laboratory director on all pathology reports is acceptable, the director's name must be distinct from the name of the reviewing cytotechnologist/pathologist, unless the director personally evaluated the case.

Laboratory Statistics

CLIA regulations specify a variety of statistics that should be maintained in the laboratory, some of which include:

- Number of gynecologic specimens
- Number of gynecologic cases in which quality control rescreening reclassified negatives as abnormal
- Gynecologic cases broken down by diagnostic category, and number of cases of high-grade squamous intraepithelial lesion (HSIL) and above that have follow-up data

Other useful statistics include the ASC-US to SIL ratio (ASC-US:SIL). This value may be more useful than the individual ASC-US and SIL statistics because it more accurately reflects reporting tendencies, is less influenced by patient populations, and enables interlaboratory comparisons. For instance, an ASC-US rate of 6% and a SIL rate of 2% don't individually provide much useful information, and each falls well within the 10th to 90th percentiles of national laboratory reporting rates. But the calculated ASC-US:SIL is 3, approaching the 95th percentile for liquid-based cytology. A high ASC-US:SIL suggests that the laboratory overuses the ASC-US category or, inversely, that it is underreporting SIL. Either way, this elevated ratio should indicate to laboratory personnel that there may be a quality issue in need of investigation.

The reporting rates tables provided in the CAP checklist comments are useful for comparing individual laboratory statistics with national laboratory percentiles. These benchmarking data are available for conventional, ThinPrep, and SurePath slides.[3] In addition to ASC-US:SIL, the percentage of HPV-positive results in ASC-US cases (particularly in the circumstance of reflex ASC-US HPV testing) may be a more objective measure of ASC-US interpretation. Providing this indicator to individual pathologists and longitudinal monitoring may be a very good quality assurance indicator for morphologic interpretation of ASC-US.[5,6] A 2007 CAP Q-Probes study reported data from 68 institutions.[7] The mean HPV-positive rate among ASC-US cases was 47%, with a range of 33% to 53% representing the 25th to 75th percentiles. An "ideal" rate of 55% has been put forward by some, because ASC-US, being a truly equivocal category, should be positive in 50% of cases, but with an additional 5% baseline HPV-positive rate in the cytologically normal population.[5]

Reviews of the correlation of ASC-US:SIL and HPV-positive ASC-US rates detail the caveats of using these two measures in tandem.[5,6]

Gynecological Cytology Quality Assurance

Screening

Primary. CLIA '88 requires that all gynecological slides should be thoroughly screened by a cytotechnologist(s)/pathologist in a CLIA-certified laboratory. All reactive/reparative, atypical, premalignant, and malignant cases must be referred to a pathologist for final interpretation. Documentation of this review process should be maintained. Written records of previous cytological/histological specimens, if available, should be reviewed prior to final reporting.

Narrative descriptive nomenclature must be used in reporting gynecological specimens. Any numerical classification (eg, Papanicolaou classification) is no longer appropriate. Acceptable methods of reporting squamous lesions in gynecological cytology include the Bethesda System (2001),[8] cervical intraepithelial neoplasia classification scheme (CIN I, II, III),[9] and the World Health Organization (WHO) nomenclature indicating degrees of dysplasia (ie, slight, moderate, severe dysplasias, and carcinoma in situ).[10] A clear, concise, and descriptive nomenclature is essential to ensure communication between the laboratory and the clinician.

Written educational comments or suggestions for further diagnostic studies are optional but can be useful. Many laboratories use educational notes to inform clinicians and patients about the limitations of Pap testing and about current guidelines for management following Pap testing results. In addition to the written report, verbal communication may be necessary in cases where further diagnostic studies are indicated. Such communication should be documented, preferably on the report, or at a minimum in the laboratory information system record or in a laboratory log book.

Discordant interpretations (between cytotechnologist[s] and pathologist[s] or between two pathologists) should be resolved, if possible, prior to final reporting. Review at a multiheaded microscope or consensus conference, with discussion of the case, is a useful educational exercise.

Rescreening and Retrospective Reviews. The 2001 Bethesda System recommends reporting cases where no preneoplastic or neoplastic process is present as "negative for intraepithelial lesion or malignancy (NILM)." There is no standard method that has been scientifically validated which specifies the percentage of negative cases that should be rescreened.

CLIA '88 regulations specify that at least 10% of negative gynecological specimens from each primary screener (cytotechnologist or pathologist) be rescreened, and that both randomly selected cases and those from "high-risk" individuals (based on available patient information) be included in the rescreened specimens. The review must be performed by a supervisory-qualified cytotechnologist or pathologist and must be completed prior to reporting. Written documentation of all rescreening efforts should be maintained. The rescreening process should allow identification of the original and rescreening cytotechnologists in the laboratory records.

At present, the only exception to this regulation is for slides primarily screened by the BD FocalPoint™ Slide Profiler (see chapter 11). In this process, a minimum of 15% of the highest scoring "review" slides must be rescreened for quality control (QC) purposes. A Centers for Medicare and Medicaid Services (CMS) waiver letter indicating this deviation from the CLIA-mandated quality control procedure is available from the manufacturer and should be included in the laboratory's procedure manual if this method of QC rescreening is used.

Rescreening of negative slides should be an integral part of the evaluation of new technologists. Many laboratories utilize a system of graduated rescreening of cases when new cytotechnologists are hired. Some laboratories have utilized a process of "rapid" rescreening of all or a portion of specimens initially interpreted as NILM. This process is not a CLIA '88 requirement but has shown utility in practice and allows "second looks" at all specimens prior to release of final reports.[11]

Previously negative cytological and relevant histologic material should be reviewed to correlate results whenever current material shows a significant abnormality that could have been overlooked in the prior specimen. The degree of abnormality that triggers such a review can be determined by the laboratory, however CLIA '88 stipulates that negative or normal cytology specimens obtained within the previous 5 years, either onsite or in storage, should be reviewed whenever an HSIL or a malignant lesion is first detected on a subsequent cytologic specimen. This review should be documented in the laboratory quality assurance records. A pathologist should also review any previous cases in which rescreening by the technologist detects possible abnormality.

The laboratory should have criteria in place regarding what constitutes a significant variance in the interpretation between the original screening and rescreening events. Using this threshold, laboratories can monitor individual performance for quality assurance and educational purposes. According to CLIA '88 regulations, if significant abnormalities that would affect current patient care are found on retrospective review, the clinician must be notified and an amended report issued. An example of this situation is if an endocervical glandular abnormality is identified on the prior Pap test, which is being retrospectively rescreened for a current Pap test interpretation of HSIL.

Measures of Cytotechnologist Performance

CLIA '88 regulations require laboratories to evaluate individuals in comparison to overall laboratory performance, and to document discrepancies and corrective action, if appropriate. Although the regulations do not specify the method of comparison, laboratories are required to use 10% random rescreening data and cytotechnologist/pathologist interpretation correlation data for cytotechnologist workload determination. Other methods that can be used to monitor performance include targeted rescreening, retrospective rescreening, calculation of sensitivity ("pick-up") rates (or percentage of abnormal specimens), and tracking of cytological/histological correlation data. These various methods of evaluating screening performance each have advantages and disadvantages, depending on a variety of factors, including laboratory size, caseload, and abnormal prevalence in the population screened. Some of the methods may be most useful as education and training devices.

Rescreening Data. Random and targeted rescreening of cases may be a useful method to compare performance in relatively large laboratories (several cytotechnologists and large, evenly distributed gynecologic case volume). This method should use a randomizing strategy to select cases. Some laboratories use this data to calculate an estimated false-negative proportion (FNP). The FNP is the percentage of women with cervical neoplastic or preneoplastic lesions who have a negative Pap test. It is defined as the number of false-negative reports divided by the total number of women with a cervical abnormality:

$$FNP = FN/(TP+FN)$$

where FN is the number of false-negative reports and TP is the number of true-positive cases.

Although the FNP is a commonly used statistic in quality assessment, it may not accurately reflect the laboratory performance because the false-negative rate of rescreening, which can be substantial, is not taken into account. Reports have suggested that this rescreening false-negative rate may be as high as 75%.[12]

Targeted rescreening of high-risk patients has also been discussed previously and is mandated under CLIA '88. It is very useful as a quality assurance mechanism. Since the population is preselected, rescreening will not be a random sample, and numerical error rate calculation is difficult.

Abnormal Pick-Up Rates. In this discussion, "pick-up" rate refers to the percentage of abnormal cases interpreted by an individual; for example, the sum of atypical, premalignant, and malignant cases is divided by the total cases examined. This method is useful in most laboratories, provided that the individual screeners and/or pathologists view a similar mix of cases. A total pick-up rate can be calculated for each individual and compared with the overall laboratory rate. Performing this type of calculation may be feasible on a quarterly basis. Alternatively, various degrees of abnormalities can be compared for individuals. Since numbers for each category will be smaller than the total abnormal pick-up rate, the frequency of performing calculations may be once or twice a year. In addition to calculating rates for squamous abnormalities, it may be useful to compare rates for unsatisfactory specimens and other nonneoplastic findings, such as candida, trichomonas, or herpes.

Cytotechnologist/Pathologist Correlation Data. Cytotechnologist/pathologist correlation data should be considered in the determination of cytotechnologist workload limits and, at the discretion of the laboratory, can be monitored in a variety of ways. An example of one method of tracking this data is by assigning diagnostic scores to calculate correlation discrepancy scores. These data can then be summarized in histograms.[13]

Cytologic interpretations or histologic diagnoses are assigned scores as follows:

Negative	0
Reactive/Repair	1
Atypical squamous cells (either of undetermined significance or cannot exclude high-grade squamous intraepithelial lesion (ASC [-US or -H])/atypical glandular cells (AGC)	1.5
LSIL/CIN I	2
HSIL/CIN II	3
HSIL/CIN III	4
Squamous cell carcinoma	5
Adenocarcinoma	5

The score of the pathologist diagnosis is subtracted from the score of the cytotechnologist and the result is the discrepancy score for that case. An example of how such a correlation can be incorporated into a screener competency assessment is illustrated in Figure 12-3.

Performance on Proficiency Tests and Interlaboratory Comparison Programs. Annual proficiency testing (PT) is now required for all individuals screening and interpreting gynecologic cytology under the regulations of CLIA '88 (starting in 2005). CMS-approved proficiency-testing programs are administered by the College of American Pathologists, the American Society for Clinical Pathology (ASCP), and the State of Maryland. In addition, CAP and ASCP have educational interlaboratory comparison programs associated with the PT exercises. These educational programs circulate slides and have online computer-based exercises that allow for comparisons of performance between individual subscribers, the pool of all peers completing the exercises, and expert referee pathologists. Such programs are suitable for quality improvement and continuing education purposes. All records of participation and results obtained should be reviewed individually and/or discussed at laboratory meetings.

Gynecologic Cytologic/Histologic Correlation. As per CLIA '88, the laboratory must compare all gynecological cytology reports with an interpretation of at least high-grade squamous intraepithelial lesion or carcinoma with the histopathology report, if available, in the laboratory (either on site or in storage) and determine the cause of any discrepancies. Although this process is mandated by CLIA '88, no methods of analysis are specified. A system-wide approach using this program may result in improved patient care.

The Pap test and the histologic specimen should be independently reviewed. As the histologic biopsy may not always be the "gold standard," reasons for discrepancy should be pursued. The latter should be adequately sectioned and oriented so that a continuous lining epithelium that includes the transformation zone is observed. In HSIL

Cytotechnologist Competency Assessment

Cytotechnologist: ______________________

	Satisfactory	Needs Improvement
Rescreen Discrepancies		
Gyn Statistics		
Pathologist/Cytotech Discrepancies		
Non-Gyn Screening		
Final Report and Billing Accuracy		
PAP Program		
FNA Adequacy Assessments		
Knowledge of Procedure Manual Contents		
Other		

Comments:

______________	______________	________
Cytotechnologist	Supervisor	Date

Figure 12-3. An example of a screener competency assessment form.

cases where initial sections show no correlating lesion, deeper sections should always be obtained prior to concluding that no lesion exists. If available, prior negative cytology cases may also be reviewed whenever the histology is positive as an adjunct to the 5-year retrospective process noted above. It is important to stress that some agreed-upon definition of diagnostic discrepancy should be established. Peer or consensus conference review of noncorrelating specimens may be helpful to achieve best representations of "accuracy standards" in such cases. Results should be summarized on a regular basis so that trends and improvements can be tracked.

While cervicovaginal cytology is appropriately regarded as a screening test, and colposcopic biopsy is often considered to be the "gold standard" confirmatory test, both tests are subject to sampling error and, in some cases, the Pap test may better represent the cervical pathology than does the biopsy. In the case of a patient with a Pap interpretation of HSIL and negative biopsy follow-up, if the cause of the discrepancy is determined to be a biopsy sampling error, and if consensus review of the Pap confirms the original interpretation, the clinician may choose to proceed to further investigation or definitive treatment (eg, loop electrosurgical excision [LEEP]). Therefore, Pap/biopsy correlation is critical for appropriate patient management, and communication of findings with clinicians is vital. An ideal practice is to correlate specimens in "real-time"—at the time of histologic sample review. When this is done, a comment referring to the correlation can be included in the histopathology report. This process allows for patient-care interventions to occur which are directly linked to the cytology-histology correlation review. Direct communication via phone calls or letters is useful to discuss individual patient follow-up. Amended cytologic reports may be necessary if screening, interpretive, or technical problems are detected that would affect current patient care. Interdepartmental committees or conferences are another avenue in which to discuss cytohistologic correlation results. Histologic follow-up may not always be available. In these cases, the findings of other follow-up studies, such as high-risk HPV testing, repeat Pap tests, and colposcopic examination, may be informative. Follow-up management is particularly important in cases of HSIL, glandular abnormalities, and carcinoma.

Continuing Education

Continuing medical education for cytotechnologists and pathologists in gynecological cytology is an integral part of quality improvement. This may include:

- Journal subscriptions with individual or group reviews (journal clubs)
- Internal conferences (such as microscopic consensus conferences, lecture review, or interactive sign-out)
- Participation in mailed education programs, such as the CAP Interlaboratory Comparison Program in Gynecologic Cytopathology (PAP), ASCP Check Samples, American Society of Cytopathology (ASC) teleconferences, and other cytology courses and meetings
- Comparison with data from other laboratories, as in interlaboratory peer comparison programs. This is an excellent and important educational and benchmarking monitor.

Documentation of participation in continuing medical education activities is often required for state licensure or certification. It is also an excellent monitor to ensure ongoing participation for the purposes of workload assessment reviews.

References

1. Nakhleh RE, Fitzgibbons PL, eds. *Quality Management In Anatomic Pathology: Promoting Patient Safety Through Systems Improvement and Error Reduction.* Northfield, Ill: College of American Pathologists; 2005.

2. Commission on Laboratory Accreditation. Laboratory Accreditation Program. *Cytopathology Checklist.* Northfield, Ill: College of American Pathologists; 2007. Available at: http://www.cap.org/apps/cap.portal?_nfpb=true&cntvwrP tlt_actionOverride=%2Fportlets%2FcontentViewer%2Fshow &_windowLabel=cntvwrPtlt&cntvwrPtlt%7BactionForm.con tentReference%7D=laboratory_accreditation%2Fchecklists% 2Fchecklist.html&_state=maximized&_pageLabel=cntvwr. Accessed April 28, 2008.

3. Clinical Laboratory Improvement Amendments of 1988. Final Rule. *Fed Reg.* 1992;57:7001-7186. Available at: http://www.phppo.cdc.gov/clia/regs/toc.aspx. Accessed April 28, 2008.

4. Solomon D, Nayar R, eds. *The Bethesda System for Reporting Cervical Cytology Definitions, Criteria, and Explanatory Notes.* 2nd ed. New York: Springer-Verlag; 2004.

5. Ko V, Nanji S, Tambouret RH, Wilbur DC. Testing for HPV as an objective measure for quality assurance in gynecologic cytology: positive rates in equivocal and abnormal specimens and comparison to the ASC-US:SIL. *Cancer (Cancer Cytopathol).* 2007;111:67-73.

6. Cibas ES, Zou KH, Crum CP, Kuo F. Using the rate of positive high-risk HPV test results for ASC-US together with the ASC-US/SIL ratio in evaluating the performance of cytopathologists. *Am J Clin Pathol.* 2008;129:97-101.

7. Tworek JA, Jones BA, Raab S, Clary KM, Walsh MK. The value of monitoring human papillomavirus DNA results for Papanicolaou tests diagnosed as atypical squamous cells of undetermined significance: a College of American Pathologists Q-Probes study of 68 institutions. *Arch Pathol Lab Med.* 2007;131:1525-1531.

8. Solomon D, Davey D, Kurman R, et al; Forum Group Members; Bethesda 2001 Workshop. The 2001 Bethesda System: terminology for reporting results of cervical cytology. *JAMA.* 2002;287:2114-2119.

9. Richart RM. A modified terminology for cervical intraepithelial neoplasia. *Obstet Gynecol.* 1990;75:131-133.

10. Frappart L, Fontainiere B, Lucas E, Sankaranarayanan R, eds. *Histopathology and Cytopathology of the Uterine Cervix. Digital Atlas.* Lyon, France: IARC Screening Group; 2004.

11. Michelow P, McKee G, Hlongwane F. Rapid rescreening of cervical smears as a quality control method in a high-risk population. *Cytopathology.* 2006;17:110-115.

12. Renshaw AA, Luzon KM, Wilbur DC. The human false-negative rate of rescreening Pap tests: measured in a two-arm prospective clinical trial. *Cancer (Cancer Cytopathol).* 2001;25:106-110.

13. Cibas ES, Dean B, Maffeo N, Allred EN. Quality assurance in gynecologic cytology: the value of cytotechnologist-cytopathologist discrepancy logs. *Am J Clin Pathol.* 2001; 115:512-516.

Billing and Coding Issues in Gynecologic Cytology: Deciphering the Alphanumeric Soup

Susan Spires, MD
Dina R. Mody, MD

Historical Background

In 1992, to ameliorate perceived inequities in reimbursement across specialties, Medicare established a standardized physician payment schedule based on the relative work for professional services. The resource-based relative value scale (RBRVS), determines payments for services based on physician work and the associated costs needed to provide them. The total relative value units (RVUs) assigned to each current procedural terminology (CPT) code is based on three inputs: physician work, physician practice expense (PE), and professional liability (PLI) cost for that code. Each component is allocated RVUs and is adjusted by a geographic practice cost index (GPCI) to account for the many regional differences in costs. Total payment for a service is calculated by multiplying the total RVUs by the annually adjusted conversion factor (CF). The CF is derived through computations by the Centers for Medicare and Medicaid Services (CMS) using the Sustainable Growth Rate (SGR). The SGR is heavily weighted by the Medicare Economic Index, which is based on the overall performance of the economy, accounting for the way it poorly reflects the effects of physician costs and inflation on payment. This system allows all physician services to be linked on a common scale through a single equation for each CPT code:

$$\text{Payment} =$$
$$\text{CF} \times [(\text{RVU}_{\text{work}} \times \text{GPCI}) + (\text{RVU}_{\text{PE}} \times \text{GPCI}) + (\text{RVU}_{\text{PLI}} \times \text{GPCI})]$$

For example, the global reimbursement for CPT code 88108 paid in Alabama at the time of this writing would be:

$$\text{88108 payment} =$$
$$\$37.90 \times [(.56 \times 1.027) + (1.21 \times 1.027) + (0.04 \times 1.027)]$$
$$= \$69.10$$

On average, the physician work component accounts for 55% of the total relative value for each service. The initial physician's work RVUs were assigned through the original Hsiao studies (also known as the Harvard-based Relative Values Studies).[1-3] The work of allocation of RVUs at present is the province of the American Medical Association (AMA)/Specialty Society RVS Update Committee (RUC), which was established in 1991 to make recommendations to CMS on RVUs for new and revised codes. The RUC then provides these recommendations to CMS, which generally accepts the inputs. (Currently, approximately 95% of RUC recommendations are unchanged in the Final CMS Rule for payment each year.)

The primary vehicle to establish new work values is through a process of RUC surveys, instruments designed to capture in RVU form the physician work it takes to perform the service. All physician services are surveyed using the same basic template that gathers data for (1) technical skill with respect to knowledge, training, and experience; (2) required mental effort and judgment; (3) physical effort; and (4) psychological stress due to the potential risk to the patient. The surveys provide a way to compare these aspects of physician work to the work of an established code currently on the physician fee schedule. It is both time and intensity of work that are the critical factors determining payment, and each is critically reviewed in comparison to the RVU of the recommended reference codes. Any inconsistencies among the three components as compared to prior data (from Harvard studies and the RUC) may create problems for RVU development.

The surveys are not administered by the AMA, but rather by a companion society to the process. The College of American Pathologists (CAP), as a founding member of the RUC, participated in initial valuation studies and remains the leading organization for pathology RUC data collection, a voluminous task that is possible only through the participation of CAP's membership. The CAP also provides information on the practice expense portion of the RUC process, via the RUC workgroup of the Economic Affairs Committee, which determines inputs for the technical component (TC) and physician work determining the professional component (PC) for most pathology codes. Practice expense inputs include technologist time, supplies, equipment, and reagents. CPT codes that describe laboratory nonphysician services are not valued as a part of the RUC process. Instead, these are placed by CMS on the Clinical Laboratory Fee Schedule (CLFS). Unlike physician services, these payment values are not formed through a consensus process. Payment is statutorily mandated by CMS as a percentage of payment from past fee schedules. Unlike Pap test interpretation, which is a physician service, Pap test screening (the technical component) is paid under the CLFS. However, CMS currently holds annual hearings to receive input from organized medicine, the laboratory industry, and manufacturers to determine CLFS pricing. In general, CMS pricing tends to reflect consensus opinions presented in these hearings, with Medicare carrier medical directors having significant input.

Current Procedural Terminology

Current Procedural Terminology (CPT) is a listing of descriptive terms and identifying codes for reporting medical services and procedures performed by physicians for payment. CPT is the intellectual property of the AMA and is copyright protected. CPT is recognized by Medicare carriers, and the bulk of the codes are also utilized as such or in a modified fashion by other third-party payers, including state Medicaid programs. The purpose of the terminology is to provide a uniform language that accurately describes medical, surgical, and diagnostic services performed, and which thereby provides an effective means for reliable nationwide communication among physicians, patients, and third-party payers.

Table 13-1 lists the Category I cytology codes from CPT 2008, which is the most recent revision at the time of this writing.[4] CPT descriptive terms and identifying codes currently serve a wide variety of important functions in the field of medical procedural nomenclature. CPT Category I codes are the primary codes used for reimbursed procedures. These codes are updated annually through the deliberations of the AMA-CPT Editorial Panel, which is ultimately responsible for the integrity of the codes. This process involves the use of CPT Advisors from many medical specialty societies, as well as input from the Pathology Coding Caucus, a group staffed and chaired by the CAP that allows laboratory-based CPT advisors and non-physician laboratory groups to work together to optimize the laboratory sections of the code set. Category II CPT codes are used for administrative purposes, such as the CMS Physician Quality Reporting Initiative, and Category III codes are used for tracking services provided prior to the establishment of their clinical utility. CPT II and III codes are therefore not used for reimbursement.

For pathology, the use of CPT modifiers is essential for Medicare billing and for some other payers in certain situations. The majority of codes are separable into professional and technical components. For those laboratories in which the component services are separately billed to Medicare, modifier −26 may be appended to the professional component and modifier −TC to the technical component. Additionally, in certain defined situations, Medicare will not pay for a particular service when another service is performed on the same patient, on the same day, by the same provider. The National Correct Coding Initiative (NCCI) system was created to provide a coding edit set that deals with these situations. Mutually exclusive and comprehensive/component edits eliminate payment on secondary codes identified in NCCI lists unless the code is billed with a modifier −59, as allowable. This modifier should not be indiscriminately used to bypass edits but rather to indicate that the procedure performed on the same patient the same day was on a separately identifiable specimen and/or was a distinct procedure. For quarterly updates on these edits, see the CMS website at www.cms.hhs.gov/physicians/cciedits for downloadable lists.

Table 13-1. Examples of CPT Codes for Gynecologic Cytology

CPT Codes

88141 Cytopathology, cervical or vaginal (any reporting system), requiring interpretation by a physician

88142 Cytopathology, cervical or vaginal (any reporting system), collected in preservative fluid, automated thin layer preparation; manual screening under physician supervision

88143 → with manual screening and rescreening under physician supervision

88147 Cytopathology, cervical or vaginal; screening by automated system under physician supervision

  (for use with conventional specimens, screened with automated devices, requiring no manual screening: FocalPoint, no further review cases)

88148 → screening by automated system with manual rescreening under physician supervision

  (for use with conventional specimens, screened with automated devices, requiring full manual screening: FocalPoint, review cases)

88164 Cytopathology, slides, cervical or vaginal (the Bethesda System); manual screening under physician supervision

88165 → with manual screening and rescreening under physician supervision

88174 Cytopathology, cervical or vaginal (any reporting system), collected in preservative fluid, automated thin layer preparation; screening by automated system, under physician supervision

  (for use with liquid based specimens, screened with automated devices, requiring no manual screening: FocalPoint, no further review cases)

88175 → with screening by automated system and manual screening or review, under physician supervision

  (for use with liquid based specimens, screened with automated devices, requiring field of view review or full manual screening: FocalPoint, review cases, ThinPrep Imaging System, all cases)

Healthcare Common Procedural Coding System

The Healthcare Common Procedural Coding System (HCPCS) Level I codes are equivalent to their corresponding CPT codes. HCPCS Level II codes are also referred to as alphanumeric codes, because they consist of a single alphabetical letter followed by four numeric digits. These codes were first developed in the 1980s. In October of 2003, the Secretary of Health and Human Services under the Health Insurance Portability and Accountability Act of 1996 (HIPAA) legislation delegated authority to CMS for maintenance and distribution of HCPCS Level II Codes.

These constitute a set of codes established to submit claims for those items covered by Medicare and other insurers that are either not included in or are insufficiently identified by CPT codes, such as screening (as to be distinguished from diagnostic) Pap tests. For conventional screening, Paps use the P30xx series; liquid-based and automated Paps use the G01xx series. See Table 13-2 for a listing of current HCPCS codes for gynecologic cytology. (For further information, go to www.cms.hhs.gov/MedHCPCSGenInfo/.)

International Classification of Disease, Ninth Revision, Clinical Modification

ICD-9 CM, The International Classification of Disease (Ninth Revision), Clinical Modification (Sixth Edition),[5] is based on the official version of the World Health Organization (WHO) International Classification of Diseases. ICD-9 classifies morbidity and mortality information for statistical purposes and for indexing of hospital records by disease and operations, and for data storage and retrieval. Physicians have been required by law to submit diagnosis code(s) for Medicare reimbursement since the passage of the Medicare Catastrophic Coverage Act of 1988. In order to document medical necessity, this act requires physician offices to include the appropriate diagnosis codes when billing for services provided to Medicare beneficiaries. CMS has designated ICD-9 as the coding system physicians must use.

It is important to assign the correct and most specific ICD-9 code, as this documents medical necessity for the procedure. For pathology, the proper ICD-9 code may be based on the results of the interpretation performed by the pathologist. If the test results are normal and the test was not for screening, a code appropriate to the indication for the test being performed is the most appropriate selection. For example, if a Pap test is submitted for follow up of a prior Pap test with atypical squamous cells of undetermined significance (ICD-9 code 795.01) and the finding is low-grade squamous intraepithelial lesion (LSIL), the code for LSIL (ICD-9 code 795.03) should be used. If the test result is negative, the submitting ICD-9 code appropriate to the indication for the test being performed, 795.01, should be submitted.

ICD codes are also required as documentation of necessity for screening tests, including the Pap test, which is covered by Medicare every two years for average-risk patients and every year for high-risk patients. At present, while there are a number of codes that govern documentation for the clinical comprehensive exam and pelvic exam that ensure clinician payment, only four are considered acceptable for documentation for payment to laboratories for screening Paps. These are V76.2 (routine cervical Pap smear, intact cervix), V76.47 (routine vaginal Pap – status post hysterectomy for nonmalignant condition), V76.49 (Pap smear, other site NOS - can also use for patients without cervix), and V15.89 (other specified personal history

Table 13-2. Examples of HPCPS Codes for Gynecologic Cytology

HPCPS Codes	
P3000	Screening cytopathology, cervical or vaginal (any reporting system), conventional smear, screening by cytotechnologist under physician supervision (analogous to 88164 for screening)
P3001	Screening cytopathology, cervical or vaginal (any reporting system), conventional smear, requiring interpretation by physician (analogous to 88141 for screening)
G0123	Screening cytopathology, cervical or vaginal (any reporting system), collected in preservative fluid, automated thin layer preparation, screening by cytotechnologist under physician supervision (analogous to 88142 for screening)
G0124	Cytopathology, cervical or vaginal (any reporting system), collected in preservative fluid, automated thin layer preparation, requiring interpretation by physician (analogous to 88141 for screening)
G0141	Screening cytopathology, cervical or vaginal (any reporting system), conventional smear, requiring interpretation by physician (analogous to 88141 for screening)
G0143	Screening cytopathology, cervical or vaginal (any reporting system), collected in preservative fluid, automated thin layer preparation, with manual screening and rescreening by cytotechnologist under physician supervision (analogous to 88143 for screening)
G0144	Screening cytopathology, cervical or vaginal (any reporting system), collected in preservative fluid, automated thin layer preparation, with automated review, under physician supervision (analogous to 88174 for screening)
G0145	Screening cytopathology, cervical or vaginal (any reporting system), collected in preservative fluid, automated thin layer preparation, with automated review and rescreening/review by cytotechnologist, under physician supervision (analogous to 88175 for screening) (for use with screening liquid based specimens, screened with automated devices, requiring field of view review or full manual screening: FocalPoint, review cases; ThinPrep Imaging System, all cases)
G0147	Screening cytopathology, cervical or vaginal (any reporting system), conventional smear, with automated review, under physician supervision (analogous to 88147 for screening) (for use with screening conventional specimens, screened with automated devices, requiring no manual screening: FocalPoint, no further review cases)
G0148	Screening cytopathology, cervical or vaginal (any reporting system), conventional smear, with automated review and rescreening by cytotechnologist, under physician supervision (analogous to 88175 for screening) (for use with screening conventional specimens, screened with automated devices, requiring full manual screening: FocalPoint review cases)

representing hazards to health – use for high-risk Pap tests).

It is important to note that ICD-9 codes for biopsy diagnosis of dysplasia are separate from those for cytologic diagnosis of squamous intraepithelial lesions (795 series for cytologic procedures, 622/233 series for biopsy procedures). In addition, changes in individual assignment for codes have been made, eg, unsatisfactory Pap is no longer 795.09 but is now 795.08. The ICD-9 codes must be coded to the highest possible degree of specificity. For example 622.1 dysplasia of cervix has been subdivided into 622.10 for dysplasia, unspecified as to grade; 622.11 for mild dysplasia; and 622.12 for moderate dysplasia.

Commonly used ICD-9 codes for gynecologic (cervical and vaginal) and anal cytology are listed in Tables 13-3 and 13-4.

Coding Rules

It is important to recognize the distinction between screening and diagnostic Pap tests, as this will determine whether to use CPT or HCPCS codes for Medicare. For diagnostic (medical) Medicare Paps and for most other third-party payer Pap tests, CPT codes are used exclusively. The designation of a Pap test as diagnostic is based on information provided by the referring physician. This may be in the form of ICD-9 codes, signs and symptoms, or a written narrative. These include (1) prior or current cancer of cervix, uterus, or vagina; (2) previous abnormal Pap smear; (3) abnormal findings in lower abdomen or gynecologic tract; (4) complaint referable to female genital tract; and (5) any sign or symptom that the clinician deems to be related to a gynecological disorder. Diagnostic Paps are not limited by frequency and are payable as submitted as long as information that documents medical necessity is included (ie, the proper ICD-9 code). In the absence of such information, it may be necessary to directly access the patient's medical record or to contact the clinician's office. Mere use of archival laboratory results on a patient is not acceptable in lieu of this information, as it does not in itself constitute evidence of the indication for the collection of the present specimen. However, archival laboratory results, which should be consulted in any case when evaluating a current specimen, can appropriately prompt recourse to more accurate coding information from the patient's medical record or clinician's office than may routinely have been submitted with the specimen.

For screening Medicare Paps, HCPCS codes are used for billing purposes (see the following and Table 13-2). A screening or routine Pap is one that is performed in the absence of signs and symptoms, and is payable only when billed with certain ICD-9 codes (see previous ICD section and Tables 13-3 and 13-4). This includes the professional interpretation (P3001 for conventional, G0124 for liquid based). Confusion may arise over ICD-9 coding when a screening Pap has findings that prompt pathologist review. The correct protocol is to document the reason for the Pap

Table 13-3. Examples of ICD-9 CM Codes for Gynecologic Cytology/Pathology

ICD-9-CM Codes
V76.2   Cervix – routine cervical Papanicolaou smear for screening purposes only
V15.89   Other specified personal history presenting hazards to health
Use when Pap is for follow up of prior abnormality or other abnormal history
795.0   Abnormal Papanicolaou smear of cervix and cervical HPV
795.00   Abnormal glandular Papanicolaou smear of cervix
Atypical endocervical cells NOS
Atypical endometrial cells NOS
Atypical glandular cells NOS
795.01   Papanicolaou smear of cervix with atypical squamous cells of undetermined significance (ASC-US)
795.02   Papanicolaou smear of cervix with atypical squamous cells, cannot exclude high-grade squamous intraepithelial lesion (ASC-H)
795.03   Papanicolaou smear of cervix with low-grade squamous intraepithelial lesion (LSIL)
795.04   Papanicolaou smear of cervix with high-grade squamous intraepithelial lesion (HSIL)
795.05   Cervical high-risk human papillomavirus (HPV) test positive
795.06   Papanicolaou smear of cervix with cytologic evidence of malignancy
795.08   Unsatisfactory sample
622.1   Dysplasia of the cervix (use only for biopsy results)
622.10   Dysplasia of the cervix, unspecified
622.11   Mild dysplasia of cervix (CIN I)
622.12   Moderate dysplasia of cervix (CIN II)
233.1   Carcinoma in situ of uterine cervix (use only for biopsy results)
Severe dysplasia (CIN III)
Squamous carcinoma in situ (CIN III)
Endocervical adenocarcinoma in situ

(eg, screening) as the first ICD code (eg, V76.2), with the interpretive findings (eg, 795.03 LSIL) as the second code. The follow-up Pap will then be a diagnostic Pap billed with 795.03 as the primary ICD-9 and will not be subject to frequency limitations. The same is true for unsatisfactory Paps (ICD-9 795.08).

In some circumstances, it may be necessary to provide, as a warning to the referring physician, an advance benefi-

Table 13-4. Examples of ICD-9 CM Codes for Vaginal and Anal Cytology Specimens

ICD-9-CM Codes	
795.07	Satisfactory cervical smear but lacking transformation zone
795.10	Abnormal glandular Papanicolaou smear of vagina
795.11	Papanicolaou smear of vagina with atypical squamous cells of undetermined significance (ASC-US)
795.12	Papanicolaou smear of vagina with atypical squamous cells cannot exclude high grade squamous intraepithelial lesion (ASC-H)
795.13	Papanicolaou smear of vagina with low grade squamous intraepithelial lesion (LGSIL)
795.14	Papanicolaou smear of vagina with high grade squamous intraepithelial lesion (HGSIL)
795.15	Vaginal high risk human papillomavirus (HPV) DNA test positive
795.16	Papanicolaou smear of vagina with cytologic evidence of malignancy
795.18	Unsatisfactory vaginal cytology smear
795.19	Other abnormal Papanicolaou smear of vagina and vaginal HPV
796.70	Abnormal glandular Papanicolaou smear of anus
796.71	Papanicolaou smear of anus with atypical squamous cells of undetermined significance (ASC-US)
796.72	Papanicolaou smear of anus with atypical squamous cells cannot exclude high grade squamous intraepithelial lesion (ASC-H)
796.73	Papanicolaou smear of anus with low grade squamous intraepithelial lesion (LGSIL)
796.74	Papanicolaou smear of anus with high grade squamous intraepithelial lesion (HGSIL)
796.75	Anal high risk human papillomavirus (HPV) DNA test positive
796.76	Papanicolaou smear of anus with cytologic evidence of malignancy
796.77	Satisfactory anal smear but lacking transformation zone
796.78	Unsatisfactory anal cytology smear

ciary notice (ABN) to allow for billing the patient if Medicare is expected to deny payment. In this case, modifier –GA is appended to the code to indicate that the beneficiary signed an ABN and the service is expected to be denied. The modifier GZ indicates that there is no signed ABN and the service is expected to be denied.

The CPT codes for interpretation and hormonal assessment are add-on codes and, at present, can only be billed when a simultaneous screening code is billed. CPT codes may be billed as Bethesda or non-Bethesda, conventional or liquid based, and those inputs will determine ultimate coding.

SNOMED Clinical Terms

SNOMED Clinical Terms® (SNOMED CT®) is a dynamic, scientifically validated, clinical health care terminology that assists in making health care knowledge more usable and accessible. SNOMED CT helps to structure and computerize the medical record, reducing the variability in the way data is captured, encoded, and used for clinical care of patients and medical research. It provides a common language that enables a consistent way of capturing, sharing, and aggregating health data across specialties and sites of care. Among the applications for SNOMED CT are electronic medical records, laboratory reporting (including the Bethesda System for reporting gynecologic specimens), clinical decision support, medical research studies, clinical trials, disease surveillance, image indexing, and consumer health information services.

When built into electronic patient records, SNOMED CT enables primary and specialty care providers and patients to share comparable data at any time, increasing opportunities for optimization of continuity of care. This is achieved through the availability of consistent, reliable information relating to patients' health history and care processes. SNOMED CT allows for family history, medications, allergies, diseases, and treatments to be shared between clinicians, sites of care, and even geographic boundaries. Access to knowledge relating to each patient will ultimately result in the delivery of better, safer care.

Examples in SNOMED CT from the Bethesda System include:

- Reactive cellular changes associated with intrauterine contraceptive device (SNOMED Concept ID: 103642003; SNOMED ID: M-67059)
- Atypical endocervical cells, favor neoplastic (SNOMED Concept ID: 373882004; SNOMED ID: M-67403)
- Atypical squamous cells of undetermined significance (SNOMED Concept ID: 39035006; SNOMED ID: M-67014)
- Endometrial cells in a woman 40 years of age or older, negative for squamous intraepithelial lesion (SNOMED Concept ID: 373885002; SNOMED ID: M-6013B)

SNOMED CT has mappings to other medical terminologies and classification systems. This avoids duplicate data capture, while facilitating enhanced health reporting, billing, and statistical analysis. It also provides a framework to manage language dialects, clinically relevant subsets, as well as concepts and terms unique to particular organizations or localities. Currently, SNOMED CT is mapped to ICD-9 CM as well as several nursing terminologies. At the time of this writing, a map between SNOMED CT and CPT is in development.

Since 1965, SNOMED versions were originally created and maintained by the College of American Pathologists. In 2007, the newly formed International Health Terminology Standards Development Organisation (IHTSDO®) acquired the intellectual property rights to SNOMED CT from the CAP, creating a milestone in the international standardization of health care data. The

IHTSDO is registered as a global not-for-profit association based in Denmark, and is responsible on a global scale for the international release of the terminology SNOMED CT. This international organization is responsible for the ongoing maintenance, development, quality assurance, and distribution of SNOMED CT. The CAP supports the IHTSDO operations and releases under an initial three-year contract and will continue to provide SNOMED-related products and services as a licensee of the terminology. A description of IHTSDO's principles and objectives, open and participatory governance process, and uniform licensing terms is available at http://www.ihtsdo.org/.

References

1. Hsiao WC, Braun P, Becker ER, Thomas SR. The Resource-Based Relative Value Scale: toward development of an alternative physician payment system. *JAMA*. 1987;258:799-802.

2. Hsiao WC, Braun P, Dunn D, Becker ER, DeNicola M, Ketchum TR. Results and policy implications of the resource-based relative value study. *N Engl J Med*. 1988;319:881-888.

3. Hsaio WC, Braun P Yntema D, Becker ER. Estimating physicians' work for a resource based relative value scale. *N Engl J Med*. 1988;319:835-841.

4. *cpt® 2008, Current Procedural Terminology*. Chicago, Ill: American Medical Association; 2007.

5. *ICD-9-CM 2008*. International Classification of Diseases, 9th Revision. Clinical Modification, 6th Edition. Los Angeles, Calif: Practice Management Information Corporation; 2007.

Acknowledgments. The authors would like to thank Dr. Mark Synovec, chair of CAP Economic Affairs Committee (EAC), for his significant input, and EAC staff, Pam Johnson and Lisa Miller, for their help in preparation of this document. The authors thank Drs. Diane Davey, William Tench, and W. Stephen Black-Schaffer, and Mary Kennedy, CT(ASCP), for their valuable contributions to this chapter.

Personnel Management in the Cytopathology Laboratory

Jonathan H. Hughes, MD, PhD
Dina R. Mody, MD
Sue Zaleski, MA, HT(ASCP), SCT(ASCP)

Introduction

Optimal management of personnel is important in the operation of a high-quality cytopathology laboratory. An understanding of the basic principles and strategies for effective personnel management will allow laboratory leadership to find, hire, and maintain an effective workforce. Further, continuing application of the topics presented in this chapter will provide methods and strategies for ensuring ongoing staff competency. Taken together, these principles will allow optimization of the workforce and hence the laboratory environment and output.

Embracing Diversity

Diversity means difference, and although there are numerous ways in which diversity has been defined, there is no definition that fully includes all the characteristics that a population may bring to the workplace. Diversity may encompass but is not limited to our differences as they relate to race, ethnicity, gender, sexual orientation, socioeconomic class, age, geographic location, national origin, religious beliefs, and physical abilities. Diversity is valued because it generates a multiplicity of ideas and viewpoints, leads to more creative and efficient problem solving, fosters an understanding and acceptance of individuals from different backgrounds, and recognizes the contributions that a variety of individuals and groups can make.

Increased generational diversity challenges today's managers who employ and direct four generations of employees working side by side. Employees of different generations have distinct workplace viewpoints. Each of these generations has different life experiences, and hence differing expectations and values, related to their careers and the workplace. The four identified generations are:
- Veterans: born before 1945.
- Baby Boomers: born between 1945 and1964.
- Generation X: born between 1965 and 1980.
- Nexters, also called Generation Y: born after 1980.

Studies of these generations have shown different views or values toward training and development, childcare assistance, retirement benefits, and a variety of other workplace issues. From a practical laboratory standpoint, the most common negative workplace conflicts arise over work hours and are often described as differences in work ethic. The younger generations value work/life balance, and this item is one of the most important factors promoting job satisfaction among younger employees. For example, managers might perceive Generation Xers and Nexters who turn down an opportunity to cover an extra shift as lacking loyalty or commitment, or not being patient centered. This is in contrast to the "workaholic" Boomer and Veteran workforce. To address the work/life balance required to satisfy an ever younger workforce, hospitals and laboratories may consider restructuring shifts to make them more flexible and appealing.

Younger employees want to be involved in the decision-making process. Nursing units are encouraging a teamwork structure that allows younger nurses an opportunity to be part of the clinical team. They expect to contribute, have their input welcomed, and be treated respectfully by older nurses and physicians.

The younger generation's experiences with computers and technology create another arena for workplace conflict. Young recruits evaluate employers on having the essential technology tools. Access to technology has become an expectation of the younger generation, and they may decide against employers who don't have these tools readily available or emphasized in the workplace.

Laboratory managers will increasingly find themselves in a multigenerational and multicultural environment. They must learn about and understand the fundamental differences between the employee populations in order to successfully recruit and retain good workers. In addition, managers must learn how to communicate important workplace information in a manner that will translate across generations. The communication needs of younger employees are less formal and more technologically savvy than older employees, who tend to value face-to-face communication.

There is a wide range of approaches, strategies, and initiatives for managing diversity in the workplace. No single initiative is comprehensive enough to successfully manage diversity in organizations; however, diversity training is one of the primary and most widely used initiatives to address these issues. Diversity in the workplace and diversity issues will continue because the world is shrinking, with companies becoming global, and laboratories, in order to meet workforce shortages, recruiting from an international applicant pool. As diversity is becoming more and more complex, diversity training will continue to be an essential element of the overall diversity strategy.[1-3]

Job Description

The job description, or position description, is a tool that clarifies the roles and responsibilities of the employee and the expectations of the employer. The job description lists the responsibilities and functions that are required of the employee to be successful in the specified position. Job descriptions are commonly made up of five sections: job title, qualifications and worker traits, job duties, responsibilities and accountabilities, and job relationships. The Clinical Laboratory Improvement Amendments of 1988 (CLIA '88) addressed the minimum requirements for laboratory personnel. These minimal requirements should be customized to meet specific environmental issues.[4]

Job descriptions are usually developed by conducting a work (job) analysis. The analysis examines the tasks and sequences of tasks, areas of knowledge, and skills needed to perform the job. Information about a position may be obtained by interviewing the incumbent; however, information is usually obtained through the use of a questionnaire. Someone thoroughly familiar with the position should complete, or assist in completing, the questionnaire.

The job description is a series of written task statements. Each task or responsibility statement should start with a verb that describes the activity. These verbs should be "standardized" or understood by those using the descriptions and the person doing the job. Job descriptions are used for advertising to fill an open position, for determining compensation, and as a basis for performance reviews.

Needs Assessment

The notice of a vacancy gives the employer an opportunity to conduct a needs assessment. A needs assessment is a process of gathering information to assist in making data-driven decisions and recommendations about staffing levels and skill mix. A thorough review of current laboratory practices, including the use of technologies, should be performed. In addition, it is important to include consideration of strategic goals that will influence future labor needs and decisions about staffing levels and skill mix. These considerations as well as productivity measurements may result in recommendations to eliminate, redefine, downgrade, or upgrade the position. It is also an appropriate time to review the job description for accuracy of the duties, skills, and education requirements.

Recruitment, Selection, and Employment of Personnel

The hiring process is generally managed by a human resources department representative who has the responsibility to ensure that the organization complies with federal, state, and local regulations; and assist with recruiting qualified candidates. Hiring and regulatory requirements that were designed to protect the civil rights and to ensure the rights of employees in the workplace are enforced by the US Equal Employment Opportunity Commission (EEOC), which was created in 1965.

The Interview and Hiring Processes

Screening Resumes

Screening resumes is an important first step in the hiring process and can be time consuming. Organizations and individuals responsible for this activity typically develop evaluation systems to manage the process. The system depends on the size of applicant pool and level of position to fill. Large organizations receiving thousands of resumes daily may use a technology-based tool and word searches to evaluate resumes. In contrast, laboratory positions generally result in a smaller applicant pool where manual review of resumes is manageable. A grid system based on the required and desired qualifications allows the reviewer to view and discern qualifications among the candidates from the resumes submitted.

The Interview Team

The interview team should remain small and reflect the department's diversity with regard to gender, ethnicity, and age. It is recommended that at least three qualified candidates be interviewed for any single position. The interview team should be structured such that the candidates are interviewed at least three times and by at least three people. If the approach is to narrow the field of candidates down to a few, schedule the second interview at times different than the original interview time. This will allow the interview team to see the candidate at different times of the day.[5] The interview team should be configured in line with the type of position being recruited. For example, an interview team for a supervisory level position might be made up of the recruit's potential supervisor, a pathologist, a peer, and a subordinate staff member.

The Interview

The EEOC restricts questions during the application or interview process that may either directly or indirectly reveal information considered protected against discrimination. The employer must be cautious about the wording of interview questions so as not to create a situation in which a candidate is set up to reveal information about themselves that could contribute to a hiring decision based upon inappropriate personal data. Examples of discrimination categories and definitions are listed below; however, complete facts and guidance may be obtained at the EEOC website, eeoc.gov.
- Height and weight
- Marital status, number of children, and child care arrangements
- English language proficiency
- Arrest record
- Military service
- Citizenship (however, in the US, all applicants must supply evidence that they are eligible to work)
- Credit history
- Availability to work on religious holidays or weekdays
- Property ownership

Interviewing and selection is critically important for the organization. There are several interviewing roadblocks that appear to be common sense; however, these road-blocks should be anticipated and avoided. They include:

- Scheduling failures. Identify good and bad times to interview.
- Lack of preparation. Evaluate the resumes and have questions prepared in advance of the scheduled interview.
- Interruptions and distractions. Eliminate distractions; post a "do not disturb" sign on the door, forward calls, and turn off cell phones and pagers.
- Pressure to hire. Adhere to the selection and interview criteria; hire right rather than hire to fill.
- Ineffective interviewing tools. Ensure the job description, interview questions, and postinterview evaluations are current.
- Preconceived assumptions. Avoid glossing over interview and selection requirements because the interviewee is well known or is an internal candidate; a properly configured interview process may yield new information relevant to the hiring process.

The purpose of the employment interview is to identify the most qualified candidate whose potential contributions, career goals, and ambitions fit those of the organization. The interview is a formal conversation that requires skillful use of questioning and listening techniques. There are several general interview goals, which include:

- Establishing a relationship
- Exchanging pertinent information
- Verifying credentials
- Comparing and contrasting candidates
- Evaluating suitability
- Predicting candidate performance and probability of success

There are several types of interview strategies: the structured or patterned interview, in which a preset group of questions are asked; the unstructured interview, in which the interview is free to progress in an unplanned, or free-form, manner; and the stress interview, in which a particular stressor, such as a complicated question, task, or puzzle, forms the basis for interaction with the interviewee. An increasing number of employers have found greater success using an alternative technique referred to as behavioral interviewing. This interviewing technique was developed in the 1970s by industrial psychologists and is based on the premise that past performance is a good predictor of future performance.

Employers use the behavioral interviewing process to evaluate a candidate's experiences and behaviors in order to determine the applicant's potential for success. The interviewer identifies job-related experiences, behaviors, knowledge, skills, and abilities that the organization has decided are desirable for the position. These skill sets may include decisionmaking and problem solving, self-confidence, professionalism, leadership, motivation, communication, interpersonal skills, planning and organization, critical thinking skills, team building, and the ability to influence others. The interviewer identifies desired skills and behaviors, and creates open-ended questions and statements in order to elicit detailed responses. A rating system is developed and criteria are evaluated during the interview.

For example, traditional interview queries such as
– Tell me about yourself.
– What are your strengths and weaknesses?
– Why are you interested in this position?
may allow the candidate to give false testimony or tell the interviewer what she/he believes the interviewer wants to hear.

In behavioral interviewing, the candidate is asked to give specific examples of when he/she demonstrated particular behaviors, or skills. The candidate is expected to describe in detail a particular event, project, experience or situation and the result or outcome. Candidates can frame their response in a three-step process called a STAR statement: (1) Situation or Task (ST); (2) Action (A); (3) Result/Outcome (R). Examples of behavioral interview questions might be:

- Describe a time when you were faced with problems or stresses at work that tested your coping skills. What did you do?
- Give me an example of a time when you had to be relatively quick in coming to a decision.
- Give me an example of an important goal you had to set, and tell me about your progress in reaching that goal.
- Give me an example of a problem you faced on the job, and tell me how you solved it.
- What have you done in the past to contribute toward a teamwork environment?[6]

Use of questions asking about specific experiences in the interviewee's past history generally tends to give the interviewer a very good vignette of not only the ability of the candidate to react to such an open-ended question, but will allow for an assessment of the depth and quality of the response as it relates to the level of job responsibility and to the actual performance of the individual in the past.

Equal Employment Opportunity Versus Affirmative Action

The ideas underlying affirmative action and equal employment opportunity are similar with respect to selection, employment, and promotion; however, affirmative action and equal employment opportunity represent different concepts. Equal employment opportunity means that all individuals must be treated equally in the hiring process, in training, and in promotion. Each person has the right to be evaluated as an individual on his or her qualifications without discrimination based on stereotypic preconceptions of members of minority groups or any other protected class. Classifications protected under federal and state equal employment opportunity laws are those of race, color, sex, national origin, religion, age, veteran status, and disability.

Affirmative action goes further than equal employment opportunity. It affirms that organizations and individuals in organizations will seek to overcome the effects of past discrimination against groups, such as women and minorities, disabled persons, and veterans, by making a positive and continuous effort in their recruitment, employment, retention, and promotion. Affirmative action also means that organizations must actively seek to remove any barriers that artificially limit the professional and personal development of individuals who are members of protected classes. Affirmative steps should be taken to attract those qualified women and minorities in the field. These efforts include recruiting, employing, and advancing qualified women, minorities, and people with disabilities who have been or who are excluded from jobs. One way to increase the number of women and minorities in the workplace is by advertising job openings in journals and publications aimed at women and minority audiences. An even more effective means of increasing the number of women and minorities is developing a network of women and minorities in the field and contacting them directly about opportunities. Affirmative action applies to all job categories and levels.

Competency Assessment

There are many different ways in which people interpret competency. Webster's dictionary defines competence as "the state or quality of being well qualified; skill; ability." Hence, a competent person is one who has the ability or skill to produce a desired effect; one who has the power to perform a task.

Competency can be observed and measured within three skill areas: psychomotor, cognitive, and affective skills. Laboratory testing requires the performance of all three skills. Psychomotor skills involve manual dexterity, that is, the physical characteristics of performing the tasks. Cognitive skills involve the information or knowledge that is necessary to correctly perform the tasks. Affective skills reflect an employee's attitude and can be observed in his/her actions and/or behaviors. These actions can include customary conduct and communication with colleagues, pathologists, and clinicians. Therefore, competency, as it relates to the laboratory, is the demonstration of the essential psychomotor, cognitive, and affective skills needed to produce accurate, efficient, and reliable results in relation to the particular laboratory task.

Assessment means gathering information and taking action that will serve a need or solve a problem. There are many ways to gather information. Some assessment methods commonly used in the laboratory setting are listed in Table 14-1.

Table 14-1. Common Laboratory Assessment Methods

Continuing education	Direct observation
Documentation	Peer review
Proficiency testing	Quality control documents
Laboratory practical	Quality assurance findings

Putting this definition of assessment together with competency, competency assessment is the systematic determination and documentation of one's abilities to accurately perform specified functions in order to achieve quality patient care. The purpose of competency assessment is to assure that all employees involved in preanalytic, analytic, and postanalytic testing processes perform their tasks and responsibilities such that the test results are accurate.

Why Do Competency Assessment?

The answer to this question may simply be to comply with regulations. However, laboratories report that competency assessment also provides a critical review of the laboratory's policies and procedures, which results in revision of outdated materials and development of new ones. The end result is better written policy and procedure manuals, hence process control. In addition, once a competency deficiency is discovered, retraining efforts are documented. Finally, once employees understand and accept the need for competency assessment, the activity helps to reaffirm knowledge and skills that promote individual confidence and enhances commitment to quality.

The problem with competency assessment is that most people do not understand how it fits into the employee evaluation system. The following analogy helps to illustrate the relationship between employee performance and competency assessment. First, imagine that a puzzle has been emptied onto a table, with the picture of the completed puzzle in full view. In this case, the completed puzzle picture is total employee performance, with competency assessment just one piece of the puzzle; the other pieces are: training and verification, performance appraisal, and performance standards.

Training and verification refers to making an individual skillful through teaching and practice (training), and then ensuring that the individual is appropriately skilled (verification). The individual's skill is measured against the performance standard, a statement of specific expected results or behaviors. If the individual fulfills the expected results or behaviors, then he or she is competent. The performance appraisal is more global, incorporating not only performance standards and competence, but also attributes such as punctuality, interpersonal skills, and compliance with rules and regulations.

The performance appraisal is a written evaluation of an employee's performance as it relates to the job or position description. An appraisal is typically performed at six months, one year, and annually thereafter. The appraisal process provides an avenue for two-way communication about the employee's performance, training needs, and professional aspirations. Goal setting to meet organizational or professional goals and needs is an expected outcome of the appraisal.

Performance appraisals generally use a scale to rate performance. Regardless of the rating system, measurement criteria should be established and uniformly applied.

Table 14-2. CLIA '88 493.1451 Standard: Technical Supervisor Responsibilities

I	Direct observations of routine patient test preparation, if applicable, specimen handling, processing, and testing.
II	Monitoring the recording and reporting of test results.
III	Review of intermediate test results or worksheets, quality control records, proficiency testing results, and preventive maintenance records.
IV	Direct observation of performance of instrument maintenance and function tests.
V	Assessment of test performance through testing previously analyzed specimens, internal blind testing samples, or external proficiency testing samples.
VI	Assessment of problem solving skills.

The technical supervisor is responsible for evaluating of the competency of all testing personnel and assuring that the staff maintain their competency to perform test procedures and report test results promptly, accurately, and proficiently. The procedures for evaluation of competency of the staff must include but are not limited to the above.

Who Needs to be Assessed?

US federal regulations specifically state that all personnel performing moderate or high complexity laboratory testing must be evaluated "to ensure that staff maintains their competency to perform test procedures and report test results promptly, accurately, and proficiently" (CLIA '88). The benefits of competency assessment in providing continuous quality improvement should be viewed as a benefit for all employees.

Who Mandates Competency Assessment?

The requirements for competency assessment are mandated by CLIA and the deemed-status accrediting agencies of the College of American Pathologists (CAP) and the Joint Commission (formerly the Joint Commission on Accreditation of Healthcare Organizations [JCAHO]). A summary of the competency assessment requirements from CLIA '88 are shown in Table 14-2, and the specific requirements of the CAP and Joint Commission checklists are shown in Table 14-3 and Table 14-4, respectively.

CLIA '88 requires a mechanism for periodically evaluating the effectiveness of policies and standard operating procedures to ensure employee competence. The periodic assessment must include evaluation procedures as defined in CLIA. The laboratory director must ensure that compe-

Table 14-3. College of American Pathologists Laboratory Accreditation Program General Laboratory Checklist (September 2007)

GEN.55500	Has the competency of each person to perform his/her assigned duties been assessed?
GEN.57000	If an employee fails to demonstrate satisfactory performance on the competency assessment, does the laboratory have a plan of corrective action to retrain and reassess the employee's competency?
GEN.58500	Is there documentation of retraining and reassessment for employees who initially fail to demonstrate satisfactory performance on competency assessment?

CAP requires a sufficient workforce with adequate documented training and experience to meet the needs of the laboratory. Periodic evaluations are required.

Table 14-4. Joint Commission: Management of Human Resources Standards

Standard HR.1.10	The laboratory provides an adequate number and skill mix of staff consistent with the laboratory's staffing plan.
Standard HR.1.20	Staff qualifications are consistent with his or her job responsibilities.
Standard HR.2.10	The laboratory provides initial orientation.
Standard HR.2.30	Ongoing education, including in-services, training, and other activities, maintains and improves staff competence.
Standard HR.3.10	Staff competency to perform job responsibilities is assessed, demonstrated, and maintained.

tent personnel are employed to perform and report tests. The technical supervisor is responsible for evaluating competency and conducting performance evaluations twice for new employees during their first year of employment, and annually thereafter. The technical supervisor may delegate these evaluations to the general supervisor. Should performance problems be discovered, a plan of corrective action must be generated (Table 14-2).

CAP requires adequate staffing levels for the workload with adequate documentation of training and experience to meet laboratory needs. Periodic evaluations are required (Table 14-3).

The Joint Commission also requires individual competency for the accurate performance of tests, with an emphasis on specific measures to prevent transfer of infection. The laboratory director must maintain competency of staff initially and continuously. The Joint Commission requires

Table 14-5. Example of Development and Implementation of the Educational Enhancement

Objectives (Upon completion, employee will be able to...)	Criteria for Successful Completion	Date to Be Completed	Achieved? (Yes/No) Comments
1. Describe the criteria that are diagnostic of HPV	Describe the criteria used for the diagnosis of HPV	Within 3 days	Yes
2. Identify HPV in a variety of backgrounds in unknown cases	Identify at least 85% of the HPV cases in the unknown	Within 1 week	Yes, difficulty in obscured and subtle cases
3. Identify HPV in routine cases	Identify HPV with an accuracy rate of 85% in routine cases	Monitor for 4 weeks	No, need to review more unknowns and monitor for 3 weeks

Goal = Upon completion, employee will be able to identify changes diagnostic of HPV with an accuracy rate of 85%.

documentation of performance evaluations and suggests areas for assessment (Table 14-4).

Although the regulatory agencies have set forth these mandates, they do not specify all of the necessary details of how to develop and implement a competency assessment plan. Specific plans are the responsibility of the individual laboratory.

Who is Responsible for Assessment?

CLIA '88 clearly places the responsibility for competency assessment on the technical supervisor. However, the technical supervisor may delegate, to the general supervisor, the responsibility for annually evaluating and documenting the performance of all testing personnel [493.1463(b)(4) Standard].

When do Assessments Need to be Performed?

The regulations mandate that this should be 6 months and 12 months for new employees and annually thereafter. To keep up with new or modified test procedures, in-service educational exercises should be conducted with employees, and their participation and understanding of the new or revised test methodology should be documented.

What Needs to be Assessed?

CLIA '88 is very specific about what is to be assessed and what the assessment methods should be. According to CLIA, the procedures for evaluation of competency of the staff must include:

(i) direct observations of routine patient test performance;

(ii) monitoring, recording, and reporting of test results;

(iii) review of worksheets, quality control records, proficiency test results, and preventive maintenance records;

(iv) direct observation of instrument maintenance and function checks;

(v) assessment of test results on previously analyzed specimens, internal masked samples, external proficiency testing samples; and

(vi) assessment of problem solving skills.

An effective assessment must be meaningful and appropriate. In addition, the criteria for competency are established ahead of time through policies and procedures. The competency assessment must have specific measures based on performance standards. Staff must be aware of the results that constitute competency as well as results that will require education and re-testing. CLIA requires that a plan of corrective action be generated should a performance deficiency be discovered. The employee cannot perform that particular test or task until competency can be demonstrated.

Developing a Performance Improvement Plan: The Educational Enhancement

Once a problem is identified, along with the reason for the problem and the individual having the problem, the laboratory leadership can begin to develop the actual educational enhancement. The enhancement has to begin with a concrete goal, which must be the laboratory standard, and with clearly stated, obtainable objectives that are worded specifically to the individual's level of understanding. Outcomes of the objectives should be measurable in concrete terms, which are not abstract or subjective and are therefore verifiable. A time frame in which the goal and objectives must be met should also be identified. An example of an educational enhancement is illustrated in Table 14-5.

Putting the Plan Into Action

The outcomes as well as the consequences, whether favorable or not, must be discussed with the employee. Always remember to include the employee in every step of the process, or at least where it's feasible, from beginning to end. The issue should be discussed fully and completely with the employee, and the reason why improving this particular skill is so critical to the laboratory and to the patient should also be discussed. It is equally important to talk at their level (ie, use appropriate terms) and avoid terms with any negative connotation.

During the entire process, reinforce positive change by providing positive feedback in other areas that are deserved. Being proactive in your approach (eg, asking the employee how he/she feels the problem can be resolved) can increase chances of success. Positive reinforcement (eg, reminding him/her that "this can be done") encourages a positive outcome.

Confidentiality of the entire process must be maintained to the best of the monitor's ability. This may be difficult in smaller laboratories. However, confidentiality is critical to the preservation of self-image as well as overall laboratory functioning. The employee may choose to reveal the situation to co-workers; however, the monitor should not discuss the issue with coworkers. Use of routine periodic educational enhancements designed for the entire laboratory cannot only help to "hide" individual programs, but it can also reinforce the importance and value of continuing education.

Following Up

The process of competency assessment should be ongoing. Once the goal has been successfully accomplished, continued performance should be encouraged. This can be done by something as simple as having periodic "chats" with the employee to see how everything is going.

Positive reinforcement and a positive educational environment are the keys to improving performance and achieving the laboratory standards of quality. Finally, the whole process, from beginning to end, needs to be documented. Accrediting agencies require documentation to ensure compliance. Verbal assurances of compliance will not be sufficient to satisfy inspectors in the modern laboratory accreditation process.

References

1. Miller S. *Generational Differences.* Alexandria, Va: Society for Human Resource Management; August 2004
2. Greene J. *Different Generations, Different Expectation.* Hospitals and Health Networks (HHN). March 2005.
3. Lewis S, Zaleski S. *Applying Generational Studies to Enhance Laboratory Student Recruitment.* Chicago, Ill: American Society for Clinical Pathology; Tech Sample CY-62005.
4. Clinical Laboratory Improvement Amendments of 1988. Final Rule. Subpart M. Personnel for moderate and high complexity testing. *Fed Reg.* 1992;57:7001-7186. Also available at: http://www.phppo.cdc.gov/clia/regs/toc.aspx. Accessed April 28, 2008.
5. Cottrell D. Hire tough. In: *Monday Morning Leadership.* Dallas, Texas: CornerStone Leadership Institute; 2002.
6. Hansen K. *Behavioral Interviewing Strategies for Job Seekers.* Available at: http://www.quintcareers.com/behavioral_interviewing.html. Accessed May 29, 2008.

CAP Interlaboratory Comparison and Proficiency Testing Programs in Gynecologic Cytology: Reliable Data About Slides and Their Interpretation

Andrew A. Renshaw, MD
Lisa A. Fatheree, SCT (ASCP)
David C. Wilbur, MD

Introduction

The Pap test is arguably the most successful cancer screening program ever devised. A unique set of circumstances allows a program geared toward the prevention of cervical cancer to be awarded this accolade. First, cervical cancer was a highly prevalent disease prior to the introduction of screening. Second, the cervix is a readily accessible organ from which cells can be easily harvested. Third, cervical cancer has a relatively long chain of preinvasive stages that allow many opportunities for detection, any of which can lead to a complete cure. Screening programs for other types of cancer are generally designed around highly sensitive detection schemes. In fact, cervical cancer screening by the cytologic method has been shown to be a relatively insensitive test.[1] It is only through the unique features interplay, as noted above, and the frequency (annually) at which the test has been traditionally performed, that obtaining cells from the cervix for microscopic examination has been so successful in the prevention of cervical cancer.

Just how insensitive is the routine Pap test for the detection of cervical neoplastic lesions? Studies have suggested that the overall sensitivity of the test may be no better than 50%, when all aspects of specimen collection, processing, screening, and interpretation are taken into account.[1] Over time, each of these areas of fault has been addressed in a variety of improvements in the technique. Improved education of clinicians regarding smear collection and immediate processing, improved sampling devices, better methods of making consistent specimens (eg, liquid-based collection), education of cytologists in criteria-based interpretation, and, finally, automated screening devices have all led to more sensitive and precise results. Despite all of these gains, the lynchpin in the entire process is the performance of the individual cytologist who evaluates the specimen and renders a final interpretation.

Measuring the performance of this practitioner in gynecologic cytology can be difficult.[2] There are many different ways of evaluating performance and defining an appropriate gold standard. In addition, although gynecologic cytology is a common procedure, there are no meaningful methods currently in use to measure performance in clinical practice.[3] Two-armed masked studies of cervical cytology practice have yielded some performance data. One large study showed that the overall screening detection rate for any type of abnormality on a Pap test hovers around 80%.[4] Fortunately, as the abnormality increases in severity, the sensitivity of detection improves considerably, going up to

an 85% detection rate for refereed cases of low-grade squamous intraepithelial lesion and above (LSIL+) and up to 93% for high-grade squamous lesions and above (HSIL+). Even further degrees of improvement have been shown with the addition of automated scanning instrumentation to the process. In this same study, at every level of abnormality, incremental improvements in detection sensitivity were noted using automation (LSIL+ at 92% and HSIL+ at 97%).[4]

However, from such studies it is clear that not all slides are created equal, and, undoubtedly, the physical and morphologic characteristics of each slide render it as a unique challenge to the cytologist. Indeed, humans being what they are, the interaction between each slide and each screener is almost certainly a unique event. Some cytologists are "better" at finding atypical glandular cells, others at HSIL, etc. That abnormal slides differ in their "detectability" has been documented in a number of studies. In one analysis of the detection of false-negative slides on quality control rescreening (slides called negative in initial manual screening), the sensitivity for classification of such slides as abnormal was found to be an amazingly low 25%.[5] Does this low level of performance reflect this specific population of slides (are false-negative slides somehow inherently different), or does it reflect relatively low attention given, on the part of cytologists, to the task of rescreening a very low prevalence (and hence low probability) population of slides? Almost certainly it is a combination of the two factors mentioned.

That cytologists all have unique operating characteristics forms the basis for the process of testing proficiency and providing continual educational challenges. The skill levels of practitioners are hypothesized to fall along a normal (bell-shaped) distribution. In order to ensure that the vast bulk of the curve falls above a defined level of disease detection (to ensure competency and hence patient safety), educational programs have been developed and proficiency testing has now been implemented.[6,7] However, as noted above, the skill of the practitioner is not the only variable in the cytology equation; the slides also follow their own "performance curves." Some slides are reliably and precisely identified and classified, while others are not.

The discussion that follows details how the College of American Pathologists (CAP) gynecologic cytology programs were developed, the methods by which they are implemented, and some of the data that has been derived from a continuing evaluation of the performance of the participants and glass slide challenges.

The College of American Pathologists Gynecologic Cytology Programs

Over the past 20 years, the CAP has provided participating laboratories with three distinct gynecologic cytology programs. Philosophically, the CAP has been committed to providing the means for laboratories to compare their screening and interpretive performance to that of other laboratories. This was accomplished through the CAP Interlaboratory Comparison Program in Cervicovaginal Cytology, using well-characterized slides with known performance ("graded" slides, described below). With the use of highly standardized challenges, this program provided a measure of overall laboratory performance and could therefore be utilized as one piece of the overall laboratory accreditation process. In addition, the CAP is committed to providing educational challenges of less well-characterized slides, more akin to those seen in daily practice. Review of such slides provides individuals with the opportunity of educational exposure to rarer or more difficult diagnostic entities, or unusual slide presentations without punitive sanctions for inaccurate interpretations. The CAP PAP educational slide review module provides this benefit. The third slide-based program developed by the CAP came into being in 2006 with the implementation of individual practitioner gynecologic cytology proficiency testing as mandated by the Clinical Laboratory Improvement Amendments of 1988 (CLIA). The CAP Interlaboratory Comparison Program in Cervicovaginal Cytology was merged into the proficiency-testing program (PAP PT) and is now administered to all eligible individual subscribers, along with the continuation of the educational PAP challenges.

Over time, the members of the CAP Cytopathology Resource Committee, the body that maintains the testing program, have analyzed much of the data from the thousands of slides and participants in the various programs. Several interesting findings related to the performance of participants and slides in the program have been identified. This review summarizes many of these findings.

The Conduct of the Programs

The PAP programs are glass-slide based. Prior to 2005, the CAP Laboratory Accreditation Program (LAP) required that all laboratories evaluating gynecologic cytology enroll in the PAP program or an equivalent interlaboratory comparison program. After 2005, CLIA-mandated proficiency testing required all cytology practitioners to participate in one of the approved PT programs. The PAP PT Program is one of three possible choices for participants. Demographics assessments have shown that a wide variety of cytology laboratories participate, with the largest number (approximately 60%) being hospital based. In addition, independent laboratories, as well as federal and government, university, and other types, such as those associated

Table 15-1. Diagnostic Menu from the College of American Pathologists Interlaboratory Comparison Program in Cervicovaginal Cytology

Reference Diagnosis			
000	Unsatisfactory	115	Cellular changes c/w herpes
101	Negative for intraepithelial lesion	120	Reparative changes
111	Fungal organisms c/w Candida	201	LSIL
113	Trichomonas vaginalis	211	HSIL
		221	Squamous cell carcinoma
		225	Adenocarcinoma

with a group practice or physician's office, also participate in the PAP exercises.[8]

Slides utilized in the programs are generously donated by participants. Submitted slides with diagnoses of low-grade squamous intraepithelial lesion (LSIL) or higher must be biopsy confirmed. After receipt and accessioning into the program, all slides are reviewed by at least three experienced cytopathologists from the CAP Cytopathology Resource Committee. Before acceptance into the program, each slide must be judged to be of good technical quality and an excellent example of the submission diagnosis. All three reviewers must agree on the exact target diagnosis, and this must agree with the submission and biopsy diagnoses prior to accepting a slide for circulation into the educational program set.

The PAP program consists of mailings of five glass slides of cervicovaginal material. Modules are available for conventional, ThinPrep, or SurePath slides, or for combinations of all three slide types. Coded answer sheets have diagnostic menus using terminology modified from the Bethesda System.[9] Prior to 2006, referenced slides were placed into one of three selection series: the 000 series for unsatisfactory slides; the 100 series for negative, infectious, and reparative conditions; and the 200 series for epithelial abnormalities and carcinoma (Table 15-1). This classification scheme grouping makes good sense from a practical biologic standpoint because all squamous intraepithelial lesions require similar initial triage, and because data clearly shows that the distinction between low-grade and high-grade dysplasias is not a highly reproducible categorization.[10] All slides are initially placed in ungraded, education-only, slide sets. In order for slides to progress to be used in the so-called graded sets, certain validation criteria indicative of reproducible interpretation must be satisfied.[11,12] Slides meeting these criteria are then eligible to be included in the proficiency-testing or accreditation-related slide challenges.

Graded (or validated) slides must meet specific performance requirements. For all so designated slides, they must have been reviewed by a statistically determined number of participants in the educational challenges and must have achieved a 95% level of agreement to the series (000, 100, 200).

Table 15-2. Example of the Number of all Cases Entered Into the Educational Component of the College of American Pathologists Interlaboratory Comparison Program in Cervicovaginal Cytology that Subsequently Fail to Complete the Field Validation Process [11]

Reference Diagnosis	# Conventional Slides Evaluated	% Failed Field Validation	# ThinPrep Slides Evaluated	% Failed Field Validation
001 Unsatisfactory	138	58	7	43
101 Negative for Intraepithelial Lesions, NOS	2227	19	350	23
111 Fungal organisms c/w Candida	448	18	227	15
113 Trichomonas vaginalis	782	13	144	13
115 Cellular changes c/w herpes	182	11	43	4
120 Reparative changes	323	50	19	52
201 LSIL	1183	26	391	25
211 HSIL	1717	14	315	18
221 Squamous cell carcinoma	822	2	42	19
225 Adenocarcinoma	753	12	98	13
226 HSIL/Carcinoma	54	48	7	14
Total	8629	18	1643	20

Data Regarding Evaluation of Slide Quality and Performance

A major finding of Program data analysis is that not all Pap slides are created equal. In some slides, it is very easy for participants to identify abnormal findings and render correct interpretations, while in other slides, it is more (or even very) difficult.[11] A major thrust of the Program has been to identify slides that can be regularly, reliably, and correctly identified—that is, slides that average cytologists would be expected to essentially always interpret correctly and, hence, would be appropriate and fair for PT challenges having potentially punitive consequences.

Interestingly, nearly half of all participant-submitted slides (41%) do not make it past the initial three cytopathologist review at enrollment, meaning that they are either judged to be not representative of the submitted diagnosis, have technical issues, or lack adequate biopsy documentation.[13]

An example of the percentages of cases that successfully complete this validation process are shown in Table 15-2. Despite the best efforts of not just one but three expert cytopathologists to identify only cases that should be regularly and reliably classified correctly, approximately 20% of all cases fail to ever achieve field validation (this includes both conventional smears and liquid-based specimens). As hypothesized above, the exact percentage of validation failure varies significantly depending upon the reference interpretation. Cases of squamous cell carcinoma on conventional smears are most likely to be validated (98%), while only half of unsatisfactory and negative slides with reparative changes will complete the validation process.[11]

In summary, these results strongly suggest that identifying slides that can be regularly, reliably, and correctly

classified is a complex process. Less than half of cases submitted by participants in the Program as representative examples from their routine practices achieve ultimate validation. Review by three expert cytopathologists is insufficient to identify slides that will achieve validation. In addition, the number of reviews necessary in order to determine if a slide is statistically acceptable varies with the diagnostic category.

These results, gained from many years of experience with glass-slide-based challenges have particular relevance to the advent of CLIA-mandated proficiency testing in gynecologic cytopathology. CLIA regulations at present only require that cases be reviewed by experienced board-certified anatomic pathologists before being used in proficiency testing challenges. The results of the CAP studies strongly suggest that this is an insufficient method for identifying cases that will perform in a fair and reproducible manner. If a cytologist fails a test composed of nonvalidated slides, does that imply lack of proficiency or lack of slide reproducibility? Undoubtedly both causes exist, but determining which it is will not be a trivial task and therefore may unfairly penalize otherwise acceptable practitioners.

Data Regarding the Cytologic Features of Slides That Can (and Cannot) be Regularly, Reliably, and Correctly Interpreted

The cytologic features of slides that performed well and slides that performed poorly in the Program have been extensively detailed; some of these results are summarized in Table 15-3.[14-21] There are several important differences between the characteristic cytologic features of different

Table 15-3. Cytologic Characteristics of Cases That Can Regularly and Reliably be Identified [14-21]

	Characteristic Features	Most Common Type of Error in Missed Cases
LSIL, CS	>250 dysplastic cells	Screening
LSIL, TP	>250 dysplastic cells	Screening
HSIL, CS	>500 single cells *	Screening and interpretation
	Large dysplastic cells [a]	
	Keratinized	
HSIL, TP	>500 single dysplastic cells and no small cells or hyperchromasia *	Screening and interpretation
Squamous cell carcinoma, CS	>1000 abnormal cells	Screening
	Keratinized	
Squamous cell carcinoma, TP	No Trichomonas vaginalis	Distraction
	No atypical repair	Interpretation
Adenocarcinoma, CS	>1000 abnormal cells	Screening
	Large cells [b]	
	Large nuclei [c]	
	Atypia	
	Hyperchromasia	
Adenocarcinoma, TP	Insufficient data for analysis to date	
Adenocarcinoma in situ	No such cases yet identified	

Abbreviations: CS, conventional smear; TP, ThinPrep.

* Hyperchromatic groups are not included in any cell counts.

a. nuclear diameter > 4 lymphocyte nuclei
b. large cells have a cell diameter more than twice a normal endocervical cell
c. large nuclei have a diameter more than twice a normal endocervical cell

reference interpretations. First, the type of error that is most common varies. While the presence of *Trichomonas vaginalis* is a consistent association (and hence an important potential distraction) in slides in which squamous cell carcinoma in liquid-based specimens is missed, other reference diagnoses do not have significant distraction patterns.[16] Instead, squamous cell carcinoma in conventional smears, and HSIL and LSIL in all studied specimen types, exhibit screening errors as being most common. Such cases appear to require a minimum number of dysplastic cells in order to be regularly and reliably identified. In addition, HSIL, on both conventional and liquid-based slides, has a consistent error attributable to misinterpretation, with hyperchromatic groups in both preparations being routinely misinterpreted as benign. Cases of adenocarcinoma in conventional smears also require a minimum number of abnormal cells that are significantly larger than normal glandular cells for an accurate interpretation.[14-20]

The overall accuracy (sensitivity/specificity) of correct interpretation depends on the reference category. As summarized in Table 15-4, using recent year-end summary statistics, there is a relatively wide range of performance, even among validated slides, ranging from 95.2% sensitivity for reparative change to 99.4% sensitivity for squamous cell carcinoma.[22]

Precision also varies, as is shown in Table 15-5. While the reference interpretations of negative for intraepithelial lesion (NILM), *Candida*, herpes, *Trichomonas*, and LSIL were very reproducible, the reference interpretations of HSIL, adenocarcinoma, and repair were less reproducible.[23]

The performance of specific reference interpretations has been further examined. The possible reasons why reparative change is consistently the least reproducible interpretation in the Program have been examined.[24] In addition, it has been shown that there is extensive overlap between the diagnoses of LSIL and HSIL, with as many as 10% of all responses in each reference category being in the other interpretation.[25] Cases with mixed LSIL and HSIL features have been shown to perform differently depending upon whether they are conventional or liquid-based specimens.[26]

As mentioned above, slide performance may also be associated with specimen type. The exact reason for these differences is not clear, and it may not be due to the specimen type alone. Selection bias in cases that are submitted to the Program, as well as variation in the experience of the participants with the various liquid-based specimens, may account for these differences. However, inherent technical and morphologic features present in conventional versus the various types of liquid-based preparations may also account for some of the performance differences. Nevertheless, the results certainly warrant further study in other data sets to try to determine what the causes of these differences are and, hence, to develop potential methods to improve the performance of both techniques.

Interestingly, the accuracy of different reference interpretations in the Program vary with specimen type.[27] Some

Table 15-4. Accuracy of Diagnosis (to Series) for Different Interpretations Using 2002 Year-End Summary Data, Laboratory Response, Validated Slides Only (%) [22]

Reference Diagnosis	Conventional Smears
000 Unsatisfactory	NA
101 Negative for intraepithelial lesion	97.2
111 Fungal organisms c/w Candida	98.2
113 Trichomonas vaginalis	98.6
115 Cellular changes c/w herpes	98.6
120 Reparative changes	95.2
201 LSIL	97.6
211 HSIL	98.9
221 Squamous cell carcinoma	99.4
225 Adenocarcinoma	98.9
Total	97.9

Table 15-5. Match Rates for Groups of Validated Slides [23]

Reference Diagnosis	% Slides with Match Rate <50	% Slides with Match Rate <100
Least Reproducible/Most Difficult		
120 Repair	19.0%	88.9%
211 HSIL	20.8%	81.6%
221 Squamous cell carcinoma	28.2%	81.7%
225 Adenocarcinoma	18.2%	72.5%
Most Reproducible/Least Difficult		
101 Negative	5.3%	50.8%
111 Candida	8.0%	58.7%
113 Trichomonas	4.7%	56.8%
115 Herpes	2.1%	27.1%
201 LSIL	3.7%	56.8%

Table 15-6. Accuracy of Diagnosis (to Series) for Different Interpretations Using 2002 Year-End Summary Data, Laboratory Response, Validated Slides Only (%) [27]

Reference Diagnosis	Conventional Smears	ThinPrep Preparations
101 Negative for intraepithelial lesion	96.1	97.9
111 Fungal organisms c/w Candida	97.8	98.9
113 Trichomonas vaginalis	97.8	98.1
115 Cellular changes c/w herpes	98.5	99.4
120 Reparative changes	94.6	Na
201 LSIL	96.6	98.5
211 HSIL	98.1	98.9
221 Squamous cell carcinoma	98.9	99.0
225 Adenocarcinoma	98.1	98.7

of these differences are summarized in Table 15-6. For validated slides only, matched to series, ThinPrep specimens perform better than do conventional smears in every reference category. However, for educational slides only, the error rates for both HSIL and squamous cell carcinoma were actually higher in ThinPrep specimens than in conventional smears. In addition, when matched to exact diagnosis rather than to series, the error rate for squamous cell carcinoma was also higher for ThinPrep specimens.

Possible reasons for the differences in accuracy of the two techniques were explored. First, it was noted that hyperchromatic groups were not reliably identified in either conventional or ThinPrep preparations in cases of HSIL.[28] Preliminary evidence suggests that these groups may be more difficult to correctly classify in ThinPrep specimens, most likely due to greater three-dimensionality. Third, associations between false-negative diagnoses and other diagnoses for HSIL slides were investigated.[29] This study showed that conventional smears of HSIL that are commonly missed are more often interpreted as a variety of abnormal lesions, including LSIL, adenocarcinoma in situ (AIS), adenocarcinoma, and squamous cell carcinoma. In contrast, cases of HSIL ThinPrep specimens that are commonly missed are only more often interpreted as AIS—again, most likely related to the greater three-dimensionality of the groups in liquid-based specimens, mimicking cells of glandular origin. Fourth, the performance of cases with mixed features appears different for the two techniques.[26] While conventional smears with mixed LSIL/HSIL features are identified to the correct series at a level between that of pure LSIL and HSIL, for ThinPrep specimens, mixed cases are correctly classified more often than either pure LSIL or pure HSIL. The reasons for this difference are as yet unknown. Finally, the effect of certification in liquid-based technique has been investigated.[30] It has been shown that in comparison to participants that

were not certified, participants that are certified performed better on liquid-based as well as on conventional smears. This finding almost certainly relates to the fact that certified practitioners most likely view more of such cases in their practices than do noncertified individuals, reflecting overall experience. However, this finding may also indicate greater educational effort being associated with improved performance across the board.

These data from the Program analyses, taken together, lead to several conclusions. The most common type of error in each category varies with the reference diagnosis. For screening errors, the number of abnormal events present on the slide can determine the outcome, and this outcome varies with the reference diagnosis. Because there is so much difference in the characteristic cytologic features of cases that are regularly and reliably identified, one cannot assume that any of these features may apply to other types of cases or specimens. The criteria are not hard and fast, and exceptions do occur. In the PAP Program, approximately 10% of cases perform more poorly than one would expect based on their cytologic features, and 10% perform better than would be expected. This finding is most likely related to the high variability of diagnostic expertise in the laboratories participating in the Program. Not every slide circulates to every participant—a circumstance that may lead to statistical outliers in the overall results.

Finally, the data that the Program generates are not a perfect reflection of real-world practice. The data reflect performance within a testing situation that may allow for "gaming" and other potential biases.[31] A number of important and highly prevalent reference categories, including atypical squamous and glandular cells, are not included in the Program, creating a potentially biased approach to the interpretation of each slide challenge (eg, if ASC-US is not a choice given, the distinction between LSIL and ASC-US falls more easily to the LSIL side). In addition, routine laboratory interpretation includes consultation with colleagues, reading, comparison to prior specimens, and/or ancillary testing. Therefore, final interpretation may not be based solely on skill, but also on judgment (eg, when to show a case around, when to read about the features). According to these facts of life, it is almost certainly true that performance in routine clinical settings may be different and should be better. However, the more appropriate question for observers of this data is whether the performance of an individual in this program, when compared to all other takers of the challenge, indicates anything about that individual's performance compared to the same group, in routine practice.

Hypothetically, CLIA-mandated proficiency testing attempts to do just that. However, based on the results from the first years of testing, it appears that the limitations that government regulations have placed on the test design, along with the problem of reproducibility inherent in the test, reduces the sensitivity of the proficiency testing program for inadequate performance. In the first year of the nationally-mandated program, some practitioners failed the first testing event, while passing subsequent challenges.[32] In the first year of nationally mandated proficiency testing (CAP did not have a program in that year), the cases were not field validated, and it is possible, and in fact likely, that some of these failures were the result of using test slides that were not reproducible, rather than any reflection on the competency of the test takers. In fact, one can closely predict how many failures will occur on the basis of slide reproducibility issues alone.[33] Estimates fall very close to the actual levels of performance noted, suggesting that failure and slide reproducibility are indeed linked to some extent in the current PT program.

After that first year, and with the introduction of field-validation for slide selection, only a small fraction of remaining cytologists have failed PT examinations, and one would expect this result to continue.[34] However, as cytologists are forced to continue to repeatedly take this test at very frequent intervals, the majority of failures will

be based on a single disagreement in a test composed of very few challenges. As would be expected, the majority of these practitioners will pass subsequent challenges based on an entirely different set of cases. Such a testing scenario stretches the statistical and practical reliability of any test and increases the chance that a failure represents a chance event rather than a measure of practitioner skill. This is particularly true when the test is based on slides that are both inherently difficult to reproducibly classify and are constantly changing their performance as they age. As a result, it remains unclear whether the practitioners who fail are really "non-proficient" or are victims of the limits of the testing program detailed herein. [35]

Conclusions

Results obtained from the College of American Pathologists Gynecologic Cytology Program (PAP PT) have both distinct advantages and disadvantages compared with those from other sources. On the one hand, the sheer number of interpretations is unmatched by any other source. As a result, trends that might not be apparent in other study sets may be identified in this setting. In addition, the national scope of the Program is also unmatched. The majority of other data sets rely on the interpretation of one or a small group of pathologists, the vast majority of whom have specialty training and/or interest in gynecologic cytology. As such, the results herein are more likely to be representative of typical pathologists and cytotechnologists across the country.

On the other hand, the Program does have its limits. It is a test, and as such, it may not exactly mirror the results one may obtain with true clinical practice. However, it is unclear if the results obtained in the program are either better or worse than those in clinical practice. The Program does not specifically control who participates; hence, there is little control over the level of experience and skill of each test-taker making up the total data set. Finally, the cases in the Program are submitted by the participants. It is entirely possible, even with the extensive selection process in place, that these results may reflect a bias in case selection.

With these caveats in mind, several general conclusions can be reached. First, this data strongly suggests that the performance of participants on slides from different reference interpretations vary significantly. There are many possible explanations, with the most likely being that different diagnoses have different cytologic criteria, and some of these are more easily recognized, well-learned, or require differing levels of experience than do others. Importantly, it appears that there are significant differences between the performance of cases of LSIL and HSIL, and taken together, these data raise significant doubts about the validity of using LSIL as a surrogate marker for HSIL either in the clinical setting or in the evaluation of new technologies. Finally, we have demonstrated that liquid-based specimens in the Program perform differently than do conventional specimens in a variety of ways. We must emphasize that there are several possible reasons for this, all of which may, or may not, be indicative of the liquid-based process in general. Nevertheless, these results warrant further analysis in other data sets.

These results also have implications for the future direction of the Program. As has been noted above, all glass slides are not created equal. With the CAP PAP Education and PAP PT programs, more than 15 years of experience using glass slides in the evaluation has shown the performance of cytologists. A major goal of the analyses performed has been to ensure that the results in the Program reflect the performance of the participants rather than deficiencies of the glass slides. No other program has the depth of documentation to support the claims made about the robust reproducibility of results obtained on included slides. As a result, the material in the Program is the best available at present to accurately and fairly measure the performance of individuals in gynecologic cytology.

Our studies have also allowed an evolution of educational offerings that reflect the current standards in practice today. Based upon the Program performance, slides that perform poorly are removed, and the reasons for the poor performance are analyzed, leading to insights into cytology practice. These insights have formed the basic core of information that the CAP Cytopathology Resource Committee has used in developing its educational efforts, both at the CAP annual meetings and through the initiation of new computer-based case studies and reviews.[36]

At the same time, programs designed to test competency will need to continue to evolve as both practice modes and the biology of cervical cancer screening change. As a glass-slide-based exercise, the current Program measures both screening and interpretation skills in the "classic" setting of manual-based techniques. Practice is moving toward more slides being screened by automated instrumentation, with presentation of highest probability fields of view only.[37,38] Such technology will potentially lessen the role of screening and increase the role of interpretation and triage-based "threshold-setting" in the day-to-day practice of cervical cytology. In addition, changes in disease prevalence—both absolute numbers and types of abnormality—will occur in the post–HPV-vaccine implementation era. Such changes will affect screening and interpretation efficiency in future screening programs and will warrant additional changes in the mode of competency assessment. Indeed, proficiency testing on well-validated slides may already be driving an increased emphasis on interpretation rather than screening. Efforts to design and implement measures of screening and interpretation skills that are applicable to future modes of testing and disease biology will need to be addressed in the future of this and other programs.

In conclusion, the data summarized in this review show how quantitative analysis of the results of programs such as that of the College of American Pathologists can demonstrate new trends and conclusions concerning the performance of slides, methods, and participants, and should serve as a springboard for further analyses in other settings. Constant reanalysis of such data will be necessary to implement new programs that continually remain relevant and aligned with the technology and biology of contemporary cervical cancer screening programs.

References

1. Renshaw AA. Measuring sensitivity in gynecologic cytology: a review. *Cancer Cytopathol.* 2002;6:210-217.
2. Renshaw AA. Rescreening in cervical cytology for quality control: when bad data is worse than no data, or what works, what doesn't, and why. *Clin Lab Med.* 2003;23:695-708.
3. Renshaw AA, Holladay EB, Geils KB. Results of multiple-slide, blinded review of Papanicolaou slides in the context of litigation: determining what can be detected regularly and reliably. *Cancer (Cancer Cytopathol).* 2005;105:263-269.
4. Wilbur DC, Prey MU, Miller WM, Pawlick GF, Colgan TJ. The AutoPap system for primary screening in cervical cytology: comparing the results of a prospective, intended-use study with routine manual practice. *Acta Cytol.* 1998;42:214-220.
5. Renshaw AA, Lezon KM, Wilbur DC. The human false-negative rate of rescreening Pap tests: measured in a two-arm prospective clinical trial. *Cancer (Cancer Cytopathol).* 2001; 93:106-110.
6. Nielsen ML. Cytopathology interlaboratory improvement programs of the Collage of American Pathologists: Laboratory Accreditation Program (CAP LAP) and Performance Improvement Program in Cervicovaginal cytology (CAP PAP). *Arch Pathol Lab Med.* 1997;121:256-259.
7. Clinical Laboratory Improvement Amendments of 1988. Final Rule. 42 USC §263a(f)(4)(B)(iv)§353(f)(4)(B)(iv) of the Public Health Service Act, 57. *Fed Reg.* 1992;7001-7186.
8. Interlaboratory Comparison Program in Gynecologic Cytopathology. *PAP 2007. Year-End Summary Report.* Northfield, Ill: College of American Pathologists; 2007.
9. Solomon D, Davey D, Kurman R, Moriarty A, et al; Forum Group Members; Bethesda 2001 Workshop. The 2001 Bethesda System: terminology for reporting results of cervical cytology. *JAMA.* 2002;287:2114-2119.
10. Stoler MH, Schiffman M; Atypical Squamous Cells of Undetermined Significance - Low-grade Squamous Intraepithelial Lesion Triage Study (ALTS) Group. Interobserver reproducibility of cervical cytologic and histologic interpretations: realistic estimates from the ASCUS-LSIL Triage Study. *JAMA.* 2001;285:1500-1505.
11. Renshaw AA, Walsh MK, Blond B, Moriarty AT, Mody DR, Colgan TJ; Cytopathology Resource Committee, College of American Pathologists. Robustness of validation criteria in the College of American Pathologists Interlaboratory Comparison Program in Cervicovaginal Cytology. *Arch Pathol Lab Med.* 2006;130:1119-1122.
12. Renshaw AA, Wang E, Mody DR, Wilbur DC, Davey DD, Colgan TJ; Cytopathology Resource Committee, College of American Pathologists. Measuring the significance of field validation in the College of American Pathologists Interlaboratory Comparison Program in Cervicovaginal Cytology: how good are the experts? *Arch Pathol Lab Med.* 2005;129:609-613.
13. Renshaw AA, Mody DR, Wang E, Wilbur DC, Colgan TJ; Cytopathology Resource Committee, College of American Pathologists. Measuring the significance of participant evaluation of acceptability of cases in the College of American Pathologists Interlaboratory Comparison Program in Cervicovaginal Cytology. *Arch Pathol Lab Med.* 2005;129:1093-1096.

243

14. Renshaw AA, Prey MU, Hodes L, Weisson M, Haja J, Moriarty AT. Cytologic features of high grade squamous intraepithelial lesion in conventional slides: comparison of cases which performed poorly and well in the College of American Pathologists gynecologic cytology program. *Arch Pathol Lab Med.* 2005;129:733-735.

15. Renshaw AA, Plott E, Dubray-Benstein B, et al. Cytologic features of high grade squamous intraepithelial lesion in ThinPrep slides: comparison of cases which performed poorly and well in the College of American Pathologists Interlaboratory Comparison Program in Cervicovaginal Cytology. *Arch Pathol Lab Med.* 2004;128:746-748.

16. Renshaw AA, Dubray-Benstein B, Cobb CJ, et al. Cytologic features of squamous cell carcinoma in ThinPrep slides. *Arch Pathol Lab Med.* 2004;128:403-405.

17. Renshaw AA, Mody DR, Lozano RL, Volk EE, Davey DD, Birdsong GG. Adenocarcinoma in situ of the cervix is significantly more difficult to identify and categorize than adenocarcinoma, high grade squamous intraepithelial lesion, or squamous cell carcinoma. *Arch Pathol Lab Med.* 2004;128:153-157.

18. Renshaw AA, Dubray-Benstein BL, Haja J, Hughes JL. Cytologic features of low grade squamous intraepithelial lesion in ThinPrep and conventional smear specimens. *Arch Pathol Lab Med.* 2005;129:23-25.

19. Renshaw AA, Schwartz MR, Wang E, Haja J, Hughes JH. Cytologic features of adenocarcinoma, not otherwise specified, in conventional smears: comparison of cases that performed poorly with those that performed well in the College of American Pathologists Interlaboratory Comparison Program in Cervicovaginal Cytology. *Arch Pathol Lab Med.* 2006;130:23-26.

20. Renshaw AA, Henry MR, Birdsong GG, Wang E, Haja J, Hughes JH. Cytologic features of squamous cell carcinoma in conventional smears: comparison of cases that performed poorly with those that performed well in the College of American Pathologists Interlaboratory Comparison Program in Cervicovaginal Cytology. *Arch Pathol Lab Med.* 2005;129:1097-1099.

21. Renshaw AA. Making the cut: what can be regularly and reliably identified in gynecologic cytology? *Diagn Cytopathol.* 2006;34:181-183.

22. Interlaboratory Comparison Program in Gynecologic Cytopathology. *PAP 2002. Year-End Summary Report.* Northfield, Ill: College of American Pathologists; 2002.

23. Renshaw AA, Davey DD, Birdsong GG, et al; College of American Pathologists Comparison Program in Cervicovaginal Cytology. Precision in gynecologic cytologic interpretation: a study from the College of American Pathologists Interlaboratory Comparison Program in Cervicovaginal Cytology. *Arch Pathol Lab Med.* 2003;127:1413-1420.

24. Colgan TJ, Woodhouse SL, Styer PE, Kennedy M, Davey DD. Reparative changes and the false-positive/false negative Papanicolaou test: a study from the College of American Pathologists Interlaboratory Comparison Program in Cervicovaginal Cytology. *Arch Pathol Lab Med.* 2001;125:134-140.

25. Woodhouse SL, Stasny JF, Styer PE, Kennedy M, Praestgaard AH, Davey DD. Interobserver variability in subclassification of squamous intraepithelial lesions: results of the College of American Pathologists Interlaboratory Comparison Program in Cervicovaginal Cytology. *Arch Pathol Lab Med.* 1999;123:1079-1084.

26. Renshaw AA, Mody DR, Styer P, Schwartz M, Ducatman B, Colgan TJ. Papanicolaou tests with mixed high-grade and low-grade squamous intraepithelial lesion features: distinct performance in the College of American Pathologists Interlaboratory Comparison Program in Cervicovaginal Cytopathology. *Arch Pathol Lab Med.* 2006;130:456-459.

27. Renshaw AA, Young NA, Colgan TJ, et al. Comparison of performance of conventional and ThinPrep gynecologic preparations in the College of American Pathologists Gynecologic Cytology Program. *Arch Pathol Lab Med.* 2004;128:17-22.

28. Renshaw AA, Mody DR, Wang E, Haja J, Colgan TJ; Cytopathology Resource Committee, College of American Pathologists. Hyperchromatic crowded groups in cervical cytology–differing appearances and interpretations in conventional and ThinPrep preparations: a study from the College of American Pathologists Interlaboratory Comparison Program in Cervicovaginal Cytology. *Arch Pathol Lab Med.* 2006;130:332-336.

29. Renshaw AA, Styer PR, Mody DR, Colgan TJ. Associations between false-negative rates and other interpretations for high-grade squamous intraepithelial lesion in conventional smears and ThinPrep specimens. *Arch Pathol Lab Med* (in press).

30. Renshaw AA, Mody DR, Walsh M, Bentz JS, Colgan TJ; Cytopathology Resource Committee, College of American Pathologists. The significance of certification in liquid-based cytology and performance in the College of American Pathologists Interlaboratory Comparison Program in Cervicovaginal Cytopathology. *Arch Pathol Lab Med.* 2006;130:1269-1272.

31. Hughes JH, Bentz JS, Fatheree LA, Wilbur DC. Changes in participant performance in the "test-taking" environment: observations from the 2006 CAP gynecologic cytology proficiency test (PT). *Arch Pathol Lab Med* (in press).

32. Centers of Medicare and Medicaid Services. Final 2005 National Cytology Proficiency Testing Results. Available at: http://www.cms.hhs.gov/CLIA/downloads/2005FinalTesting Results080906MDMIME.pdf. Accessed August 20, 2008.

33. Young NA, Moriarty AT, Walsh MK, Wang E, Wilbur DC. The potential for failure in gynecologic regulatory proficiency testing with current slide validation criteria: results from the College of American Pathologists Interlaboratory Comparison in Gynecologic Cytology Program. *Arch Pathol Lab Med.* 2006;130:1114-1118

34. Bentz JS, Hughes JH, Fatheree LA, Schwartz MR, Soures RJ, Wilbur DC; Cytopathology Resource Committee, College of American Pathologists. Summary of the 2006 College of American Pathologists Gynecologic Cytology Proficiency Testing Program. *Arch Pathol Lab Med.* 2008;132:788-794.

35. Nagy GK, Naryshkin S. The dysfunctional federally mandated proficiency test in cytopathology: a statistical analysis. *Cancer Cytopathol.* 2007;111;467-476.

36. View rare cases, earn CME credits online. *CAP Today.* October 2006.

37. Dziura B, Quinn S, Richard K. Performance of an imaging system vs. manual screening in the detection of squamous intraepithelial lesions of the uterine cervix. *Acta Cytol.* 2006;50:309-311.

38. Wilbur DC, Parker EM, Foti JA. Location guided screening of liquid-based cervical cytology specimens: a potential improvement in accuracy and productivity is demonstrated in a preclinical feasibility trial. *Am J Clin Pathol.* 2002;118:399-407.

Abbreviations

ACOG	American College of Obstetricians and Gynecologists		FOV	fields of view
AGC	atypical glandular cells		HCG	hyperchromatic crowded group
AIS	adenocarcinoma in situ		HPV	human papillomavirus
ANSC	anucleated squamous cells		hrHPV	high-risk human papillomavirus
ARC	anal-rectal cytology		HSIL	high-grade squamous intraepithelial lesion
ASC	American Society of Cytopathology		HSV	herpes simplex virus
ASC	atypical squamous cells		hTERT	human telomerase reverse transcriptase
ASCCP	American Society for Colposcopy and Cervical Pathology		IUD	intrauterine device
ASC-H	atypical squamous cells, cannot exclude HSIL		IUO	investigational use only
ASC-US	atypical squamous cells of undetermined significance		LAP	Laboratory Accreditation Program
			LBC	liquid-based cytology
ASCP	American Society for Clinical Pathology		LEEP	loop electrosurgical excision
AV	atrophic vaginitis		LIS	laboratory information system
BV	bacterial vaginosis		LSIL	low-grade squamous intraepithelial lesion
CAP	College of American Pathologists		LUS	lower uterine segment
CDC	Centers for Disease Control and Prevention		N:C	nuclear to cytoplasmic ratio
CFC	chronic follicular cervicitis		NG	*Neisseria gonorrhea*
CIN	cervical intraepithelial neoplasia		NILM	negative for intraepithelial lesion or malignancy
CIN II/III	cervical intraepithelial neoplasia grade 2/3		PCR	polymerase chain reaction
CIS	carcinoma in situ		PK	parakeratotic (cells)
CLIA '88	Clinical Laboratory Improvement Amendments of 1988		RUO	research use only
			SCC	squamous cell carcinoma
CMS	Centers for Medicare and Medicaid Services		SIL	squamous intraepithelial lesion
CMV	cytomegalovirus		TBM	tingible body macrophage
CT	*Chlamydia trachomatis*		TM	tubal metaplasia
DUB	dysfunctional uterine bleeding		TV	*Trichomonas vaginalis*
EC/TZ	endocervical/transformation zone		TZ	transformation zone
FIGO	International Federation of Gynecology and Obstetrics		VLP	virus-like particle
			WHO	World Health Organization

Index